KU-226-922

Evidence-based Paediatric Oncology

Edited by

Ross Pinkerton
Professor of Paediatric Oncology, Institute of Cancer Research and Royal Marsden Hospital, London and Sutton

Thierry Philip
Director of Standards, Options and Recommendations, President, Federation Nationale des Centres de Lutte Contre le Cancer (FNCLCC), Paris, France

Beatrice Fervers
Coordinator of Standards, Options and Recommendations, Federation Nationale des Centres de Lutte Contre le Cancer (FNCLCC), Paris and Centre Leon Berard (CLB), Lyon France

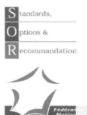

© BMJ Books 2002
BMJ Books is an imprint of the BMJ Publishing Group

All rights reserved. No part of this publication may be reproduced, stored in a retrieval
system, or transmitted, in any form or by any means, electronic, mechanical, photocopying,
recording and/or otherwise, without the prior written permission of the publishers.

First published in 2002
by BMJ Books, BMA House, Tavistock Square,
London WC1H 9JR

www.bmjbooks.com

British Library Cataloguing in Publication Data

A catalogue record for this book is available from the British Library

ISBN 0 7279 1440 5

Typeset by SIVA Math Setters, Chennai, India
Printed and bound by MPG Books, Bodmin, Cornwall

Contents

Contributors

Joann Ater
Division of Paediatrics, University of Texas Medical Department, Anderson Cancer Center, Texas, USA

Archie Bleyer
Head, Division of Paediatrics, University of Texas Medical Department, Anderson Cancer Center, Texas, USA

Judith Chessells
Department of Haematology, Institute of Child Health, London

Alan Craft
Head of Department of Child Health, Royal Victoria Infirmary, Newcastle upon Tyne

Anne Davidson
Consultant Paediatrician, The Royal Alexandra Hospital for Sick Children, Brighton

Tim Eden
Professor of Paediatric Oncology, Academic Unit of Paediatric Oncology, Christie Hospital NHS Trust, Manchester

Dan Green
Department of Paediatrics, Roswell Park Cancer Institute, New York, USA

Beatrice Fervers
Coordinator of Standards, Options and Recommendations, Federation Nationale des Centres de Lutte Contre le Cancer (FNCLCC), Paris and Centre Leon Berard (CLB), Lyon, France

Katherine Matthay
Professor of Pediatrics, Chief Pediatric Oncology, Department of Pediatrics, University of California, San Francisco, USA

Thierry Philip
Director of Standards, Options and Recommendations, President, Federation Nationale des Centres de Lutte Contre le Cancer (FNCLCC), Paris, France

Ross Pinkerton
Professor of Paediatric Oncology, Institute of Cancer Research and Royal Marsden Hospital, London and Sutton

AG Shankar

Department of Paediatric Haematology and Oncology, The Royal London Hospital, London

Michael Stevens

Paediatric Oncology Unit, Institute of Child Health, Royal Hospital for Children, Bristol

Introduction

Ross Pinkerton, Thierry Philip, Beatrice Fervers

The introduction of effective chemotherapy in the early 1960s led to a dramatic improvement in the outcome of childhood leukaemia and solid tumours. Cure rates have been further improved by the judicious use of surgery and radiotherapy and the application of appropriate staging systems based on sophisticated imaging techniques. In recent years, the rate of improvement has tended to reach a plateau and it has become increasingly important to design trials that ask explicit questions, are powered to be reliable and will provide answers in a reasonable time. Excellent examples where this has been the case include the series of trials in Wilms' tumour run by the National Wilms Tumour Study Group (NWTS) and International Society of Paediatric Oncology (SIOP) Groups and the IRS trials. Much has also been learned in acute leukaemias and lymphoma from the American Children's Cancer Group (CCG), the French Society of Pediatric Oncology (SFOP), Pediatric Oncology Group (POG) and UK Medical Research Council (MRC) trials. Trial design is a complex procedure starting with an individual idea and ultimately brought through a multidisciplinary group to a formal study protocol. This is a time consuming process often involving contentious issues and compromise on the part of participants who may have their own ideas about priorities. Moreover, because of concerns over late sequelae, long term follow up is required in many studies. It is easier often to design simpler, limited centre studies which are under-powered or ask unclear questions.

Consequently, the paediatric oncology literature is littered with small single arm "studies" and reports of what is essentially "best standard practice", which, whilst of interest, often fail to take things forward. Similarly, there is a temptation in patients with poor prognoses to apply investigational regimens in the hope that if there is an improvement this will become evident when compared with historical controls. Such an approach has in many ways delayed progress.

Reluctance to run large randomised trials has resulted in the overuse of inappropriate strategies and the slow application of effective ones. Differences in outcome not only between continents, but even within Europe – highlighted by the Eurocare project – emphasise the need for standardised, evidence-based treatments[1].

The aim of this book is to review the surprisingly sparse information that is available for randomised trials in childhood cancer. These data should not only provide a rational evidence base for current practice but also indicate where there are gaps in our knowledge and new studies are a priority.

The inspiration for this book was the Standards, Options and Recommendations (SOR) project of the National Federation of French Cancer Centres. This ambitious project sets out to review clinical trials – both randomised and non-randomised – in adult and childhood cancer and provide evidence-based guidelines for clinical practice[2]. In the absence of randomised trials the presentation

Table 1 Definition of Level of Evidence (Standards, Options and Recommendations)

Level A	There exists a meta-analysis of high standard or several randomised therapeutic trials of high standard which give consistent results
Level B	There exist studies, therapeutic trials, quasi-experimental trials, or comparisons of populations, of which the results are consistent when considered together
Level C	There exist studies, therapeutic trials, quasi-experimental trials or comparisons of populations, of which the results are not consistent when considered together
Level D	Either the scientific data does not exist or there is only a series of cases
Expert agreement	The data does not exist for the method concerned but the experts are unanimous in their judgement

of "best available evidence" helps to guide practice.

For this book the initial searches through the electronic databases were carried out by SOR staff, Sylvie Guillo, in particular, and subsequently expanded by Susan Sugden, in the library of the Institute of Cancer Research. The sources of data are those used in the SOR project, namely Medline, Cancerlit and Embase, searching from 1980.

Guidelines are ideally based on systematic reviews that follow the Cochrane methodology. These are very labour intensive, requiring exhaustive searches for both published and unpublished data. The body of data in childhood cancer does not lend itself to this approach.

Similarly, because of the small number of randomised trials in most childhood solid tumours, formal meta-analysis is not possible. Only in acute lymphoblastic leukaemia are there sufficient studies asking comparable questions for this approach to be followed. There are, however, solid tumours, such as Wilms' tumour

and rhabdomyosarcoma where meta-analysis should be attempted. Moreover, there may be a place for pooling data from single arm studies to learn more about prognostic factors.

If the criteria for defining the quality of evidence used by SOR are applied (Table 1), there is only one report to level A and most are, at best level B. Using the SIGN criteria, as recommended by the UK Royal College of Paediatrics and Child Health Quality of Practice Committee[3] (Table 2), most are level 1+ or 1– in the case of the smaller studies.

Much current practice is based on protocols that appear to produce the most favourable results in single arm studies. Many are associated with significant early and late morbidity which subsequent randomised evaluation proves to have been unjustified. It is, therefore, of importance that novel strategies are adequately evaluated before they become accepted as standard practice. It is hoped that the data in this book will provide useful background information for those involved in trial design and also be of value to those early in their oncology careers who should be aware of what

Table 2 Levels of Evidence (Scottish Intercollegiate Guideline Network)

Level	Type of evidence
1++	Evidence from high quality meta-analyses, systematic reviews of RCTs, or RCTs with a very low risk of bias
1+	Evidence from well conducted meta-analyses, systematic reviews of RCTs, or RCTs with a low risk of bias
1–	Evidence from meta-analyses, systematic reviews of RCTs, or RCTs with a high risk of bias
2++	Evidence from high quality systematic reviews of case-control or cohort studies or high quality case–control or cohort studies with a very low risk of confounding, bias or chance and a high probability that the relationship is causal
2+	Evidence from well conducted case–control or cohort studies with a low risk of confounding, bias, or chance and a moderate probability that the relationship is causal
2–	Evidence from case–control or cohort studies with a high risk of confounding, bias, or chance and a significant risk that the relationship is not causal
3	Evidence from non-analytic studies, e.g. case reports, case series
4	Evidence from expert opinion

studies have been done but find that current text-books provide only minimal details of these trials. From short summary tables it is impossible to assess the quality of the study or the strength of the conclusions.

We have been fortunate to have persuaded many well known figures in children's cancer to add short commentaries to each section. These are aimed to focus on the major conclusions from the studies presented and also on future research priorities.

Textbooks are often criticised for becoming obsolete almost as soon as they are published. Inevitably, some of the studies published in

2001/2002 will be missing from this text. To avoid this problem, we have arranged that study reviews in the same format as the text will appear at regular intervals on the book's website www.evidencebased_paediatriconcology.com Interested readers will be able to find a review of more recently published randomised studies in each of the categories within a few months of their being published.

References

1   Childhood Cancer Survival in Europe 1978–1992: the Eurocare study. *Eur J Cancer* 2001;**37**:671–816.

2   Clinical practice guidelines for cancer care from the National Federation of French Cancer Centres. *Br J Cancer*, 2001;**84** (Supplement 2).

3   Royal College of Paediatrics and, Child Health *Standards for development of clinical guidelines in paediatrics and child health*, 2nd edn, 2001. (www: rcpch.ac.uk)

Part I
Solid Tumours

Ross Pinkerton

1

Rhabdomyosarcoma

Commentary – Michael Stevens

Background

Soft tissue sarcoma (STS) account for about 8% of all childhood malignancies. As a diagnostic category this represents a rather heterogeneous group of tumour types, some of which are more frequently found in adult life and many of which are very rare in childhood. Rhabdomyosarcoma (RMS) is the single most common diagnosis (accounting for approximately 60% of all STS) and in view of its rarity in adults it is characteristically viewed as a paediatric malignancy. It is consequently the tumour which is best defined, and although there are important differences in behaviour between RMS and some of the non-RMS soft tissue sarcomas (e.g. in their metastatic potential, chemosensitivity, etc.), most of the experience of treatment for non-RMS STS in childhood is derived either from experience of managing the same diagnoses in adult practice or is based on the principles derived from the management of rhabdomyosarcoma.

Potential difficulties in reviewing clinical trials in RMS

Attempts to compare the results of clinical trials involving RMS in childhood are confused by the lack of use of standard terminology for staging and treatment stratification. Although there is now good communication between the major international collaborative groups, and even an attempt to define standard criteria for staging

and pathological classification, the experience of reviewing the literature can be confusing. Furthermore, as there are important differences in the philosophy of treatment, careful consideration is required of the optimal measure by which outcome is defined.

Most of the important differences relate to the method and timing of local treatment, and, more specifically, to the place of radiotherapy in guaranteeing local control for patients who appear to achieve complete remission with chemotherapy, with or without significant surgery. This represents an important philosophical difference between the International Society of Paediatric Oncology (SIOP MMT) studies and those of the Intergroup Rhabdomyosarcoma Study Group (IRSG) and, to some extent, those of the German (CWS) and Italian (ICG) Co-operative Groups. Local relapse rates are generally higher in the SIOP studies than those experienced elsewhere although the SIOP experience has also made it clear that a significant number of patients who relapse may be cured with alternative treatment. In the context of such differences, *overall* survival rather than *disease free* or *progression free* survival becomes the most important criterion for measuring outcome and, ultimately, there should be some measure of the 'cost' of survival which takes into account the total burden of therapy experienced by an individual patient and the predicted late sequelae that may result.

Treatment: the general approach

Experience in all studies has confirmed that a surgical–pathological classification which groups patients according to the extent of residual tumour after the initial surgical procedure predicts outcome. The great majority of patients (approximately 75%) will have macroscopic residual disease (IRS Clinical Group III) at the primary site at the start of chemotherapy (this is equivalent to pT3b in the SIOP post surgical staging system). The variability with which RMS presents at different anatomical sites has a particularly strong influence on strategies for treatment. The additional prognostic influence of tumour size, histological subtype and patient age adds to the complexities of treatment stratification. More recently IRSG have extended the concept of the Group to define a new IRS staging system which, by including information about tumour site and size, provides further refinement to the assignment of risk based chemotherapy. All current clinical trials utilise some combination of the best known prognostic factors to stratify treatment intensity for patients with good or poor predicted outcomes and the impetus for this approach comes as much to avoid overtreatment of patients with a good prospect for cure, as to improve cure rates for patients with less favourable disease.

The importance of multi-agent chemotherapy, as part of coordinated multi-modality treatment, has been clearly demonstrated for RMS. Cure rates have improved from approximately 25% in the early 1970s when combination chemotherapy was first implemented, and now overall 5 year survival rates of more than 70% are generally achieved. Nevertheless, it is interesting to see how relatively little the results of randomised controlled trials have actually contributed to decision making in the selection of chemotherapy and to the development of the design of the sequential studies which have shown this improvement in survival over those years.

Lessons from studies of rhabdomyosarcoma

IRSG was formed in 1972 as a collaboration between the two former paediatric oncology groups in North America (Children's Cancer Group and Pediatric Oncology Group) with the intention of investigating the biology and treatment of RMS (and undifferentiated sarcoma) in the first two decades of life. This group, whose work and publications have been pre-eminent in the field, now forms the Soft Tissue Sarcoma Committee of the Children's Oncology Group (COG). Results of treatment of more than 4000 eligible patients have improved significantly over time. The percentage of patients alive at 5 years has increased from 55% on the IRS-I protocol (Study 1) to approximately 71% on the IRS-III and IRS-IV protocols (Studies 3, 6).

Combinations of vincristine, actinomycin D and cyclophosphamide (VAC) have been the mainstay of chemotherapy in all IRS studies. Actinomycin D was originally given in a fractionated schedule but subsequent experience, including a randomised study from Italy (Study 5), showed no advantage in terms of outcome and have suggested that fractionation may increase toxicity; single dose scheduling is now standard across all studies. There have never been any results that challenge the use of these drugs as first line therapy and the results of all randomised studies which compare other drugs with, or against, VA or VAC have failed to show significant advantage.

Alternative agents of particular interest include doxorubicin, which has been evaluated in a number of IRSG studies. A total of 1431 patients with Group III and IV disease were randomised to receive or not receive doxorubicin in addition to VAC during studies in IRS-I to IRS-III. The results did not indicate any significant advantage for those who received doxorubicin (Adriamycin). Furthermore, also in IRS-III, patients with Group II (microscopic residual) tumours were randomised between VA alone and VA + doxorubicin without any significant difference in survival. Despite these results, and the lack of historical phase II data for the use of doxorubicin in RMS, many paediatric oncologists continue to ponder the value of anthracyclines in the treatment of rhabdomyosarcoma and both the SIOP MMT and the German–Italian cooperative studies continue to treat some patients with chemotherapy combinations that include anthracycline drugs. Current European studies (MMT 95 and CWS–ICG 96) both include randomisations between their ifosfamide based standard chemotherapy options (ifosfamide, vincristine and actinomycin D (IVA) in MMT 95 and ifosfamide, vincristine, actinomycin D and doxorubicin (VAIA) in CWS–ICG 96) and an intensified six drug combination which includes epirubicin (with carboplatin and etoposide). The first results of these studies should be available by late 2002 and although the study designs cannot specifically address the anthracycline question, the absence of any benefit from the intensified chemotherapy arm would further reinforce the message that patients may not benefit from anthracycline as part of first line therapy. This is especially important given the risk of significant cardiotoxicity, which was seen in 4% of patients who received doxorubicin in IRS-III.

One of the most significant differences between IRSG and the European studies has been in the choice of alkylating agent which provides the backbone of first line chemotherapy. Ifosfamide was introduced into clinical practice earlier in Europe than in the United States and phase II data are available which supports its efficacy in RMS. IRS-IV (Study 6) attempted to answer the question of comparative efficacy by randomising VAC (using an intensified cyclophosphamide dose of $2 \cdot 2$ g/m^2) against VAI which incorporated Ifosfamide at a dose of 9 g/m^2. A third arm in this randomisation included ifosfamide in combination with etoposide (VIE). No difference was identified between the higher dose VAC and the ifosfamide-containing schedules and VAC remains the combination of choice for future IRSG (now COG) studies. The rationale for this is explained by the lesser cost and easier (shorter) duration of administration required for cyclophosphamide, and concern about the nephrotoxicity of ifosfamide. Nevertheless, the European groups are almost certain to retain IVA as their standard combination as the experience of significant renal toxicity at cumulative ifosfamide doses < 60 g/m^2 is now very small and there is some suggestion (yet to be established with certainty) that the gonadal toxicity of ifosfamide may be significantly less than that of cyclophosphamide.

Experience of the value of other drugs in IRSG studies has been relative slim. IRS-III included the addition of cisplatin and etoposide in a three-way randomisation between VAC, VAC + doxorubicin and cisplatin, and VAC + doxorubicin, cisplatin and etoposide. No advantage was seen in selected Group III and all Group IV patients and there were concerns about additive toxicity. IRS-IV (and an earlier IRS-IV pilot) explored the value of melphalan in a three way randomisation which compared initial treatment for metastatic (Group IV) patients with vincristine/melphalan (VM), ifosfamide/etoposide (IE) and ifosfamide/doxorubicin (ID). Patients who received IE did

5

best and those who received VM did worst. This was almost certainly due to enhanced myelotoxicity which reduced tolerance of subsequent treatment but there was the additional anxiety that this combination also produced the highest rate of second malignancy (7·2% at 5 years).

Radiotherapy (RT) has been a standard component of therapy for the majority of patients in the IRSG studies from the outset. Randomisation studies within IRS-I to III have established that RT is unnecessary for Group I (completely resected) patients with embryonal histology. Analyses from the same studies suggest that RT does offer an improved failure-free survival in patients with completely resected alveolar RMS or with undifferentiated sarcoma. Studies from the European groups have attempted to relate the use of RT to response to initial chemotherapy, the most radical approach being used by the SIOP group who have tried to withhold RT in patients with Group III (pT3b) disease if CR is achieved with initial chemotherapy ± conservative second surgery. This approach has produced evidence that it is possible to avoid local therapy in some children who would otherwise receive RT but there is a need to try to define such favourable patients at the outset so as to reduce the risk of relapse requiring second treatment within the whole group. Doses of RT have, somewhat pragmatically, been tailored to age, with reduced doses in younger children, although there is no defined threshold below which late effects can be avoided and yet tumour control is still achieved. In IRS-IV, a pilot study established the feasibility of hyperfractionated (twice daily) RT treatment (an approach also explored by the European groups) but, so far, no data about the advantage of such an approach are available although data should emerge from the randomised study in IRS-IV. Unless this confirms the superiority of hyperfractionated treatment, most studies will probably continue to offer conventional fractionation, if only for logistical reasons.

Although considerable progress has been made in improving overall survival, progress has been as much incremental and intuitive, based on careful treatment planning, the coordination of chemotherapy with surgery and radiotherapy and better prognostic treatment stratification. Relatively little has been learned about improving treatment from randomised studies although important lessons have been learned about the place of doxorubicin, the avoidance of RT in very good risk patients and the lack of benefit of increased treatment intensity using some additional agents. The challenge for the future requires the development of a greater ability to selectively reduce treatment for some groups of patients with a high chance of cure and to identify better forms of therapy for those with a very poor prognosis. Patients with metastatic disease, for example, continue to have a very poor survival rate. Successful randomised studies in this group of patients will probably require transatlantic collaboration in order to achieve the power necessary to draw any conclusion; the idea has been mooted and needs to be pursued. It is also gratifying that there is now outline agreement for a joint European study for non-metastatic patients which will harness the resources of the SIOP and the CWS–ICG collaborations to produce a study base of similar size to that currently enjoyed by IRSG/COG.

Lessons from studies of non-RMS soft tissue sarcoma

Although this chapter refers to two studies that include patients with non-RMS STS (Studies 7, 8), Study 7 is the only published study which was specifically designed to answer a randomised question about the value of chemotherapy in this difficult and heterogeneous group of patients. Unfortunately, the power of this study was limited and further work needs to be undertaken to better understand optimal therapy. Perhaps the most important immediate question is to ascertain whether the treatment of children with non-RMS STS, particularly with the diagnoses more frequently seen in adults, should be assessed any differently than for adults with the same

condition. If not, combined studies, particularly of new agents, could be productive.

Conclusion
Despite progress made, children with soft tissue sarcoma continue to have an outcome that is unsatisfactory in terms of overall cure. Wider international collaboration is the key to providing a patient base that will allow timely and valid randomised studies.

Studies

Study 1

Maurer HM, Beltangady M, Gehan EA, Crist W, Hammond D, Hays DM, Heyn R, Lawrence W, Newton W, Ortega J.
The Intergroup Rhabdomyosarcoma Study-I. A final report.
Cancer 1988;**61**:209–20,

This study was carried out between 1972 and 1978 by the US Intergroup Rhabdomyosarcoma Study Group.

Objectives

- To evaluate the role of local radiotherapy in IRS Group I patients who received vincristine, actinomycin D (dactinomycin), cyclophosphamide (VAC) chemotherapy.
- To determine whether the addition of cyclophosphamide to vincristine and actinomycin (VA) was of benefit in Group II patients who received local irradiation.
- To document the complete remission rate achieved by pulsed VAC plus local irradiation in patients with Group III and IV disease.
- To evaluate the role of adding doxorubicin (Adriamycin) to VAC in Group III and IV patients.

Details of the study

Patients eligible were under 21 years with rhabdomyosarcoma or undifferentiated sarcoma.

The treatment regimens were as shown in Figure 1.1. Local irradiation was given at the start of treatment in Group I/II patients and after 6 weeks of chemotherapy for all other patients. Radiation dose was 50–60 Gy, reduced to 40 Gy for those under 3 years of age. Patients with lung metastases received 18 Gy bilateral lung irradiation.

The randomisation method is not described in detail. The study was designed to detect a doubling of the median disease free survival time for both Group I and II patients, with 90% power at the 5% level, requiring 87 patients in each arm in both of these studies.

For Group III and IV it was predicted that there would need to be 100 patients in each arm to detect a 20% improvement in response rate, with 90% power at the 5% level. A response rate of 50% was assumed for the control group.

Outcome measures were disease free survival (DFS), overall survival (OS) and local and distant response.

Outcome

A total of 799 patients were registered, of whom 686 were eligible for inclusion. After review of all pathology, radiology and treatment flow sheets 575 were deemed evaluable, but all 686 eligible patients are included in the outcome analysis on an intention to treat basis.

Group I

Regimen A: 43 patients, 81% 5 year DFS, 93% 5 year OS.
Regimen B: 43 patients, 79% 5 year DFS, 81% OS.

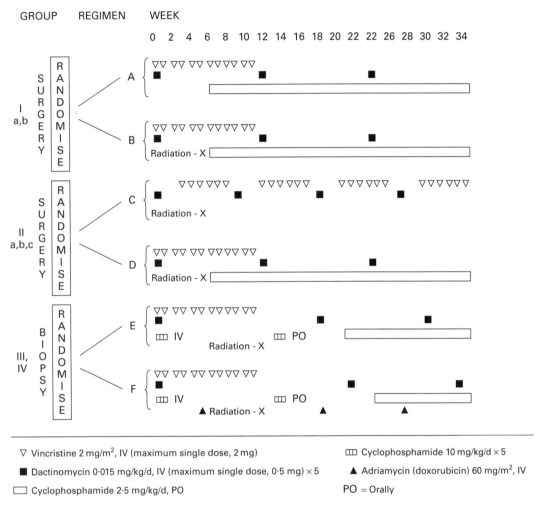

GROUP   REGIMEN   WEEK

0 2 4 6 8 10 12 14 16 18 20 22 22 26 28 30 32 34

Figure 1.1 Treatment regimens. Copyright © 1988 American Cancer Society. Reprinted and adapted by permission from Maurer HM *et al* (full reference p 8) of Wiley-Liss, Inc., a subsidiary of John Wiley & Sons, Inc (full reference on p 8).

▽ Vincristine 2 mg/m², IV (maximum single dose, 2 mg)

▥ Cyclophosphamide 10 mg/kg/d × 5

■ Dactinomycin 0·015 mg/kg/d, IV (maximum single dose, 0·5 mg) × 5

▲ Adriamycin (doxorubicin) 60 mg/m², IV

▭ Cyclophosphamide 2·5 mg/kg/d, PO

PO = Orally

No significant difference between the two arms. No difference was noted in the site of relapse in the two groups with regard to local or distant metastases.

Group II

Regimen C: 87 patients, 72% 5 year DFS, 72% OS at 5 years.

Regimen D: 98 patients, 66% DFS at 5 years, 72% OS.

No significant difference between the two arms.

Group III

Regimen E: 146 patients, complete response rate 67%, median time to achieve complete

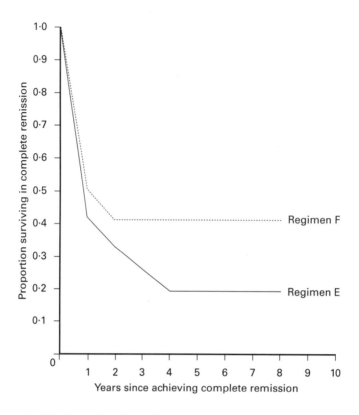

Figure 1.2 Event free survival for Group IV patients. Duration of complete remission curves among complete responders in Group IV by randomised treatments: "pulse" VAC + radiation (regimen E) and "pulse" VAC + Adriamycin (doxorubicin) + radiation (regimen F). Copyright © 1988 American Cancer Society. Reprinted and adapted by permission from Maurer HM *et al* (full reference p 8) of Wiley-Liss, Inc., a subsidiary of John Wiley & Sons, Inc (full reference on p 8).

remission (CR) 12 weeks, event free survival (EFS) at 5 years 49%, OS 69%.

Regimen F: 134 patients, complete response rate 72%, median time to CR 13 weeks, DFS 50%, OS 68%.

No significant difference between the two arms.

Group IV

Regimen E: 61 patients, complete response rate 51%, median time to CR 15 weeks, EFS 19%, OS 14%.

Regimen F: 68 patients, complete response rate 50%, median time to CR 10 weeks, EFS 41%, OS 26%.

No significant difference between the two arms.

Figure 1.2 – shows event free survival for Group IV patients.

Toxicity

There was a 2% treatment-related death rate, all occurring on regimen E or F. There were three severe cardiac toxicities in patients receiving anthracyclines.

Conclusions

- Group I patients achieved no benefit from local irradiation.
- The addition of cyclophosphamide did not add to the efficacy of VA in Group II patients who received local irradiation.
- Doxorubicin did not add to VAC in Group III patients who received local irradiation.

- Although there was a trend to benefit from doxorubicin in Group IV with regard to a more rapid complete response rate and a lower relapse rate in those achieving a complete response, there was no significant difference overall in event free survival or overall survival.

Study 2

Maurer HM, Gehan EA, Beltangady M, Crist W, Dickman PS, Donaldson SS, Fryer C, Hammond D, Hays DM, Herrmann J.
The Intergroup Rhabdomyosarcoma Study-II.
Cancer 1993;**71**:1904–22.

This study was carried out between 1978 and 1984 by the Intergroup Rhabdomyosarcoma Study Group, with participation of the United Kingdom Children's Cancer Study Group (UKCCSG).

Objectives

The aims of the study were:

- To determine the value of cyclophosphamide in favourable site/pathology IRS Group I patients.
- To evaluate the role of pulsed VAC (vincristine, actinomycin D, cyclophosphamide), compared to VA in favourable Group II patients.
- To evaluate the role of doxorubicin (Adriamycin) in Group III and IV patients, excluding special pelvic sites.

In addition, in the non-randomised component of the trial, the value of local meningeal irradiation in parameningeal tumours, the potential reduction in cystectomy rates using primary chemotherapy and the value of pulsed VAC in extremity alveolar tumours was evaluated using comparisons with IRS-I data.

Details of the study

Patients below the age of 21 with rhabdomyosarcoma, soft tissue Ewing's sarcoma and undifferentiated sarcoma were eligible.

All IRS Group I and II patients were included, except those with extremity alveolar tumours.

The dose of local irradiation in Group II patients was 40–45 Gy. For Group III patients under 6 years of age with tumours < 5 cm the dose was 40–45 Gy, over 5 cm 45–50 Gy; for those over 6 'years of age with tumours < 5 cm 45–50 Gy, over 5 cm 50–55 Gy.

Group IV patients with lung disease received 18 Gy bilateral lung irradiation and those with other soft tissue deposits received 50–55 Gy.

For details of the treatment regimens, referenced as numbers 21–26, see Figure 1.3.

Primary outcome measures were disease free survival (DFS) and survival with documentation of response rates.

The method of randomisation was not described.

For Group I and II patients there was a 1 : 2 stratification standard : study regimen. It was estimated that for the Group I patients 25 and 50 patients respectively were required. For Group II, 38 and 75 respectively, and for Groups III and IV, a total of 186 patients. The difference between the curves was analysed using log-rank tests and generalised Wilcoxon tests. The *P* values obtained from statistical tests were used as a measure of the strength of the evidence against the null hypothesis being tested, p < 0·05 indicating a statistically significant result with moderate evidence against the null hypothesis, and p < 0·01 indicating a highly significant result with strong evidence against the null hypothesis.

Outcome

A total of 1115 patients were registered, of whom 116 were excluded, 100 due to unconfirmed

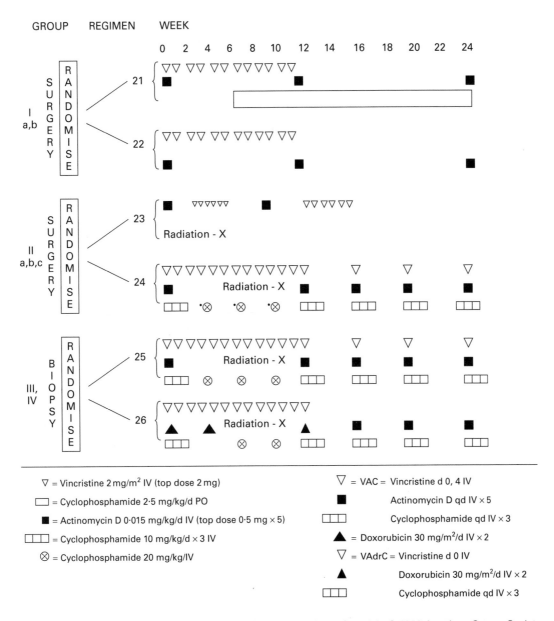

Figure 1.3 Intergroup Rhabdomyosarcoma Study II Treatment regimen. Copyright © 1993 American Cancer Society. Adapted and reprinted from Maurer HM *et al* (full reference p 12) with permission from Wiley-Liss, Inc., a subsidiary of John Wiley & Sons, Inc.

eligible pathology on review. The allocation to treatment group by local centre was confirmed on review in 92% of cases. Of the 999 patients, 776 were regarded as evaluable. Reasons to be non-evaluable included wrong treatment assignments, protocol violation or inadequate data collection. All 999 patients were included in the analysis on an intention to treat basis.

Group I

Regimen 21: 37 patients, 5 year DFS 80%, OS at 5 years 85%.

Regimen 22: 64 patients, DFS 70%, OS 84%.

There appeared to be more local recurrences in the arm not receiving cyclophosphamide – 14 versus 5% – but this was not statistically significant.

Group II

Regimen 23: 45 patients, DFS 69%, OS 88%.

Regimen 24: 85 patients, DFS 74%, OS 79%.

No significant difference between the treatment arms.

Group III

Regimen 25: 211 patients, complete remission rate 74%, continued clinical remission (CCR) at 5 years 75%, OS in complete remission (CR) patients 66%.

Regimen 26: 197 patients, CR 78%, CCR at 5 years 70%, OS 65%.

No significant difference between the treatment arms, but significantly better than in IRS-I.

Group IV

Regimen 25: 83 patients, CR 52%, median time to CR 13 weeks, CCR of CR patients at 5 years 38%.

Regimen 26: 88 patients, CR 53%, median time to CR 15 weeks, CCR at 5 years 38%.

Overall progression free survival of all patients at 5 years 21% for Regimen 25 and 25% for Regimen 26.

No significant difference.

Toxicity

There were 21 fatalities associated with treatment, overall 1–4% by regimen. There were five severe cardiac toxicities. The precise details by regimen were not specified.

Conclusion

Vincristine and actinomycin given for 1 year is equivalent to 2 years of VAC in Group I patients not given local irradiation.

Cyclophosphamide does not add benefit to VA in Group II patients who receive local irradiation.

The addition of doxorubicin to a VAC based combination does not significantly improve either complete response rate or ultimate outcome in patients with Group III or IV disease.

Comments

Womer has noted some reservations about the comparability of the regimens (Womer RB. The Intergroup Rhabdomyoma studies come of age. *Cancer* 1993;**71**:1719–21). For Group II patients, Regimen 23 had three times the vincristine and half the actinomycin dose, compared to Regimen 24 which contained cyclophosphamide. Moreover, it is possible that the addition of doxorubicin could have had an impact on the different pathological subgroups within Groups III and IV, but insufficient patient numbers were recruited to determine whether there was a difference between embryonal or alveolar rhabdomyosarcoma.

Study 3

Crist W, Gehan EA, Ragab AH, Dickman PS, Donaldson SS, Fryer C, Hammond D, Hays DM, Herrmann J, Heyn R.
The Third Intergroup Rhabdomyosarcoma Study.
J Clin Oncol 1995; **13**:610–30.

This study was carried out between 1984 and 1991 by the Intergroup Rhabdomyosarcoma Study Group.

Objectives

The aims of the study were to determine the role of doxorubicin (Adriamycin) in addition to VAC (vincristine, actinomycin D, cyclophosphamide) chemotherapy in Group II patients and, secondly, the role of the addition of either cisplatin/ doxorubicin or cisplatin/ doxorubicin and etoposide in Group III and IV patients. Non-randomised comparisons were made with IRS-II for all other patient groups.

Details of the study

Eligible patients were under the age of 21 years with rhabdomyosarcoma, undifferentiated sarcoma and extraosseous sarcoma and extra-osseous Ewing's sarcoma. Treatment had to be started within 42 days of tumour biopsy and 21 days of definitive primary surgery.

Outcome measures were progression free survival (PFS) and overall survival (OS), in addition to local and metastatic response.

It was estimated that for Group II patients, to demonstrate a 15% increase in endpoint from 80% to 95% with 73% power at the 5% level would require 92 patients. It was planned to include comparable non-randomised patients from IRS-II who received the identical standard comparator regimen.

For Group III patients, in order to detect an increase from 70% to 80%, with 76% power at the 5% level, would require a total of 472 patients. Again, it was planned to include comparable patients from the IRS-II who required the identical standard regimen.

The precise methods of randomisation were not detailed.

Details of the chemotherapy and radiotherapy regimens are given in Figure 1.4.

Group II favourable histology patients received either VA + radiotherapy or VA/doxorubicin + radiotherapy for a total of one year. Patients with testicular, orbit or head and neck non-parameningeal primaries were excluded from the randomised study.

Group III patients, with the exception of special pelvic sites and parameningeal tumours, either received the standard regimen of pulsed VAC + radiotherapy or a regimen including doxorubicin and cisplatin or doxorubicin/cisplatin/etoposide. All three regimens incorporated second line chemotherapy for patients who achieved partial response. For the standard VAC regimen this comprised doxorubicin and DTIC, for the doxorubicin/cisplatin regimen, actinomycin D/etoposide, and for the four-drug regimen, actinomycin D and DTIC.

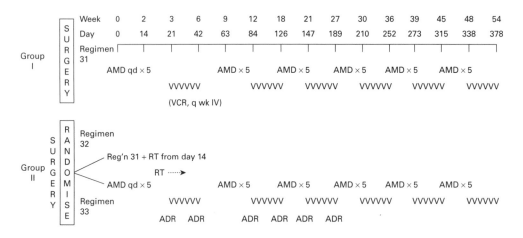

Figure 1.4a Intergroup Rhabdomyosarcoma Study III treatment regimen for Groups I and II (AMD, actinomycin D; ADR, doxorubicin; VCR, vincristine; RT, radiotherapy)

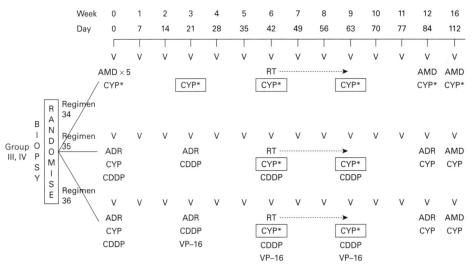

*Favourable histology

**Excluding Group III favourable histology, orbit and non-parameningeal head tumours

Figure 1.4b Intergroup Rhabdomyosarcoma Study III treatment regimen for Groups I and II (CYP, cyclophosphamide; CDDP, cisplatin; VP-16, etoposide; other abbreviations as Figure 1.4a)

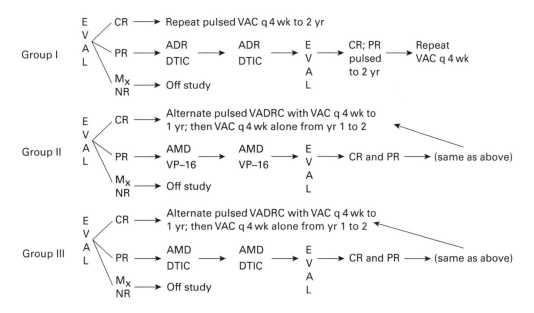

Figure 1.4c Figure 14b Intergroup Rhabdomyosarcoma Study III treatment regimen (CR, complete remission; PR, partial remission; NR, no remission; other abbreviations as Figure 1.4a)

Outcome

A total of 1194 patients were enrolled, of whom 132 were excluded, 79 due to incorrect pathology. Of the 1062 eligible patients, 235 were regarded as non-assessable for a variety of reasons, on central review of grouping, radiotherapy, chemotherapy and surgical details. All patients eligible and randomised were included in the subsequent analyses on an intention to treat basis. Overall, there was pathological agreement with the Central Review Panel in 79% of alveolar cases and 77% of embryonal cases.

Group II

Regimen 32: 23 patients, 5 year PFS 56%, OS at 5 years 54%.

Regimen 33: 51 patients, 77% PFS and 89% OS. With the addition of the identical IRS-II Regimen 23 patients, PFS in the control arm was 63% and OS 73%.

No statistical difference between the two treatment arms.

Group III

Regimen 34: 58 patients, complete remission (CR) rate at week 20 39%, with an eventual CR rate of 79%. Five year PFS 70% and OS 70%.

Regimen 35: 113 patients, week 20 CR 45%, final CR 78%, PFS 62%, OS 63%.

Regimen 36: 118 patients, week 20 CR 48%, final CR 84%, PFS 56%, OS 64%.

No statistical significant difference in the initial response, final CR or ultimate outcome.

Group IV

Regimen 34: 29 patients, week 20 CR 42%, final CR 50%, PFS 27%, OS 27%.

Regimen 35: 65 patients, week 20 CR 30%, final CR 57%, PFS 27%, OS 31%.

Regimen 36: 56 patients, week 20 CR 38%, final CR 62%, PFS 30%, OS 29%.

Comparing with IRS-II, the Group III patients did significantly better, $p < 0.01$, with 61% versus 52% PFS. This was concluded to be due to the value of second line chemotherapy achieving complete response.

Toxicity

Overall 5% fatalities. Morbidity of individual regimens was not detailed. Overall, there were 9% cardiac toxicities, of which 5% were severe. There were five cases of secondary acute myeloid leukaemia – 4 on Regimen 36.

Conclusion

It was concluded that although the overall results were superior to IRS-II, no particular subgroups benefited directly from the intensification of chemotherapy within the randomised comparison.

Study 4

Flamant F, Rodary C, Voute PA, Otten J.
Primary chemotherapy in the treatment of rhabdomyosarcoma in children. Trial of the International Society of Pediatric Oncology (SIOP) preliminary results.
Radiother Oncol 1985;**3**:227–36.

The study was run from 1975 to 1983 by the European collaboration group SIOP.

Objectives

The aim of the study was to determine whether to use of chemotherapy radiotherapy prior to surgery could minimise treatment sequelae without jeopardising survival rate.

Details of the study

Eligible patients included those aged 1–15 years with embryonal or alveolar rhabdomyosarcoma, deemed initially unresectable, with either incomplete removal or biopsy only. Patients had to have had equal or greater than 25% reduction in tumour volume after one course of VAC (vincristine, actinomycin D, cyclophosphamide) chemotherapy. Patients were also excluded if there was a major intolerance to this initial course of chemotherapy.

The method of randomisation is not specified. Randomisation was performed on day 28, with pairing according to the localisation. Ear, nose and throat primaries were also paired according to age and bone involvement of the base of the skull.

Patients received regimen A or regimen B. (see Figure 1.5). Regimen A was continuation of VAC, followed by vincristine doxorubicin (VAD)

chemotherapy, alternating for an 18 month period. If a complete clinical response was achieved, no other treatment was given. If a partial response was achieved, chemotherapy was given to maximum effect, followed by surgery and/or radiotherapy. If there was no response after two VAC/VAD, surgery and/or radiotherapy was given. With regimen B systematic radiotherapy was given to the initial tumour volume, even if the tumour had regressed after pre-trial chemotherapy. A dose of 45 gray (Gy) was used accompanied by daily actinomycin on each of the first seven radiotherapy sessions and vincristine every 2 weeks during radiotherapy. Following radiotherapy, VAC/VAD was given for 18 months, as in regimen A. In the case of bladder and prostate tumours, anterior exenteration was done followed by radiotherapy if the surgery was not microscopically complete.

Outcome at 3 years was analysed in paired cases. Using a closed pragmatic design the probability of preferring one treatment when in reality the other was better in 65% of the untied pairs was 5%. Under these conditions the number of pairs required was estimated to be 37, i.e. 74 patients. If the accrual rate was 25 patients per year, 3 years would have been needed, and the results of the last pair treated would have been available 6 years after the study started.

In the analysis the best result of the pair was chosen. If both patients died, neither treatment was preferable and this pair resulted in a tie. When only one of the pair was dead, the treatment given to the living patient was counted as preferable, even if the patient was living with a relapse. If both were living, the treatment which had given the best results, taking into consideration the

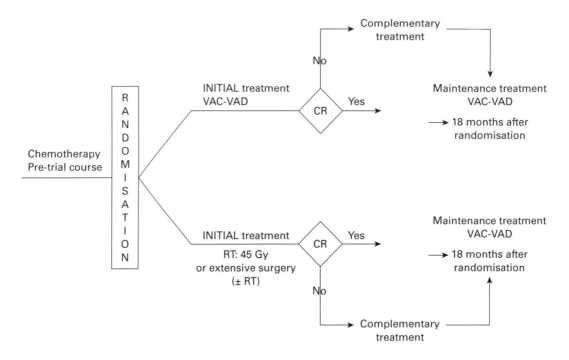

Figure 1.5 Design of the trial

existing and expected therapeutic sequelae, was preferred. When the results were equal, the less heavy treatment was chosen.

Outcome

Eighty-one patients were entered. Fifteen failed to show a sufficient response to course 1 and three were excluded due to protocol violation or pathological error. Local complete response was achieved in 21 of 32 in arm A and 21 of 31 in arm B.

The final assessment at 3 years was estimated for 22 pairs of patients. No difference was seen between the arms; the overall survival rate was 40% at 3 years. Of 56 patients with more than 2 years' follow up, 41% in arm A were in complete clinical remission compared with 48% of arm B.

It was noted that in all children with bladder primaries cystectomy was eventually performed in both treatment arms.

Conclusion

It was concluded that primary chemotherapy could avoid many late sequelae with no adverse effect on outcome, although overall disease free survival was poor in both arms. The numbers were too small to conclude unequivocally whether disease free survival differed between the two arms. This study was stopped prematurely due to poor results in those with parameningeal localisation and the refusal by doctors and the families to allow patients with bladder and prostate primaries to undergo anterior pelvectomy.

Study 5

Carli M, Pastore G, Perilongo G, Grotto P, De Bernardi B, Ceci A, Di Tullio M, Madon E, Pianca C, Paolucci G.
Tumour response and toxicity after single high-dose versus standard five-day divided-dose dactinomycin in childhood rhabdomyosarcoma. *J Clin Oncol* 1988;**6**:654–58.

The study was run from 1979 to 1985 by the Italian Multicentre Collaborative Group.

Objectives

The study aimed to compare two methods of administration of actinomycin, as part of VAC.

Details of the study

Eligible patients with a rhabdomyosarcoma included those under 15 years of age with one of the following: a tumour > 5 cm in size, primary of bladder, prostate, vagina, uterus and orbit, and included those with distant metastases.

Randomisation was carried out centrally using a closed envelope method. It was balanced for primary site, clinical group and centre size. A projected accrual rate of 15–20 patients per year was planned to achieve around 50 patients in each arm to show a 30% difference in response or toxicity, α 0·05, β 0·2.

Actinomycin, as part of VAC, was given at 0·45 mg/m^2 daily for 5 days, the combination repeated every 28 days for three courses. This schedule was compared with 1·7 mg/m^2 on day 8 only

and the regimen was repeated every 21 days for four courses.

The major outcome measure was response to treatment prior to course 4, 3 weeks after the second course.

Outcome

Thirty-six patients received split dose VAC and 42 single dose VAC. Eight patients were excluded, due to early death in 4, 2 refused after randomisation and 2 had prior chemotherapy.

Complete or partial remission was 67% on the split dose VAC and 70% for the single dose VAC. Overall survival at 3 years and 5 years with split dose was 48% and 38% and single dose 43% and 43%.

Toxicity

The split dose VAC was more myelosuppressive, although not statistically significant. There was significantly more stomatitis with split dose VAC (p < 0·01). There were two severe episodes of sepsis, both in the split dose arms.

Conclusion

It was concluded that the fractionated regimen was somewhat more toxic and no more effective in achieving an initial response than the simpler single dose regimen. In particular, there was no evidence of any increase in liver toxicity associated with the single dose regimen.

Study 6

Baker KS, Anderson JR, Link MP, Grier HE, Qualman SJ, Maurer HM, Breneman JC, Wiener ES, Crist WM.

Benefit of intensified therapy for patients with local or regional embryo- nal rhabdomyosarcoma: results from the Intergroup Rhabdomyosarcoma Study-IV.

J Clin Oncol 2000;**18**:2427–34.

The study was carried out by the US Intergroup Rhabdomyosarcoma Study between 1991 and 1997 (IRS-IV).

Objectives

The study was designed to compare three induction and continuation chemotherapies based on the VAC regimen, with the substitution of ifosfamide for cyclophosphamide or the replacement of actinomycin and cyclophosphamide with ifosfamide and etoposide.

Details of the study

Eligible patients were under 21 years of age with either rhabdomyosarcoma or undifferentiated sarcoma. Chemotherapy was to start within 42 days of initial surgery.

No details of randomisation method are given, nor the predicted number of patients required to address the issue of differences in efficacy of the respective chemotherapies.

The regimens are shown in Figure 1.6. The cyclophosphamide dose of 2·2 g/m^2 is higher than in previous IRS regimens and this was replaced by 9 g of ifosfamide infused over 5 days and the same dose combined with etoposide 500 mg/m^2 over 5 days.

Excluded from the study were patients felt to be at risk of renal problems, namely those with raised creatinine, single kidneys or pre-existing hydronephrosis. Also excluded were the good risk Group I patients with testis, orbit or eyelid primaries who received only vincristine and actinomycin D.

The primary outcome measure was failure-free survival.

Outcome

A total of 894 patients were registered with locoregional disease. For the chemotherapy comparisons no details of patient numbers or disease group are provided in this report, just the outcome. The 3 year failure-free survivals for VAC, VAI and VAE were 74%, 74% and 76% respectively, with overall survivals of 81%, 83% and 87%, i.e. no significant difference between the three arms.

No details of toxicity between the three treatments are provided.

Conclusion

Overall, the results in IRS-IV were no different from IRS-III, except for the subgroup of patients with intermediate risk embryonal histology, where there was a significant improvement in event free and overall survival. This was claimed to be due to the increase in the dose of alkylating agent in IRS-IV, compared to IRS-III.

It was concluded that none of the novel regimens had any advantage over the VAC protocol containing a higher dose of cyclophosphamide.

Regimen	INDUCTION: Treatment week 0–16									EVAL									EVAL	CONTINUATION: Treatment week 20–46								
	0	1	2	3	4	5	6	7	8		9	10	11	12	13	14	15	16		20	21	22	23	24	25	26	27	28
VAC	V	V	V	V	V	V	V	V	V	E	V	V	V	V	–	–	–	V	E	V	V	V	V	V	V	–	–	–
	A		A		A					V	C		C					A	V	A		A						
	C		C		C					A		Radiation therapy*						C	A	C		C						
VAI	V	V	V	V	V	V	V	V	V	L	V	V	V	V	–	–	–	V	L	V	V	V	V	V	V	–	–	–
	A		A		A					U	I		I					A	U	A		A						
	I		I		I					A		Radiation therapy*						I	A	I		I						
VIE	V	V	V	V	V	V	V	V	V	I	V	V	V	V	–	–	–	V	I	V	V	V	V	V	V	–	–	–
	I		I		I					O	I		I					I	O	I		I						
	E		E		E					N		Radiation therapy*						E	N	E		E						

V, vincristine 1·5 mg/m² (2 mg maximum);

A, actinomycin D 0·015 mg/kg/d (0·5 mg maximum daily dose), days 0–4;

C, cyclophosphamide 2·2 mg/m², day 0;

I, ifosfamide 1·8 mg/m²/d, days 0–4;

E, etoposide 100 mg/m²/d, days 0–4

Figure 1.6 Treatment plans for IRS-IV patients at intermediate risk of failure

(The two unshaded vertical columns — between weeks 8–9 and weeks 16–20 — read downward as EVALUATION, i.e. E V A L U A T I O N, with the letter "T" falling between the VAI and VIE blocks.)

Study 7

Pratt CB, Pappo AS, Gieser P, Jenkins JJ, Salzberg A, Neff J, Rao B, Green D, Thomas P, Marcus R, Parham D, Maurer H.
Role of adjuvant chemotherapy in the treatment of surgically resected pediatric nonrhabdomyosarcomatous soft tissue sarcomas: a Pediatric Oncology Group Study.
J Clin Oncol 1999;**17**:1219–26.

This study was carried out by the Pediatric Oncology Group (POG 8653) between 1986 and 1992.

Objectives

The study was designed to evaluate whether administration of chemotherapy following surgical resection of non-rhabdomyosarcomatous soft tissue sarcomas improved local or systemic control.

Details of the study

Patients were under 21 years of age, previously untreated and pathologies that were excluded comprised rhabdomyosarcoma, extraosseous Ewing's sarcoma, fibromatosis, undifferentiated sarcoma, angiofibroma, dermatofibrosarcoma protuberans and mesothelioma.

The randomisation method is not given, but it was balanced for clinical group status. The initial design specified a sample size of 112 patients would be required to detect a 20% improvement in 2 year event free survival (70% versus 50%) with an 80% power. A 5%, one-sided significance level was assumed. Overall survival and event free survival (EFS) were the primary outcome measures. All pathology was centrally reviewed.

The treatment schema is given in Figure 1.7. Children with Group I disease received no postoperative irradiation and were randomly assigned to be observed or receive adjuvant chemotherapy with vincristine 1·5 mg/m², doxorubicin (Adriamycin) 60 mg/m² and cyclophosphamide 750 mg/m²(VAdrC), alternating every 3 weeks with vincristine 1·5 mg/m², cyclophosphamide 750 mg/m² and actinomycin D 1·25 mg/m² (VAC) for a total of 31 weeks. Children with clinical Group II disease, i.e. microscopic residual tumour, received age-adjusted postoperative radiotherapy to the tumour bed at a dose between 35 and 45 Gy. After completion of irradiation, patients were randomly assigned to receive or not receive chemotherapy. Patients with clinical Group III disease underwent second-look surgery 6–12 weeks after completing radiation therapy. If complete tumour regression was documented, these patients were also randomly assigned to receive or not receive adjuvant chemotherapy.

Outcome

Ninety-nine patients were enrolled, 18 were excluded due to ineligible pathology. Thirty of the 81 remaining were randomised. Reasons for the high non-randomisation rate are not given, but 19 were electively treated with chemotherapy and 32 with observation alone. Overall, most patients in Group I had extremity primaries: synovial sarcoma was the commonest pathology (36%) followed by malignant fibrous histiocytoma (12%), malignant peripheral nerve sheath tumour (10%) and fibrosarcoma (10%); 47% had grade 3 tumours.

For the randomisation cases, the 5 year EFS was 87% for those observed, versus 41% for those receiving chemotherapy (p = < 0·01) and overall

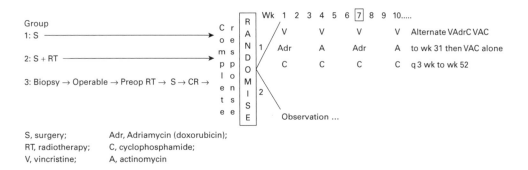

S, surgery;   Adr, Adriamycin (doxorubicin);
RT, radiotherapy;   C, cyclophosphamide;
V, vincristine;   A, actinomycin

Figure 1.7 Treatment schedule for POG-8653

survival was 93% and 69% respectively (p = < 0·016). These differences were, however, due to an imbalance in histological grade, with 73% of grade 3 in the chemotherapy arm, compared to 40% in the observation arm. Histological grade 3 included the following diagnoses: pleomorphic or round-cell liposarcoma, mesenchymal chondrosarcoma, extraskeletal osteogenic sarcoma, malignant triton tumour, alveolar soft part sarcoma and a group of tumours with a high level of necrosis and mitotic activity.

Conclusion
It was concluded that this study failed to show any significant benefit from chemotherapy but the low randomisation rate and ultimately small numbers limit the conclusions that can be drawn.

Study 8

Pratt CB, Maurer HM, Gieser P, Salzberg A, Rao BN, Parham D, Thomas PRM, Marcus RB, Cantor A, Pick T, Green D, Neff J, Jenkins JJ.
Treatment of unresectable or metastatic pediatric soft tissue sarcomas with surgery, irradiation and chemotherapy: a Pediatric Oncology Group Study.
Med Ped Oncol 1998;**30**:201–9.

The study was carried out by the Pediatric Oncology Group (POG 8654) between 1986 and 1994.

Objectives

The objective of the study was to compare two chemotherapy regimens in children with either gross residual disease at presentation following surgery or distant metastases, either at presentation or as recurrent disease after initial treatment with surgery alone.

Details of the study

Details of patient eligibility are not given with regard to age, pathology etc.

The randomisation technique is not reported. It was assumed that there would be a 25% response rate for standard chemotherapy with vincristine, doxorubicin, cyclophosphamide and actinomycin D and 94 patients would be required to document an increase to 40% with the addition of DTIC, with 80% power using Type I error.

The study outline is shown in Figure 1.8. All patients received VACA – vincristine 1·5 mg/m², actinomycin D 1 mg/m², cyclophosphamide 750 mg/m², doxorubicin (Adriamycin) 60 mg/m² – and were randomised to receive, or not receive,

additional DTIC of 500 mg/m². All received local radiotherapy at week 6, with an age-adjusted dose with maximal tumour dose of 55–65 Gy. Sites of metastases were also irradiated.

Delayed surgery was performed on Group 3 patients 6–12 weeks after radiotherapy.

Infants under 12 months received half-dose chemotherapy and the 3-weekly schedule was delayed one week if the absolute neutrophil count (ANC) was < 0·5 per microlitre and platelets < 50 per microlitre at any time. If the ANC was $< 0.25 \times 10^9/\ell$ and platelets $< 10 \times 10^9/\ell$, doses were decreased by 25%.

Primary outcome measures were response at 6 weeks and relapse free survival.

Outcome

Seventy-five patients were accrued prior to premature closure of the study. This was due to slow accrual, accompanied by investigator bias related to randomisation. Among the 75 patients, 14 were ineligible due to problems with pathology on review. These included rhabdomyosarcoma, lymphoma, fibromatosis, osteosarcoma and thymoma. Of the 61 eligible patients there were 13 malignant peripheral nerve sheath tumours, 8 synovial sarcomas, 5 alveolar soft part sarcomas, 5 malignant fibrous histiocytomas and 6 non-specified sarcomas. Twenty-five patients received VACA and 25 patients received VACA plus DTIC. Eleven received VACA electively, in part due to a lack of DTIC availability for a 12 month period during the study.

Overall response rate for VACA was 56% (35–76%) and with the addition of DTIC, 44%

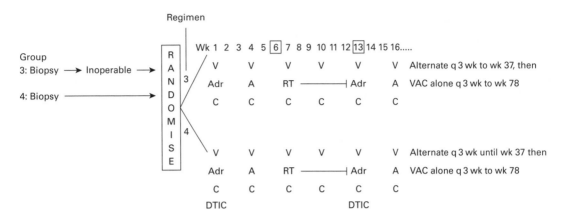

Figure 1.8 Treatment schema for POG-8654 (abbreviations as in Figure 1.7)

(24–65%). For Group 3 patients there were 14 complete responses and 5 partial responses out of 36 overall. For Group 4 patients, 3 complete responses and 6 partial responses in 25 patients. For the randomised VACA patients, there were 4 complete responses and 6 partial responses out of 25. For the DTIC arm, 7 complete responses and 4 partial responses out of 25. Event free survival for VACA was 36% at 2 years, with DTIC it was 26%. The difference was not significant.

Conclusion

In conclusion, there appeared to be a high initial response rate but poor overall event free survival and there appeared to be no benefit from the addition of DTIC.

2

Osteosarcoma

Commentary – Alan Craft

The history of the introduction of the chemotherapy in the management of osteosarcoma is one which should be studied by all new recruits to oncology and indeed those running clinical trials. It is a classic story of the need for good randomised controlled trials (RCTs) before the introduction of a new treatment and of many of the pitfalls in trying to establish a meaningful RCT.

Unfortunately the reports of the RCTs as detailed here do not give any real idea of the chronology and the excitement of the story. The studies included here are the definitive papers, which usually appeared several years after the results had been presented at major meetings and were available in abstract form.

Prior to the chemotherapy era, osteosarcoma could be cured by amputation alone in about 20% of patients. The remaining 80% of patients died, almost exclusively from lung metastases over the next 18 months or so. There were many papers in the literature confirming the 20% figure. Chemotherapy was introduced in the late 1960s and methotrexate seemed to be the drug which had the most activity. Following descriptive reports of significant improvements in survival the Mayo Clinic undertook a RCT of high dose methotrexate against no chemotherapy in osteosarcoma (Study 2). Although it was a very small study, both progression free survival and overall survival were the same in both groups. Very surprisingly, the 50% survival without

chemotherapy was more than twice that which would have been expected from historical controls.

The initial conclusion was that the natural history of osteosarcoma must have changed and that surgery, at least in the hands of the Mayo Clinic, was as good as chemotherapy. There was much speculation as to the reasons for this unusual result but the seeds of doubt had been sown regarding the efficacy of chemotherapy and for several years there was much scepticism and reluctance, particularly by orthopaedic surgeons, to refer their newly diagnosed patients to an oncologist. After all, one of the world's leading orthopedic centres, the Mayo Clinic, had shown that good surgery was all that was required.

The other main possibility for this bizarre result was that somehow the Mayo Clinic patients were not the same as the general population of osteosarcoma, that some type of selection had taken place. Two of the possibilities considered were that the Mayo was one of the first places in the world to have CT scanning and that by using a more sophisticated imaging system they were able to select out only those who really did hot have obvious pulmonary metastases, thereby improving the overall prognosis.

Another possibility was that the Mayo is a tertiary if not quaternary referral centre and in order to get there, a considerable number of steps have to be gone through, all of which takes time. A patient who did not have pulmonary metastases by the time he or she got to the Mayo maybe had a tumour which had a better natural history.

None of these possible biasing factors would have mattered in the RCT as they would have been likely to be acting in both arms. The real explanation emerged some years later when the histological type of osteosarcoma was revealed. By then it was recognised that almost a quarter of the patients had grade 2 or 3 osteosarcoma. High grade osteosarcoma is usually classified as grade 4. It appears that the surgery only arm, by chance, included more randomised patients with an inherently good prognosis because of lower grade histology.

In the meantime, Rosen, working at the Memorial Sloan–Kettering Hospital in New York, had devised a new regimen of treatment which was based on the *in vivo* response of the osteosarcoma to chemotherapy. All patients received initial chemotherapy, mainly high dose methotrexate, the tumour was then surgically resected and subsequent treatment was based on the histological response. Good responses received more methotrexate and poor responses switched to a cisplatin/doxorubicin regimen.

The early results of this "T10" protocol suggested a 90% survival and these were reported in *Cancer* in 1982. This dramatic paper is probably one of the most cited in paediatric oncology. According to Science Citation Index, between 1982 and 1995 it had been cited 378 times and not surprisingly T10 had become the gold standard of treatment.

So, in the late 1970s, investigators faced the dilemma of many people thinking that chemotherapy was of no value, the Mayo "camp",

whilst others became disciples of Rosen. Fortunately two other groups had the courage to undertake RCTs which included a no chemotherapy arm. The Multi Institutional Study (MIOS), run under the auspices of POG by Michael Link (Study 4) convinced the sceptics that chemotherapy was of value. The no chemotherapy arm had a relapse free survival of 17%, identical to the historical series in the literature. The natural history of osteosarcoma had not changed! Interestingly, the overall survival on long term follow up was not different in the two arms, suggesting that to delay chemotherapy until the appearance of metastases was not detrimental.

The other study with a no chemotherapy control arm was that reported by Eilber from UCLA (Study 5). Perhaps they had learnt the lesson from the Mayo study because they excluded all patients with low grade pathology. Disease free survival (DFS) in the no chemotherapy arm was again as expected from history – 20%. The T10 regimen had a DFS of 55% at 2 years, but considerably less than that reported by Rosen.

By the early 1980s, therefore, it seemed that chemotherapy was of value and most orthopedic surgeons began to send their patients to an oncologist. However, there was considerable scepticism about the Rosen results from New York. In Europe this was probably of greater intensity than in the US. The EORTC had undertaken an RCT between 1978 and 1983 (Study 6) in which there was no significant difference between the various treatment groups, but overall the results were disappointing at around 40–50%. They had used methotrexate but in a much lower dose than Rosen. The European Osteosarcoma Intergroup (EOI) was formed with the explicit aim of devising a simpler regimen than the T10 and then comparing it in an RCT with T10. The other major European groups, the German COSS group and the Italian Institute Rizzoli group, did not take part in the EOI, and although the French initially were going to be included, they were so convinced of the success of the T10 protocol that they wanted to replicate it.

The first EOI study (Study 7) started out as a randomised phase II study but accrual was so successful that the 60 patients needed was rapidly exceeded. The two drug cisplatin/doxorubicin regimen was superior to that also containing methotrexate but the only real conclusion that could be drawn was that increased dose intensity of cisplatin/doxorubicin was important. It could not answer any questions about methotrexate. This led on to the second EOI study (Study 10), which was the formal comparison of the best treatment from the first study against the T10 regime. This study showed no significant difference between the two treatments. It has been criticised on the grounds that many patients in the T10 arm stopped treatment early but it probably does reflect what happens in the real world in a multi-institutional setting. For economic and patient convenience reasons cisplatin/doxorubicin is now more widely used, although many groups still follow a methotrexate bases T10 type of regimen.

The COSS group (Study 1) showed no benefit for the addition of interferon, which had been suggested by Strander in the early 1970s as being a worthwhile adjuvant. They also showed no benefit for the addition of other drugs to their standard methotrexate, doxorubicin regimen.

The Italian group (Study 8) showed that high dose was better than moderate dose methotrexate perhaps providing an explanation for the overall poor results obtained with the EORTC (Study 6), which used only moderate doses.

The mode of delivery of chemotherapy – intra-arterial versus intravenous – has also received study. From a theoretical point of view it seems possible that direct delivery of the effective drug into the tumour could be of value. However it does add an additional technical complexity to the treatment. The COSS group showed no difference for IA v. IV (Study 9). Most of the other reported RCTs in osteosarcoma have looked at varying combinations of the same drugs in different intensities. Overall it seems that dose intensity is important. The only new and possibly effective drugs to appear in the Past 15 years have been ifosfamide and etoposide. These have been tested in an RCT by the CCG in the US but only preliminary somewhat confusing results are available. There was a double randomisation to ± ifosfamide and ± MTTPE. (The latter is a form of immunotherapy.) Theoretically no interaction was predicted between MTTPE and ifosfamide. Unfortunately, the results suggest that there was.

The logical next step for the EOI was to undertake a dose intensity study and that is currently almost complete. The standard two drug cisplatin/doxorubicin given every 3 weeks is being compared with the same drugs given every 2 weeks with the addition of GCSF.

What then are the main questions which remain to be answered in osteosarcoma? Survival has improved little over the past 20 years and new drugs or new modalities of treatment are needed. Of the existing drugs, the place of methotrexate is not proven. It is undoubtedly an active agent but whether it is an essential part of other combinations is not clear. An RCT with ± high dose methotrexate (HDMTX) as the only randomisation would be of interest but unfortunately, because HDMTX interferes with the dose intensity of other drugs, it has not been possible to design such a clean study.

As with many concers occurring in children and young people, it is likely that further progress will not be made with existing therapies. Targetted radiotherapy with samarium and other bone seeking isotopes may be one possibility, perhaps as an additional therapy.

Non-specific immunotherapy with MTTPE appears in the recently closed CCG study to be of some benefit, so perhaps some more specific ideas in this area would be worth considering.

The biology of osteosarcoma is beginning to be unravelled but there does not appear to be any specific gene rearrangement associated with the majority of tumours. However, potential drug targets have been identified and drugs designed to interact with these. Herceptin which interacts with $cErbB_2$ was designed to be used for breast cancer patients but may well be effective in osteosarcoma.

Whichever new therapies look promising, they will have to be tested in RCTs. Osteosarcoma is rare and in order to complete an RCT in a timely fashion it will be necessary to have multinational studies.

Finally, we have learnt a number of very important lessons from the reported RCTs in osteosarcoma which are applicable more widely. The lessons to be learnt from these studies are:

- The natural history of a condition does not change.
- In an RCT make sure that both arms contain the same type of patients.
- If the RCT is entirely conducted in a specialist hospital, the randomised comparison may be valid but the overall result may not be applicable to the general population.
- Beware of double randomisations where the two might interact.

Studies

Study 1

Winkler K, Beron G, Katz R, Salzer-Kuntschik M, Beck J, Beck W, Brandeis W, Ebell W, Erttmann R, Gobel U, Havers W, Henze G, Hinderfeld L, Hocker P, Jobke A, Jurgens H, Kabisch H, Preusser P, Prindull G, Ramach W, Ritter J, Sekera J, Treuner J, Wust G, Landbeck G.
Neoadjuvant chemotherapy for osteogenic sarcoma: results of co-operative German–Austrian study.
J Clin Oncol 1984;**2**:617–24.

This study (Coss-80) was designed and run by the German COSS group between 1979 and 1982.

Objectives

The study addressed two questions: whether the addition of either cisplatin or bleomycin/cyclophosphamide/actinomycin D (BCD) improved the efficacy of a doxorubicin/high dose methotrexate (HDMTX) based regimen and also if interferon was of benefit when given to patients following initial chemotherapy.

Details of the study/outcome

A sequential series of patients with non-metastatic high grade classic central osteosarcoma were recruited. Technetium bone scan and chest *x*-ray were used to exclude distant metastases. CT scan was used in 39% of cases.

Patients were randomised at a central base in Hamburg, using prepared random lists, with stratification for age, sex, site and local extent (relative to normal bone).

Treatment outline and drug doses are given in Figure 2.1. To address the secondary question interferon was given for a 22 week period starting in week 16.

Disease free survival (DFS) was the main outcome measure.

A total of 214 patients were registered, 56 were excluded due to incorrect diagnosis, prior chemotherapy or alternative pathologies. Of 158 entered, a further 42 were excluded due to delayed chemotherapy or a wide variety of protocol violations. One hundred and sixteen patients were available for analysis.

There was no significant difference in DFS with the addition of either cisplatin (73%) or BCD (77%) or between patients given interferon (77%) or no interferon (73%).

Overall, 55% proceeded to conservative surgery, with no difference between the chemotherapy groups. As expected, there was an increase in renal toxicity in the cisplatin based arm. There were five treatment related deaths, two due to methotrexate and three due to infection.

Conclusion

It is concluded that the two regimens were of comparable efficacy and improved overall survival compared to the previous COSS-77 trial was noted. The improvement was particularly marked in the under-12s and it was postulated this was due to the higher methotrexate given to younger patients.

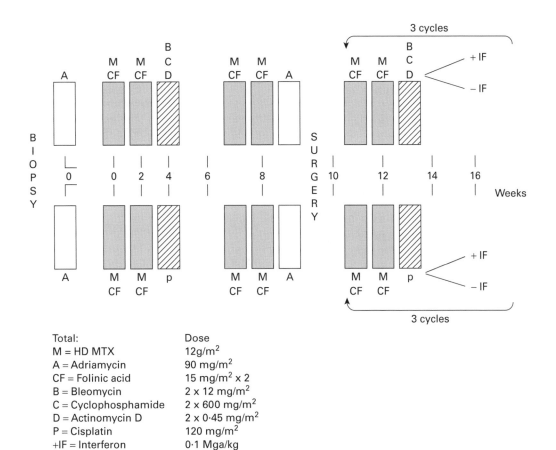

Figure 2.1 Outline of chemotherapy regimen of the COSS-80 study

Total: | Dose
M = HD MTX | 12g/m²
A = Adriamycin | 90 mg/m²
CF = Folinic acid | 15 mg/m² x 2
B = Bleomycin | 2 x 12 mg/m²
C = Cyclophosphamide | 2 x 600 mg/m²
D = Actinomycin D | 2 x 0·45 mg/m²
P = Cisplatin | 120 mg/m²
+IF = Interferon | 0·1 Mga/kg
−IF = No interferon

Study 2

Edmonson JH, Green SJ, Ivins JC, Gilchrist GS, Creagan ET, Pritchard DJ, Smithson WA, Dahlin DC, Taylor WF.

A controlled pilot study of high-dose methotrexate as postsurgical adjuvant treatment for primary osteosarcoma.

J Clin Oncol 1984;**2**:152–6.

The study was designed and run by the Mayo Clinic between 1976 and 1980.

Objectives

This study evaluated the role of adjuvant postoperative chemotherapy using regimen based on high dose methotrexate and vincristine (MTX/VCR).

Details of the study/outcome

Ninety-five eligible patients were considered who were free of distant metastases using technetium scan and CT scan. Eighty-seven were approached, and of these 41 consented to be randomised. Thirty-eight patients had osteosarcoma, three had other pathologies. The median age was 17. Twenty received chemotherapy and 21 follow up alone. Randomisation was done at the Mayo Clinic using a sequential treatment assignment, with balance of prognostic factors by "dynamic allocation". Only the 38 osteosarcoma were subsequently analysed.

Post-surgical follow up comprised six-weekly visits during year 1 and every 3 months during year 2 and the same follow up was applied after chemotherapy treatment. Chemotherapy details and doses are given in Figure 2.2.

VCR 2 mg/m^2

MTX	3·0 g/m^2	course 1	over 6 hours
	6·0 g/m^2	course 2	
	7·5 g/m^2	course 3	

further 10% escalation if MTX level <10–7 mmol/l within 5 days

Folinic acid rescue from 2 hours after completion of MTX

At relapse: cyclophosphamide 1·2 g/m^2
doxorubicin 75 mg/m^2

Figure 2.2 Chemotherapy regimen

Major outcome measures were progression free survival (PFS) and overall survival (OS).

Analysis showed a PFS of 40% in both groups and 5 year OS of 50%.

Toxicity

The toxicity was inevitably higher in the chemotherapy arm, with predictable myelosuppression, dermatitis and diarrhoea. No treatment related deaths were reported.

Conclusion

It was concluded that there was no benefit to adjuvant chemotherapy. It was, however, noted that the estimated survival of 52% 5 years after surgery exceeded all reasonable survival expectation based on historical reports. This inexplicably high cure rate with surgery alone may have accounted for the lack of any demonstrable benefit from chemotherapy.

Study 3

Jaffe N, Robertson R, Ayala A, Wallace S, Chuang V, Anzai T, Cangir A, Wang Y-M, Chen T. Comparison of intra-arterial cis-diamminedichloroplatinum II with high-dose methotrexate and citrovorum factor rescue in the treatment of primary osteosarcoma.
J Clin Oncol 1985;**3**:1101–4.

The study was designed and carried out at the MD Anderson Hospital between 1980 and 1984.

Objectives

This trial compared the efficacy of intra-arterial cisplatin with high dose intra-arterial or intravenous methotrexate.

Details of the study

Thirty patients with non-metastatic osteosarcoma (staging methods not detailed) were allocated to receive either intra-arterial cisplatin or high dose methotrexate, given by intra-arterial route in 9 patients and by intravenous route in 6. The decision to change from intra-arterial to intravenous was unclear. This was said to be for logistical reasons and also that during the course of the investigations "pharmacological studies" showed no significant differences in terms of response if the drug was administered by the intra-arterial or intravenous route. Post surgical chemotherapy depended on response and included MTX and doxorubicin (Adriamycin). Patients were aged 2–16, median 12 years.

The method of randomisation used is not described.

Details of drugs and doses are given in Figure 2.3.

The main outcome measures were clinical response after one course of chemotherapy and pathological response defined at time of surgery at 2–3 months. Complete response (CR) was defined as more than 90% of non-viable tumour, partial response (PR) 60–90%.

Outcome

Following high dose methotrexate there were 4/15 responses, 3 CR, 1 PR; with cisplatin there were 9/15 responses, 7 CR and 2 PR, p = 0·06. There was said to be more rapid pain relief with the cisplatin regimen.

Toxicity

There was one toxic death associated with high dose methotrexate.

Conclusion

It was concluded that cisplatin was superior.

Response was, however, assessed at a variable stage after between two and seven courses of chemotherapy. The distribution of assessment timing between the two arms was not detailed. The number of patients was also very small to show significant difference between the two regimens.

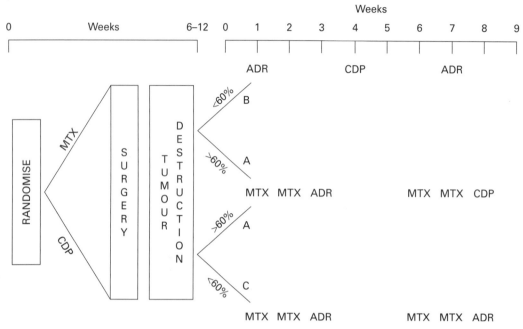

Figure 2.3 Treatment schema

MTX = Methotrexate 12·5 g/m² over 6 hours
         Folinic acid started at 12 hours after the end of MTX
CDP = Cisplatin 150 mg/m² over 2 hours
         both given every 14–21 days
ADR = Doxorubicin

Study 4

Link MP, Goorin AM, Miser AW, Green AA, Pratt CB, Belasco JB, Pritchard J, Malpas JS, Baker AR, Kirkpatrick JA, Ayala AG, Shuster JJ, Abelson HT, Simone JV, Vietti TJ.
The effect of adjuvant chemotherapy on relapse free survival in patients with osteosarcoma of the extremity.
N Engl J Med 1986;**314**:1600–6.

The study was designed and run by the multi-institutional Osteosarcoma Study Group under the auspices of the Pediatric Oncology Group and took place between 1982 and 1984.

Objectives

This trial addressed the issue whether multi-agent chemotherapy would improve the outcome when given as adjuvant therapy after amputation.

Details of the study

Non-metastatic patients (staged using CT scan and bone scan) under the age of 30 years with high grade osteosarcoma which was completely excised were eligible. Chemotherapy was started less than 4 weeks from the time of surgery.

Randomisation was through the POG statistical office, but the precise methodology is not detailed.

Chemotherapy comprised cyclophosphamide, methotrexate, doxorubicin (Adriamycin) and cisplatin given over a 4–5 week period. Methotrexate dose was modified in each patient in order to achieve a target of 1×10^3 µmol concentration. Dose details are given in Figure 2.4.

The primary outcome measure was relapse free survival (RFS) and it was predicted that 196 patients would need to be registered to show a 20% increase in two year RFS, i.e. 60 versus 40%, 80% power.

Out of 156 patients registered, 113 were eligible. Ineligibility included low grade lesions, metastases, axial primary, incomplete resection, prolonged interval from diagnosis, prior history of cancer and inappropriate staging. Only 36 patients accepted randomisation: 18 were randomised to chemotherapy and 18 to observation alone.

Follow up of patients in both adjuvant chemotherapy and control groups included monthly chest x-rays and CT scanning every 4 months. Bone scan was performed 6-monthly and x-ray of the primary site every 4 months for 2 years after surgery. During the third year after diagnosis chest x-rays were obtained every 2–3 months.

Outcome

Analysis revealed a 2 year RFS of 17% for those not receiving chemotherapy, compared with 66% in those receiving chemotherapy, p = < 001. Overall survival was in the region of 70% and did not differ between the two arms.

Predictably, chemotherapy was associated with complications and significant sepsis occurred in one-third of patients. There were two chemotherapy related deaths.

Distribution of patients between the two arms was relatively well balanced, a slightly higher percentage in the observation arm being over 12 years of age (12 v 10), and having a distal femur primary (9 v 5). More patients on the chemotherapy arm had a proximal tibial primary (6 v 2). The same number had resection, as opposed to amputation, at presentation.

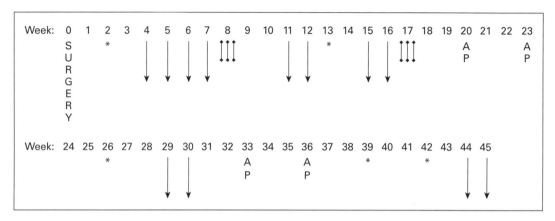

Adjuvant chemotherapy was begun 2 weeks after definitive surgery of the primary tumour

* = Cyclophosphamide 600 mg/m²
    Bleomycin 15 mg/m² $\Bigg\}$ × 21 days
    Actinomycin 0·6 mg/m²

↓ = Methotrexate 12 g/m²
    escalated to achieve serum level of 10^3 micromol

↕ = Doxorubicin 30 mg/m² × 3 doses

AP = Doxorubicin 50 mg/m²
      Cisplatin 100 mg/m²

Figure 2.4 Chemotherapy regimen of the multi-institutional osteosarcoma study. Adapted with permission, 2002 from Link MP *et al*, *N Engl J Med* (full reference on p 37). Copyright © 1986 Massachusetts Medical Society.

Conclusion

It was concluded that adjuvant chemotherapy produced a highly significant improvement in relapse free survival but the encouraging initial salvage rate following relapse reduced any effect on overall survival.

Study 5

Eilber F, Giuliano A, Eckardt J, Patterson K, Moseley S, Goodnight J.
Adjuvant chemotherapy for osteosarcoma. A randomised prospective trial.
J Clin Oncol 1987;**5**:21–6.

This study was planned and carried out by UCLA, between 1981 and 1984.

Objectives

This study evaluated of the role of the Rosen T10 regimen as adjuvant chemotherapy following preoperative intra-arterial doxorubicin and local irradiation followed by definitive surgery.

Details of the study/outcome

All patients with high grade osteogenic sarcoma and non-metastatic disease on CT and technetium bone scan staging were eligible. Of the 112 bone tumours considered, 78 were osteogenic sarcoma. Nineteen patients were excluded due to metastases or low grade pathology. Of the 59 remaining, 32 received adjuvant chemotherapy and 27 observation alone.

Randomisation was done using a file of sequential cards generated from a set of random numbers. They were balanced by treatment in blocks of 10. Randomisation was done centrally at UCLA.

Intra-arterial doxorubicin was given for 3 days followed by 1750 cGy local radiation (RT) on 5 days to the whole bone. This was followed in 44 patients by limb sparing surgery with prosthesis and in 15 by amputation.

Chemotherapy comprised high dose methotrexate (MTX), vincristine (VCR), doxorubicin and BCD, and the details are given in Figure 2.5.

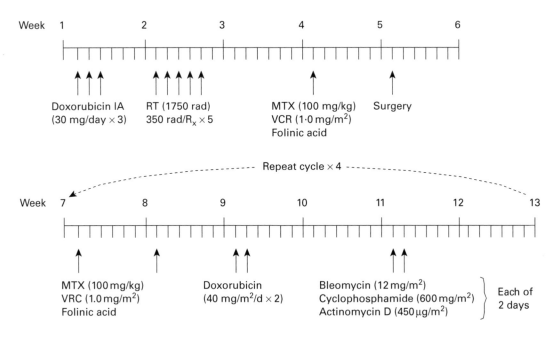

Figure 2.5 Treatment schedule

The primary outcome measures were disease free and overall survival.

Twenty-eight of 32 patients allocated chemotherapy received the full regimen. Overall, 55% were disease free at 2 years of those allocated to chemotherapy, compared with 20% who did not receive chemotherapy, $p < 0.01$. Eighty per cent receiving chemotherapy were alive, compared with 48%, $p < 0.001$. Median time to relapse was 11 months in the chemotherapy arm, compared to 5 months in the observation alone group.

Conclusion

It was concluded that there was a significant benefit in the addition of T10 Rosen chemotherapy following surgery.

Study 6

Burgers JMV, Van Glabbeke M, Busson A, Cohen P, Mazabraud AR, Abbatucci JS, Kalifa C, Tubiana M, Lemerle JS, Voute PA, van Oosterom A, Pons A, Wagener T, Van Der Werf-Messing B, Somers R, Duez AN.
Osteosarcoma of the limbs. Report of the EORTC-SIOP 03 trial 20781 investigating the value of adjuvant treatment with chemotherapy and/or prophylactic lung irradiation.
Cancer 1988;**61**:1024–31.

This study was designed and executed by the EORTC between 1978 and 1983.

Objectives

The study compared three different approaches to the treatment of undetectable lung metastases at presentation. Lung radiotherapy, chemotherapy alone, or a combination of chemotherapy and radiotherapy were randomly compared.

Details of the study/outcome

Two hundred and forty patients below the age of 30 years were registered, of whom 205 were evaluable. Exclusions were due to low grade histology, lung metastases and inadequate data. Staging comprised technetium bone scan and lung tomography. CT scan was not routinely used.

The initial surgical approach was amputation in 168 patients and local radiotherapy alone in 37.

The details of randomisation method are not given. Groups were, however, well balanced by age and site.

Sixty-five patients were allocated to chemotherapy alone and received vincristine and methotrexate, alternating with doxorubicin (Adriamycin), followed by cyclophosphamide, alternating with doxorubicin or methotrexate. Details of chemotherapy are given in Table 2.1. Seventy-three patients were allocated to receive 20 Gy bilateral lung irradiation and 67 patients received 9 weeks of initial chemotherapy, followed by 20 Gy lung irradiation.

The outcome measures considered were disease free and overall survival, metastases free survival, time to recurrence and toxicity.

Disease free survival at 5 years was 40% for chemotherapy alone, 44% for lung irradiation alone and 45% for combination therapy. There were 3 deaths, all in the chemotherapy alone arm. Lung function was impaired in 14% of those receiving irradiation.

Conclusion

The conclusion was that there was no significant difference between these approaches but a control arm with no adjuvant therapy was not included in the study design.

Reservations about the study mentioned by the investigators were the poor compliance with regard to guidelines for the administration of lung irradiation. There was also an imbalance in the nature of initial surgery prior to the study protocol.

Table 2.1 Schedule of adjuvant chemotherapy

Weeks	Induction						Consolidation		
	1	3	5	7	9	11	13	15	17
CYP						|		|	
ADR		|		|			|		
VCR/MTX/CF	|		|		|				|

Cycles of consolidation chemotherapy to be given for a total of four times, up to week 41.

MTX = methotrexate (600 mg/m²/6 hour infusion)

CF = citrovorum factor (15 mg 6 wkly x12)

VCR = vincristine (1·5 mg/m² IV max 2 mg)

ADR = Adriamycin (doxorubicin) 70 mg/m² IV

CYP = cyclophosphamide (1200 mg/m² IV)

Study 7

Bramwell VHC, Burgers M, Sneath R, Souhami R, van Oosterom AT, Voute PA, Rouesse J, Spooner D, Craft AW, Somers R, Pringle J, Malcolm AJ, van der Eijken J, Thomas D, Uscinska B, Machin D, van Glabbeke M.

A comparison of two short intensive adjuvant chemotherapy regimens in operable osteosarcoma of limbs in children and young adults: the first study of the European Osteosarcoma Intergroup.

J Clin Oncol 1992;**10**:1579–91.

The study was designed and carried out by the Medical Research Council (MRC), United Kingdom Children's Cancer Study Group (UKCCSG) and European Organisation for Research into Treatment of Cancer (EORTC) between 1983 and 1986.

It was initially started as a randomised phase II study, but because of good recruitment was extended to a formal phase III comparative study.

Objectives

This was a comparison of two chemotherapies: doxorubicin/cisplatin in one arm and high dose methotrexate combined with reduced dose intensity doxorubicin and cisplatin in the other arm.

Details of the study

Patients under 40 years of age with non-metastatic extremity high grade tumours were eligible. Staging including CT scan and technetium bone scan. The chemotherapy could be given either pre or post surgery but had to commence less than 35 days following diagnostic biopsy.

The randomisation was carried out at the EORTC/MRC centres by telephone call. Patients were randomised in such a way that a balance between the number of patients who received each treatment was maintained throughout the trial within each collaborating centre. To maintain approximately equal number of patients for each treatment, with respect to creatinine clearance, age less than 15 years, type of surgery, preoperative or postoperative chemotherapy, a minimisation procedure was used.

Regimen A comprised doxorubicin (DOX) and cisplatin (CDP) given three-weekly for six courses and regimen B, high dose methotrexate (HDMTX) 10 days prior to doxorubicin/cisplatin, which was given approximately four-weekly. Details are given in Figure 2.6. The trial was designed to detect an increase in survival of 20% from 50–70% with 80% power.

The primary outcome measures were metastatic and disease free survival, overall survival and comparative toxicities.

Outcome

Three hundred and seven patients were registered, of whom 25 were excluded due to inadequate data. These came from one cooperative group and two additional centres. From the text it is unclear whether 307 patients were registered and randomised or whether these 25 were excluded from randomisation. A further 54 were excluded because of the presence of metastatic disease, an axial primary and locally recurrent disease. A further 35 were ineligible for analysis due to excessive delay between biopsy and chemotherapy or other protocol deviations. The study finally included 198 patients, 99 patients in each arm (114 excluded from 307 should leave only 193). The two groups appeared well balanced, although there were more humeral primaries in regimen B (19 *v* 7).

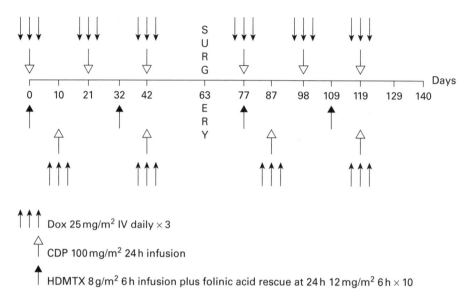

Figure 2.6 Chemotherapy regimens

Full details of the delivered intended dose and timing in both arms is given. A higher percentage of patients in arm B received intended dose, on time, and completed full therapy. There was one toxic death in arm A. There was a higher incidence of hepatic complications in arm B, associated with high dose methotrexate, and more neurological and audiometric toxicity in arm A, associated with a higher cisplatin dose and dose intensity. Pathological response was documented in only 66 of 179 possible patients. A good response, i.e. over 90% necrosis, was noted in 41% of arm A and 22% of arm B. This was not statistically significant largely due to the small number evaluable.

Local recurrence rate was similar in both arms and there was no difference between the ultimate surgery, i.e. amputation, or prosthesis.

Overall, there were fewer metastatic recurrences in those having conservative surgery.

At 5 years, 39% of group A and 53% of group B were free of metastases. The disease free survival was 57% for group A, 41% for group B, p = 0.05. Overall survival was 64% and 50% respectively, which was not statistically significant.

Conclusion

The conclusion was that the lower dose intensity cisplatin/doxorubicin arm was probably inferior, despite the addition of high dose methotrexate. It appeared that the addition of methotrexate, whilst reducing platinum related toxicity, did not compensate for a reduction in efficacy due to reduced dose and dose intensity.

Study 8

Bacci G, Picci P, Ruggieri P, Mercuri M, Avella M, Capanna R, Brach Del Prever A, Mancini A, Gherlinzoni F, Padovani G, Leonessa C, Biagini R, Ferraro A, Ferruzzi A, Cazzola A, Manfrini M, Campanacci M.
Primary chemotherapy and delayed surgery (neoadjuvant chemotherapy) for osteosarcoma of the extremities.
Cancer 1990;**65**:2539–53.

This study was carried out at the Instituto Rizzoli between 1983 and 1986.

Objectives

The study compared two doses of methotrexate in combination with cisplatin, given preoperatively.

Details of the study

The study involved patients less than 50 years old with high-grade osteosarcoma at extremity sites. They were non-metastatic on CT and technetium staging and had received no prior chemotherapy.

The randomisation method is not described, but patients were stratified for site.

The two regimens comprised high dose (HD) methotrexate 7·5 g/m^2 and moderate dose (MD) methotrexate 750 mg/m^2 followed by intra-arterial cisplatin (full details are given in Figure 2.7a).

The primary outcome measure was histological response, defined as good – more than 90% necrosis; fair – 60–89% necrosis; and poor – < 60% necrosis. There was central pathological review in all cases.

Outcome

Two hundred and forty-two patients were diagnosed in the study period, of whom 178 were eligible. The reasons for exclusions were detailed and included the presence of metastases, low grade tumours and para- or periosteal sarcoma. Thirty-two patients refused randomisation. A further 11 were not evaluated due to refusal to receive the allocated chemotherapy. A total of 127 were therefore included in the final analysis. Sixty-seven were randomised to HDMTX and 60 to MDMTX.

Good histological response was seen in 41 of 66 evaluable patients receiving HDMTX (62%), compared to 25/60 receiving MDMTX (42%) (p = < 0·04). There were 3 patients with clinically progressive disease. The clinical and radiological features were not always consistent with pathology and these were not formally compared. Despite the difference in response, there was no difference in ultimate local control rates. The subsequent chemotherapy depended on initial treatment. Those with a good response were initially continued on methotrexate and cisplatin alone, but initially poor outcome led to a change in strategy, with the addition of doxorubicin (Adriamycin) in all cases. In patients with a fair response doxorubicin was added and those with a poor response switched to a doxorubicin/ BCD combination (see Figure 2.7b).

The overall 5 year disease free survival for the HDMTX arm was 58%, and 42% for the MDMTX arm (p = 0·07). Overall, the response predicted outcome with 65% versus 40% versus 10% overall survival for good, fair and poor responders respectively (p = 0·01). No significant difference in toxicity was noted between the two arms.

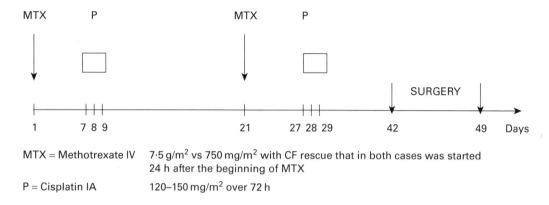

MTX = Methotrexate IV $7.5\,g/m^2$ vs $750\,mg/m^2$ with CF rescue that in both cases was started 24 h after the beginning of MTX

P = Cisplatin IA $120–150\,mg/m^2$ over 72 h

Figure 2.7a Chemotherapy protocol. Copyright © 1990 American Cancer Society. Adapted and reprinted from Bacci G *et al* (full reference p 45) by permission of Wiley-Liss, Inc., a subsidiary of John Wiley & Sons, Inc.

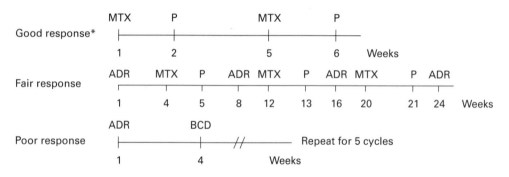

* After 12/83 Patients with good response had the same treatment as the patients with fair response

MTX, P = The same doses used preoperatively, IV
ADR   = Adriamycin (doxorubicin) $45\,mg/m^2$ IV × 2 days
BCD   = Bleomycin $15\,mg/m^2/d$
             Cyclophosphamide $600\,mg/m^2/d$
             Actinomycin D $600\,mg/m^2/d$ IV × 2 days

Figure 2.7b Subsequent chemotherapy protocol according to response to initial treatment. Copyright © American Cancer Society (as Figure 2.7a).

Conclusion

It was concluded that high dose methotrexate was significantly better than moderate dose methotrexate in achieving a good histological response but within the current study did not lead to a significant improvement in outcome.

Study 9

Winkler K, Bielack S, Delling G, Salzer-Kuntschik M, Kotz R, Greenshaw C, Jurgens H, Ritter J, Kusnierz-Glaz C, Erttmann R, Gadicke G, Graf N, Ladenstein R, Leyvraz S, Mertens R, Weinel P. Effect of intraarterial versus intravenous cisplatin in addition to systemic doxorubicin, high dose methotrexate, and ifosfamide on histologic tumour response in osteosarcoma (study COSS-86). *Cancer*, 1990;**66**:1703–10.

This study was designed and executed by the COSS group between 1986 and 1988.

Objectives

This was a comparison of intra-arterial with intravenous cisplatin given preoperatively following initial standard chemotherapy, using doxorubicin and high dose methotrexate.

Details of the study

Eligible patients were those defined as high risk on the basis of extent of tumour greater than one-third of total bone, more than 20% chondroid, less than 20% reduction in early/late phase bone scan following initial chemotherapy, including both metastatic and non-metastatic patients.

It was estimated that 100 patients should be included to detect a 25% increase of good response from 50% to 75%, with an 80% power.

Randomisation was planned to be done centrally, with stratification for age, sex, site, size, condroid and bone scan response. For reasons not entirely clear in the text, strict randomisation was not always feasible, due to some institutions' refusal to give intra-arterial cisplatin. Most patient were therefore "allocated" centrally, striving to balance all risk factors. Moreover, a number of patients

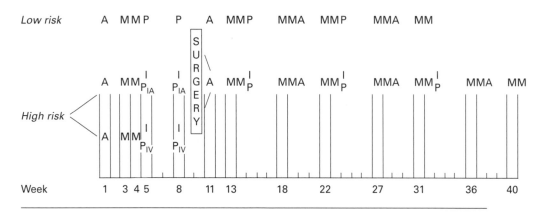

Figure 2.8 Outline of chemotherapy (*see text p. 48). Copyright © 1990 American Cancer Society. Adapted and reprinted from Winkler K *et al* (see full reference above) by permission of Wiley-Liss, Inc., a subsidiary of John Wiley & Sons, Inc.

were non-evaluable due to protocol violations (not further specified).

The treatment comprised initial doxorubicin (Adriamycin), followed by methotrexate and then a third course with ifosfamide and cisplatin, the latter given either intra-arterial or intravenously. Surgery then followed (for full details see Figure 2.8). The dose of cisplatin initially was 150 mg/m² but this was reduced to 120 mg/m² because of a high incidence of toxicity, and the infusion time was also increased to 5 hours.

The primary outcome measure was pathological response. A favourable response was defined as > 90% tumour destruction.

Outcome

Of 241 patients enrolled in the study 27 were low risk. Of the high risk patients, 94 were excluded,

38 had early surgery, 15 late surgery and 9 no surgery. There were protocol violations in 11 and 21 had missing data.

Of the 109 "randomised" patients who were evaluable there was an overall balance of risk factors, except the patients who received intravenous cisplatin were somewhat older and there were more with proximal tibial lesions. The IA route led to a 68% good response rate and the IV route to a 69% good response rate. There were no major differences in toxicity and these are detailed in the study text.

Conclusion
It was concluded that the intra-arterial route does not add to the efficacy of cisplatin when given in combination with other active agents.

Study 10

Souhami RL, Craft AW, Van der Eijken JW, Nooij M, Spooner D, Bramwell VHC, Wierzbicki R, Malcolm AJ, Kirkpatrick A, Uscinska BM, Van Glabbeke M, Machin D.

Randomised trial of two regimens of chemotherapy in operable osteosarcoma: a study of the European Osteosarcoma Intergroup.

Lancet 1997;**350**:911–17.

This study was designed and run by a collaborative group, combining the EORTC, MRC and UKCCSG plus other centres. It ran between 1986 and 1991.

Objectives

The study addressed the issue as to whether a short intensive chemotherapy regimen with doxorubicin and cisplatin would produce survival of patients with operable non-metastatic osteosarcoma, similar to that obtained with a complex and longer duration regimen, based on the Rosen T10 protocol.

Details of the study

The study was a prospective, randomised trial. Eligible patients were under the age of 40 years, had high grade osteosarcoma and had received no prior chemotherapy. They had non-metastatic disease detected on CT scan and technetium bone scan. The time from biopsy to randomisation had to be less than 35 days.

Randomisation was done by telephone or fax via the EORTC or other centralised data centre offices. The minimisation procedure was used and patients were stratified for site, age and planned surgery. The study was designed to exclude a difference of 15% in 5 year survival, a significance of 5% in a two-sided test, with 80% power. It was predicted to require 400 patients overall. Interim analysis was planned every 6 months but there were no formal stopping rules.

Outcome measures were response rates, survival and progression free survival.

Patients were randomised to receive either an 18 week regimen, including doxorubicin/cisplatin (arm A), or a 44 week multidrug regimen (arm B), based on Rosen T10 (see Figure 2.9). Surgery was at 9 weeks and 7 weeks respectively.

Outcome

The estimated source population was 600 patients and 407 were randomised. No formal record was kept of patients refusing randomisation. Of the 407, 15 were ineligible due to other pathology, secondary deposits or non-limb primaries. Three hundred and ninety-one were therefore included on the trial and were well balanced for prognostic subgroups. The minimum follow up was 4·5 years, median 5·6 years. Overall compliance was good. With regard to surgical timing, 84% of the two-drug arm were on time and 72% of the multidrug arm. Median time to surgery was 75 days in the two-drug arm and 57 days in the multidrug arm. There was a high degree of dose reduction in both arms, with about two-thirds of the planned dose intensity given in both treatment arms. This was due both to toxicity and early relapse, the latter particularly in the multiagent, longer duration arm B.

Toxicity

Toxicity was more severe in the two-drug arm, including grade 4 leucopenia (75% *v* 19%), thrombocytopenia (46% *v* 3%) and severe infection (21% *v* 3%) when comparing the two-drug versus six courses of the multidrug regimen. No statistical comparison is presented.

- **Two-drug regimen**
  Doxorubicin 25 mg/m^2 × 3
  Cisplatin 100 mg/m^2
    6 cycles at 21 day intervals

- **Multidrug regimen**
  Preoperative: Vincristine 1·5 mg/m^2
    Methotrexate 8 g/m^2
      (12 g/m^2 for < 12 yr)
    Folinic acid rescue started
      at 18 h after end of MTX

    VCR/MTX given weekly × 4
    Doxorubicin 25 mg/m^2 × 3

  Postoperative: Bleomycin 15 mg/m^2 ⎤
    Cyclophosphamide
      600 mg/m^2 ⎬ × 2 days
    Actinomycin D
      0·6 mg/m^2 ⎦
    Doxorubicin 30 mg/m^2 ⎤ × 2 days
    Cisplatin 120 mg/m^2 ⎦

Figure 2.9 Chemotherapy doses

The type of surgery ultimately carried out was compared in the two arms. Fewer amputations were performed than planned in arm A (22/40) compared with arm B (27/41). Where conservative surgery was planned, it was achieved in 87% arm A and 83% in arm B.

Clinical response in arm A was 59% and in B, 42% (odds ratio 2·02). All initial pathology was reviewed centrally but only 66% of resection samples were ultimately centrally reviewed. For pathological response, a good response was defined as at least 90% necrosis of the tumour, and poor response as any degree less than this. In arm A there was a 30% good response and in arm B, 29%.

Progression free survival and overall survival were identical in both arms: 65% at 3 years and 55% at 5 years for arm B. The outcome for good pathological responders was 75% at 5 years, compared to 45% for bad responders. There was the same difference for both study arms.

Conclusion

There was no difference between the two-drug and the multidrug regimens, although a difference of 10% or less would not be detectable in the trial. The two-drug regimen is cheaper, of shorter duration and concluded to be the treatment of choice despite its higher early toxicity.

Comments

The inevitably increased late effects of doxorubicin and cisplatin in children are not given specific consideration when discussing the merits of the two regimens.

Study 11

Winkler K, Beron G, Delling G, Heise U, Kabisch H, Purfurst C, Berger J, Ritter J, Jurgens H, Gerein V, Graf N, Russe W, Gruemayer ER, Ertelt W, Katz R, Preusser P, Prindull G, Brandeis W, Landbeck G. Neoadjuvant chemotherapy of osteosarcoma: results of a randomized cooperative trial (COSS-82) with salvage chemotherapy based on histological tumor response.
J Clin Oncol 1988;**6**:329–37.

The trial was designed and run by the German COSS Group between 1982 and 1984.

Objectives

The study asked the question whether a combination of bleomycin, cyclophosphamide and actinomycin D (BCD) could replace the more toxic cisplatin and doxorubicin combination as preoperative chemotherapy, reserving cisplatin/doxorubicin for poor responders.

Details of the study

This was a prospective, randomised trial. Patients eligible had any primary classic osteosarcoma of the extremities, were free from detected metastases, under the age of 40 years, and had started chemotherapy less than 3 weeks after biopsy.

The method of randomisation was not specified. Patients were stratified on the basis of age, above and below 12 years, sex, site and size of tumour (more or less than one-third of total bone). It was assumed that the 2 year metastatic free survival would be 80%. To detect a 20% difference, a total of 150 patients were planned, with 80% power, 5% significance. A stopping rule was included, so that if metastatic free survival was equal or more than 15% worse than in the previous COSS-80 study in the first 50 patients the trial would be stopped.

Patients were randomised to receive high dose methotrexate in combination with either BCD or cisplatin and doxorubicin (see Figure 2.10). Poor responders on the BCD arm were treated with cisplatin and doxorubicin and poor responders on the cisplatin/doxorubicin arm received a combination of cisplatin, ifosfamide and BCD.

The major outcome measure was metastatic free survival (MFS).

Outcome

Two hundred and fifty-nine patients were registered, of whom 118 were excluded for a variety of reasons, including over the age of 40 years, flat bone primary, presence of metastases, surgery at diagnosis or delayed chemotherapy. Of 141 entered on the trial, 16 were non-evaluable, predominantly due to chemotherapy violations.

Overall, clinical response showed a poor correlation with histological response. Of 81 patients, 42% of good responders had poor pathological response. There were 5 events other than metastases, 3 local relapses and 2 toxic deaths. Of 125 patients evaluable, the favourable pathological response defined as $\geq$90% tumour cell destruction was seen in 15 of 57 patients (26%) with BCD compared to 35 of 58 patients (60%) with doxorubicin/cisplatin ($p = < 0.001$). The 4 year MFS was 49% for BCD versus 68% for doxorubicin/cisplatin ($p = 0.1$), but 5 year MFS was 45% versus 68% ($p = < 0.05$).

Overall, the 4 year MFS for poor responders was 44%, compared to 77% for favourable responders

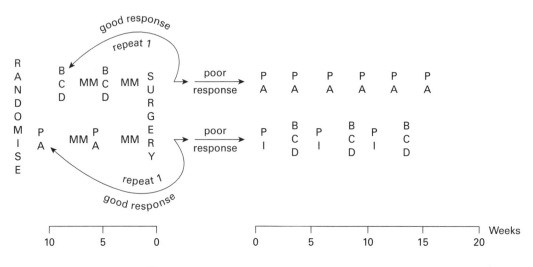

P = Cisplatin 120 (90) mg/m^2
A = Doxorubicin 30 mg/m^2/d $\times$ 2
M = Methotrexate 12 g/m^2
B = Bleomycin 15 mg/m^2/d $\times$ 2
C = Cyclophosphamide 600 mg/m^2/d $\times$ 2
D = Dactinomycin 0·6 mg/m^2/d $\times$ 2
P = Cisplatinum 20 mg/m^2/d $\times$ 5
I = Ifosfamide 2 g/m^2/d $\times$ 5

Figure 2.10 Treatment protocol

($p = < 0.001$). The outcome in poor responders following BCD was 41%, compared to 53% following doxorubicin/cisplatin, when the appropriate second line chemotherapy was given (not significant).

The trial was stopped early due to the appearance of a significant difference in MFS. The number recruited when the study was discontinued was not specified.

Toxicity

There were two toxic deaths, one in each treatment arm. There was no significant difference in delays to chemotherapy in the two arms but in poor responders those given the ifosfamide based regimen had the greatest delays between courses.

There appears to have been a higher incidence of renal toxicity where cisplatin was combined with doxorubicin, compared to cisplatin alone than in the COSS-80 study. The cause of this was unclear.

Conclusion
Doxorubicin/Cisplatin is significantly more effective than BCD in achieving a good response and metastasis free survival.

Comments
Full data regarding the stopping rule decision are not given. Overall, the follow up of patients was comparatively short.

Study 12

Meyers PA, Gorlick R, Heller G, Casper E, Lane J, Huvos AG, Healey JH.
Intensification of preoperative chemotherapy for osteogenic sarcoma: results of the Memorial Sloan–Kettering (T12) protocol.
J Clin Oncol 1998;**16**:2452–8.

The study was designed and performed at the Memorial Sloan–Kettering Cancer Center between 1986 and 1993.

Objectives

The aim was to determine whether intensification of preoperative chemotherapy with the addition of cisplatin and doxorubicin improved the histological response and outcome following conservative surgery.

Details of the study

All new untreated patients with high grade osteogenic sarcoma of any age who were referred to Memorial Sloan–Kettering (MSK) were eligible. Patients were randomised centrally in the trials office at MSK using block randomisation by the envelope method. Fifteen patients were non-eligible due to prior surgery and 10 refused randomisation. No predicted differences or numbers required is given.

Regimen 1 was based on the Rosen T10 protocol, with high dose methotrexate 8–12 gram/m^2 for four courses, combined with BCD (see Figure 2.11). The more intensive regimen 2 added two blocks of cisplatin/doxorubicin. Patients on regimen 1 who were poor responders had treatment intensified by the addition of cisplatin/doxorubicin, whereas good responders received the addition of doxorubicin alone. On regimen 2 the same chemotherapy was continued irrespective of histological response.

Primary outcome measures were histological response following preoperative chemotherapy and event free survival.

Outcome

Seventy-three patients were entered, aged 4–36 years. Distal femur was the commonest primary site. Twelve patients presented with lung metastases. Thirty-seven patients were treated with regimen 1 and 36 with regimen 2.

A difference in histological response was observed. With regimen 1 there were more poor responders, grade 1 (9 *v* 4 patients), with regimen 2 there were more good responders, grade 4 (12 *v* 5). Overall, the event free survival was inferior for those with grade 1 responses (EFS 30%) compared to 82% for grade 4 responses. The trial contained too few patients for statistical comparison within the two trial regimens and no statistical analysis was done for the initial histological response. No details of toxicity for the two regimens was presented.

Conclusion

The authors emphasised the limitations of conclusions that can be drawn partly due to the small numbers but also because the longer preoperative treatment in the multiagent intensive regimen 2 (10 weeks *v* 6 weeks for regimen 1). Also, the fact treatment was changed for poor responders in regimen 1, with no change in regimen 2, all emphasise the lack of evidence for this strategy having a significant impact on outcome.

Study 13
Krailo M, Ertel I, Makley J, Fryer CJH, Baum E, Weetman R, Yunis E, Barnes L, Bleyer WA, Denman Hammond G.
A randomized study comparing high-dose methotrexate with moderate-dose methotrexate as components of adjuvant chemotherapy in childhood nonmetastatic osteosarcoma: a report from the Children's Cancer Study Group.
Med Ped Oncol 1987;**15**: 69–77.

The study was carried out by the American CCG group between 1978 and 1981.

Objectives
The aim was to determine whether the doses of methotrexate given as adjuvant therapy following surgery in non-metastatic osteosarcoma influenced outcome.

Details of the study
Patients under the age of 21 years were eligible who had received no prior treatment and had extremity primaries with localised disease that was completely resected at presentation.

No details of randomisation method are given in the study and no predicted difference or numbers required are presented.

Following surgical resection and perioperative doxorubicin patients were randomised to receive either high dose methotrexate 7 g/m² every 6 weeks for 12 doses, or moderate dose methotrexate, 690 mg/m² 6-weekly for 12 doses, both in combination with doxorubicin 90 mg/m² and vincristine 2 mg/m². Chemotherapy was started 3 weeks following surgery.

The main outcome measure was disease free survival.

Outcome
A total of 234 patients were registered on the study. Sixty-eight were excluded: 39 had non-localised disease; 11 had non-extremity primaries; 16 were electively given one or other regimen; there were 2 other clinical ineligibilities. Of the 166 completely resected, 83 were randomised to high dose methotrexate and 83 to moderate dose.

Overall, relapse free survival was 38% at 4 years, with no difference between the two regimens. Relative risk of failure, high versus moderate dose, was 1·68–1·49.

Toxicity
There were 4 toxic deaths, 3 cardiac, all in the moderate dose, and one due to sepsis following high dose methotrexate. No difference was documented in grade 3 or 4 toxicity between the two regimens.

Conclusion
It was concluded that in combination with doxorubicin/vincristine the dose of methotrexate may not influence outcome.

3

Ewing's sarcoma

Commentary – Alan Craft

James Ewing's original patient presented with a spontaneous fracture of the ulna and very soon the appearance of a tumour. It was initially suspected to be an osteogenic sarcoma and was treated with a radium pack with dramatic results – the tumour had completely regressed in 5 weeks. However, 18 months later the tumour recurred and eventually Ewing decided after histological examination of the tumour that it was a "diffuse endothelioma of bone". The patient subsequently developed pulmonary metastases from which she died.

The problems encountered by Ewing are exactly those that we face today, that is, the dual control of the local tumour and micrometastatic spread. Historically, amputation alone could cure less than 5% of patients whilst radiotherapy to the primary does little better. The vast majority of patients must, therefore, have metastases at the time of diagnosis. The majority of these are in the lungs but a few patients have bone or bone marrow metastases.

In the late 1960s, early 1970s chemotherapy began to be used with dramatic effect. The survival went up from 5% to almost 50%. Mark Nesbit, one of the pioneers in the development of paediatric oncology in the United States, initiated the first randomised trial in this condition whose aim was to determine whether chemotherapy really was as good as it seemed from descriptive studies and secondly to evaluate whether doxorubicin,

radiotherapy to the lungs, or both was superior (Study 1). Nesbit recognised the need for large studies and had the vision, and the leadership skills, to bring together the different children's cancer study groups in the United States to undertake the Intergroup Ewing's Sarcoma Study (IESS).

The original "no chemotherapy" arm was quickly dropped because of an excess of deaths. There has thus never been a completed RCT of chemotherapy versus no chemotherapy in this condition. However, the consistent historic survival of 5–10% without chemotherapy compared to at least 45–50% with makes it unnecessary to demand an RCT.

IESS1 was a pioneering study undertaken between 1973 and 1978. It is not surprising therefore when the late results were reported in 1990 that they discovered that some of the important prognostic factors were imbalanced between the randomised groups. Nevertheless, for 342 eligible patients to be entered into a study of a very rare tumour was a triumph in itself. It was quite clear from the results that doxorubicin was an essential drug but lung irradiation was almost as good. Almost 30 years after the initiation of this study the basic design of treatment is similar. Ifosfamide has now replaced cyclophosphamide in most treatment schedules but otherwise we have advanced very little with survival rates, now perhaps only 10% higher than they were for patients presenting in 1975. The second IESS study, which ran from 1978 to 82, compared a pulsed, more intensive, regime than that used in IESS-1. A significant improvement was found for the intensive treatment (Study 2).

Until 1980 there was little coordinated clinical trial activity in Europe. As far as Ewing's sarcoma is concerned, the United Kingdom Children's Cancer Study Group (UKCCSG), the German Cooperative Ewing Sarcoma Study (CESS), the French Paediatric Oncology Group (SFOP) and the Rizzoli Institute in Bologna all developed separate protocols and studies with the aim of improving survival but none had sufficient patients to be able to mount a randomised controlled trial. However, the CESS group did study the effect of hyperfractionated irradiation and found no difference when compared to its conventional delivery (Study 3).

A most important contribution came from Sara Donaldson and her Pediatric Oncology Group colleagues, who showed that the previously perceived wisdom that successful treatment of the primary tumour required irradiation to the whole bone was in fact wrong and standard treatment now is for the field to include only the tumour and a surrounding safe margin but sparing the epiphysis at the growing end of the bone wherever possible. Although survival was not influenced by this trial, the late morbidity on the bone certainly has been (Study 4). The third IESS study has not yet been fully reported (Study 5), however, it does appear to show a survival benefit for the addition of ifosfamide and etoposide to standard therapy.

In 1990 the Europeans belatedly woke up to the need to cooperate outside of their traditional boundaries. The UKCCSG/MRC and CESS formed the European Intergroup Collaborative

Ewing's Sarcoma Study Group (EICESS). At last they had sufficient patients to ask a randomised question. They set up two parallel studies, one for high risk (tumours > 200 ml in original volume) and the other for standard risk. The question for standard risk was a toxicity one: could the toxicity be reduced by substituting cyclophosphamide for ifosfamide in the later part of treatment. For high risk it was a dose intensity question: would the addition of a fifth drug, etoposide, improve survival? In spite of running for almost 8 years, only the high risk arm accrued sufficient patients to answer the question posed. Early results suggest that the addition of etoposide slightly improves survival, although the differences are not significant and the median follow up is still too short to make definitive statements.

The success of the EICESS-92 study in terms of patient accrual has prompted several other major trial groups to join with EICESS for the next EUROEWING'S study. SFOP, Swiss Institute for Applied Cancer Research (SIAK) and European Organisation for Research and Treatment of Cancer (EORTC) are all entering patients into the latest study. In EICESS-92 stratification into standard and high risk was on the basis of tumour volume. For EUROEWING'S, some 8 years later, it is now known that the response of the primary tumour to initial chemotherapy is a much more powerful prognostic factor. The latest trial is investigating the role of high dose chemotherapy and autologous stem cell rescue for tumours that do not respond well to initial very intensive chemotherapy. For those who do have a good response a toxicity question is again being asked, similar to that in EICESS-92.

In the United States the CCG-7942 study opened for patient accrual in 1995. This is an RCT comparing a 5 day regimen given over 48 weeks to an intensified treatment using the same drugs over a 30 week period. Results are awaited.

There is general agreement that we are reaching the limit of improvements that we might expect from existing therapy. There may be a place in the future for RCTs to refine existing treatments, for example, timing of surgery, amount and timing of chemotherapy or different methods of delivery of radiotherapy. Although whole lung radiation was studied in the first IESS study its role is not clear with modern intensive chemotherapy. There is now almost universal consensus that ifosfamide is the alkylating agent of choice but there has never been an RCT of maximally tolerated doses of cyclophosphamide and ifosfamide.

The past 10 years have seen a huge increase in our knowledge about the basic biology of Ewing's tumour. Virtually all carry an 11:22 chromosomal translocation and we know that there

are several different genes and their products involved. EWS:Fli.1 is the commonest gene rearrangement but there are several others. Work is continuing to elucidate how these very specific gene rearrangements contribute to the production of a Ewing's sarcoma. Prospects for the future include the identification of tumour-specific targets and then the design of highly specific drugs to interact with these sites. There is also considerable work on the immunology of this tumour and in the future immunotherapy may well have a role to play.

Randomised controlled trials have allowed us to reach the position where 65–70% of Ewing's tumours can now be cured. Further improvements will either be in very small incremental steps or a bigger jump if a highly specific therapy is identified. Whichever is the case, any RCT in this tumour in the future is going to have to be very large and certainly multinational.

Studies

Study 1

Nesbit ME Jr, Gehan EA, Bergert EO Jr, Vietti TJ, Cangir A, Tefft M, Evans R, Thomas P, Askin FB, Kissane JM, Pritchard DJ, Herrmann J, Neff J, Makley JT, Gilula L.
Multimodal therapy for the management of primary, nonmetastatic Ewing's sarcoma of bone. A long-term follow-up of the First Intergroup Study. *J Clin Oncol* 1990;**8**: 1664–74.

The study was carried out between 1973 and 1978 by the Intergroup Ewing's Sarcoma Study collaboration between the American cancer study groups CCG, SWOG and CLGB.

Objectives
- To determine the value of VAC chemotherapy as post surgical adjuvant therapy.
- To determine the role of lung irradiation to prevent lung metastases.

Details of the study

The eligibility criterion was localised, previously untreated Ewing's sarcoma, with no age limit. Patients who had initial amputation of the primary lesion were ineligible for randomisation.

Centres were to initially choose between one of two concurrent randomised studies, the randomisation was a three-to-two balance between treatments 1 and 2 and treatments 2 and 3 (see below). No details of randomisation method or location are given. No detailed statistical predictions with regard to differences sought or numbers of patients required are given. Full details of statistical analytical methods are given.

Study 1 was a comparison of VAC (vincristine, actinomycin D and cyclophosphamide) chemotherapy versus no adjuvant chemotherapy. However, after a 7 month recruitment, two of the three patients who were randomised to receive no chemotherapy had relapsed and the study was therefore closed. The design was modified to be a comparison of VAC versus VAC plus doxorubicin (Adriamycin) (VACA).

Study 2 was a randomised comparison of VAC versus VAC plus bilateral lung irradiation (see Figure 3.1). Bilateral lung irradiation consisted of a midplane dose of between 15 and 18 Gy through the anteroposterior and posteroanterior ports immediately following local therapy for the primary tumour. Five fractions were delivered each week, 1.5–2 Gy daily dose.

After 3 years, entry of patients into treatment 2 was closed because of a significantly high early relapse rate compared with other treatments, and randomisation continued between treatments 1 and 3, i.e. VACA versus VAC plus lung radiotherapy. Local irradiation to the primary site was given during weeks 1–6 concurrently, with weekly vincristine 1·5 mg/m^2 and cyclophosphamide 500 mg/m^2. Lung irradiation was given during weeks 4–6. This was followed by a 7 week block, comprising actinomycin 15 µg/kg IV on 5 consecutive days during week 1, followed by vincristine and cyclophosphamide weekly for 5 weeks. Doxorubicin, where used, was given during week 7 at a dose of 60 mg/m^2.

Primary outcome measures were survival and time to relapse. All pathology was centrally reviewed,

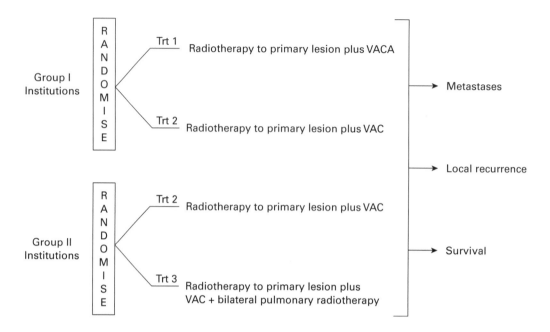

Figure 3.1 Randomisation for institutions in Groups I and II

as were the chemotherapy details and both initial imaging and radiotherapy planning films.

Of the 372 patients entered, 342 were eligible. Eighteen were excluded due to metastatic disease, 8 had wrong diagnosis and 4 had an unconfirmed diagnosis. 148 received treatment 1, VACA; 74 treatment 2, VAC; and 109 treatment 3, VAC plus lung irradiation. Four patients were subsequently excluded from the analysis because of major violations.

Outcome

Despite randomisation there was some imbalance between groups. More had an initial surgical complete remission (CR) in treatment 1 than treatment 2. There were more girls and initial surgical CR in treatment 3, than treatment 2. Five year relapse free survival was 60% for those receiving VACA, compared to 24% for those receiving VAC (p = < 0·01) for the randomised

study, and (p = < 0.001) when all patients receiving these two regimens are considered (Figure 3.1). Five year survival was 60% versus 28% (p = < 0·02) for the randomised group (Figure 3.2).

Treatment 3, VAC plus lung irradiation, was superior to treatment 2, VAC alone, both with respect to relapse free survival and overall survival. Five year RFS was 44% and overall survival 53%. For the comparison of treatment 3, VAC plus radiotherapy, versus treatment 1, VACA, the patients receiving VACA had a superior outcome, 60% versus 44% 5 year relapse free survival, although this did not quite reach statistical significance (p = 0·06 for the randomised group). For all eligible patients p = 0·001.

The above differences were not apparent when patients with pelvic primaries alone were considered. This was claimed to be due to an

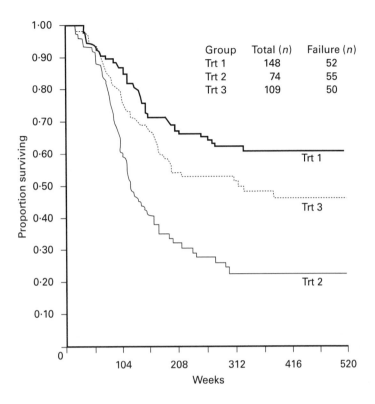

Group	Total (*n*)	Failure (*n*)
Trt 1	148	52
Trt 2	74	55
Trt 3	109	50

Figure 3.2 Survival curves for eligible patients by treatment

underestimate of the soft tissue extension taken into account for local radiotherapy planning. Fifty-one per cent of those that relapsed had lung secondaries. The incidence of lung metastases was 20% in treatment 2, versus 15% in treatment 3, i.e. no significant difference.

Toxicity

Details of toxicity were somewhat limited, but severe toxicity was reported to have occurred in 70%, 57% and 61% of treatment 1, 2 and 3 respectively and severe leucopenia in 21%, 4% and 11% respectively. There was one severe cardiac toxicity in treatment 1.

Conclusion

It was concluded that VAC alone was an inferior treatment for localised Ewing's sarcoma, and although bilateral lung irradiation appeared to improve outcome, the addition of doxorubicin to VAC produced the best relapse free and overall survival in this patient group.

An initial analysis was published by Nesbit ME, Jr, Perez CA, Tefft M, Burgert EO Jr., Vinetti TJ, Kissane J, Pritchard DJ, Gehan EA. Multimodal therapy for the management of primary, nonmetastatic Ewing's sarcoma of bone: an Intergroup Study. *Natl Cancer Inst Monogr.*1981;**56**:255–62.

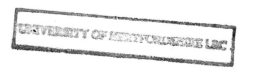

Study 2

Bergert EO, Nesbit ME, Garnsey LA, Gehan EA, Herrmann J, Vietti TJ, Cangir A, Tefft M, Evans R, Thomas P, Askin FB, Kissane JM, Pritchard DJ, Neff J, Makley JT, Gilula L.

Multimodal therapy for the management of non-pelvic, localized Ewing's sarcoma of bone: Intergroup Study IESS-II.

J Clin Oncol 1990;**8**:1514–24.

This study was carried out between 1978 and 1982 by the Intergroup IESS and included 64 institutions.

Objectives

The aim of the study was to determine whether a moderate dose continuous chemotherapy or a higher dose intermittent pulsed regimen was superior in localised Ewing's sarcoma.

Details of the study

Patient eligibility included those with non-pelvic primaries and only bone involvement. They were to have had no previous treatment and be less than one month from initial diagnosis. Excluding

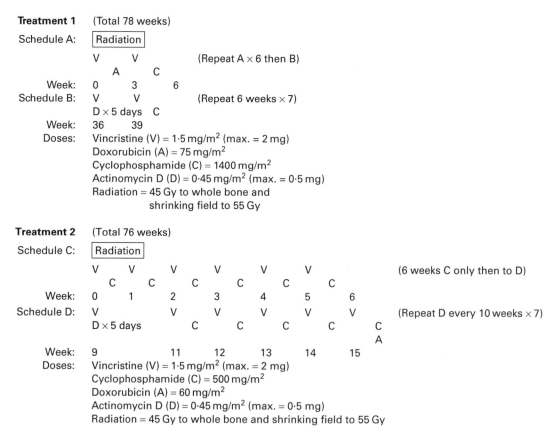

Figure 3.3 Details of radiotherapy and chemotherapy schedules

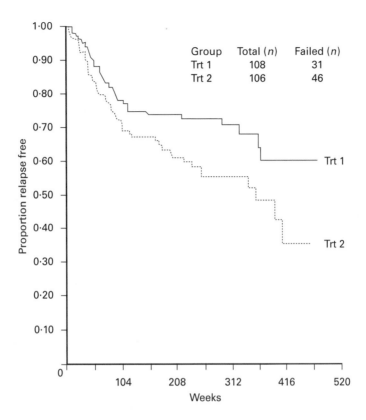

Figure 3.4 Relapse free survival by treatment group

features were node positivity, pleural or ascitic fluid, CSF positivity, soft tissue involvement only or distant metastases.

No details of randomisation method or location are given. Patients were stratified by site, sex and initial surgery. It was projected that 80 patients per randomised group would be required to detect a 15% increase in disease free survival at 2 years at 5% significance and 80% power.

All clinical data were centrally reviewed, 72% were fully assessable, 10% were non-assessable on review. All patients were included for analysis. Local radiotherapy at 55 Gy was given unless there was an initial surgical complete remission (CR) (15% of cases).

Treatment 1 included vincristine and doxo-rubicin (Adriamycin), alternating with vincristine and cyclophosphamide (see Figure 3.3). This was given 3 weekly for a total of 12 courses. The doxorubicin dose was 75 mg/m^2 and cyclophos-phamide 1·4 gm/m^2. This was then followed by seven courses of low dose continuing chemotherapy. Treatment 2 comprised weekly vincristine and cyclophosphamide for a total of six courses, followed by lower dose therapy adapted from IESS-I.

Outcome measures were survival and time to relapse.

Outcome

Following initial surgery 15 patients had a complete response, 16 a partial response and 50 had a biopsy only. Twelve per cent had initial amputation. A total of 234 patients were entered into the study, of whom 214 were eligible. Twenty were excluded, there no data in 10, secondaries in 5, a wrong diagnosis in 4 and one refused treatment. One hundred and eight patients were randomised on to treatment 1 and 106 on treatment 2.

Five year event free survival was 73% and 56% respectively for treatments 1 and 2 (p = < 0·03). Five year overall survival was 77% versus 63% (p = < 0·05). A similar number achieved a complete response (84% versus 78%), local relapses occurred in 7% versus 10% and lung relapses in 11% versus 22% for treatments 1 and 2 respectively.

Toxicity

There were three cardiac toxic deaths, all on treatment 1, but overall severe toxicity was comparable (68% and 67% respectively). The only significant difference was in significant cardiac toxicity (8% versus 2%, p = <0·03), being higher in treatment 1.

Conclusion

It was concluded that the pulsed intensive regimen was superior to the lower dose regimen used in the prior IESS-I study.

Comments

It is of note, that the 5 year relapse free survival for the non-pelvic tumours on IESS-I was 70%. The figure quoted of 57% for non-pelvic patients in IESS-I was the overall survival for all three study groups, not those on the VACA regimen. It appears, therefore, that the outcome in the control, i.e. less intensive, arm was poorer in this comparative study than in the previous trial. Reasons for this are unclear.

Study 3

Dunst J, Jurgens H, Sauer R, Pape H, Paulussen M, Winkelmann W, Rube C.
Radiation therapy in Ewing's sarcoma: an update of the CESS-86 trial.
Int J Rad Oncol Biol Phys 1995;**32**:919–30.

This study was carried out between 1986 and 1991 by the German CESS group, involving collaboration between 60 centres.

Objectives

The study addressed the issue of whether fractionated radiotherapy achieved comparable or better local control than conventional fractionation.

Details of the study

Eligibility criteria comprised Ewing's tumour of bone, including bone primitive neuroectodermal tumour (PNET); patients were under the age of 25, with localised tumours, who commenced treatment 4 weeks or less from the time of diagnosis.

No details are given regarding the randomisation method or where this was done. No statistical predictions are given with regard to differences sought or numbers required.

The study involved initial stratification of patients on the basis of tumour volume, those with volume < 100 cm³ receiving VACA (vincristine/actinomycin D/cyclophosphamide/doxorubicin), whereas those > 100 cm³ received VAIA (vincristine/actinomycin/ifosfamide/doxorubicin).

Surgery was performed, if possible, at around week 10 from diagnosis. If not possible, patients were randomised to either receive conventional radiotherapy or hyperfractionated split course irradiation simultaneous with continued chemotherapy.

The radiotherapy target volume included the pretreatment tumour volume, with a safety margin of at least 2 cm in lateral width and depth and at least 5 cm in the proximal and distal extension in extremity tumours. In the case of non-infiltrating extension of tumours in preformed cavities, e.g. pelvis or thorax, the target volume included only the actual tumour volume after chemotherapy with a 1–2 cm safety margin. The target area received a dose of up to 45 Gy and patients who received definitive radiotherapy, that is, as the only locally directed therapy, were given up to 60 Gy to the actual tumour volume with a 1–2 cm safety margin. Radioplanning programmes were centrally reviewed as part of the protocol.

Conventional irradiation was given in daily fractions of 1·8–2 Gy five times per week, with no simultaneous chemotherapy. Hyperfractionated split course irradiation was given at a dose of 1·6 Gy twice a day in two separate courses, each totalling 22·4 Gy. In the case of definitive radiotherapy without surgery a further boost of 16 Gy was given (see Figure 3.4).

Study outcome measures were relapse free survival, local control and overall survival. It was also planned to determine if it was feasible to give split dose radiotherapy with concomitant chemotherapy.

Outcome

One hundred and seventy-seven patients were registered: 111 Ewing's sarcoma, 34 bone PNET

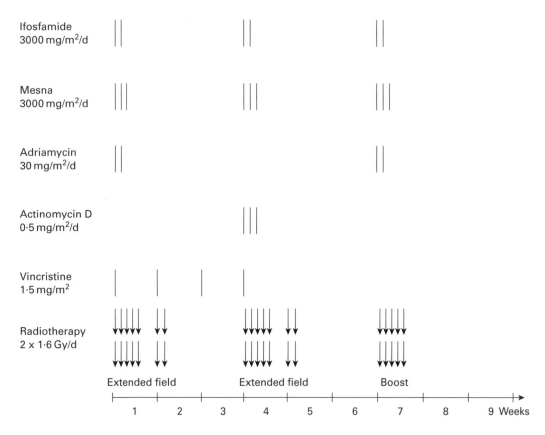

Figure 3.4 Hyperfractionation split-course irradiation with simultaneous VAIA (or VACA, not shown) chemotherapy. Reprinted from Dunst J *et al, Int J Rad Oncol Biol Phys* (full reference p 65) with permission from Elsevier Science.

(neurone specific enolase positive) and 32 non-specified tumours.

A total of 123 patients appear to have been randomised. The reasons for non-randomisation are not given in detail. The overall 5 year survival of the whole group of patients registered was 69% and the frequency of relapse was not influenced by the type of local treatment. Relapse rate was 30% after definitive radiotherapy, 26% after radical surgery and 34% after combined local treatment. After definitive irradiation 14% local failures occurred, either isolated or combined. The frequency of distant metastases was higher after surgery (26%) and resection plus radiotherapy (29%) as compared to definitive radiotherapy (16%). No statistical analysis is given.

The type of fractionation appeared to have no impact on local tumour control. When the randomised patients alone are considered, 43 received definitive radiotherapy – 21 conventional, 22 hyperfractionated – with a relapse free survival rate of 53% and 58% respectively. Local control rates were 82% versus 86% respectively. Of the 80 patients receiving postoperative radiotherapy, 40 received conventional and 40 received hyperfractionated. Relapse free survival in the two groups was 58% and 64% respectively.

Toxicity

Toxicity did not appear to be influenced by fractionation. There were two patients who developed significant proctitis, although the radiation schedule is not detailed.

Conclusion

It was concluded that radiotherapy scheduling with concomitant chemotherapy is feasible, but appeared to be of no short term benefit. The follow up was too brief to conclude whether there is any difference with regard to late sequelae. The overall reduced local failure rate compared to the previous CESS-81 study was put down to improved planning, with routine central review.

Study 4

Donaldson SS, Torrey M, Link MP, Glicksman A, Gilula L, Laurie F, Manning J, Neff J, Reinus W, Thompson E, Shuster JJ.
A multidisciplinary study investigating radiotherapy in Ewing'ssarcoma: end results of POG #8346.
Int J Rad Oncol Biol Phys 1998;**42**:125–35.

This study was carried out by the Pediatric Oncology Group between 1983 and 1988.

Objectives

The aim was to determine whether involved field irradiation was equivalent to standard whole bone irradiation in achieving local control.

Details of the study

Eligible patients were less than 30 years of age with bone Ewing's sarcoma. Extraosseous Ewing's and primitive neuroectodermal tumour were excluded and no prior treatment was allowed.

The randomisation method is not detailed, nor where this was done. Although analytical statistics are described, no anticipated patient number or predicted differences in outcome are detailed.

The protocol is as in Figure 3.5. All patients initially received a combination of cyclophosphamide 150 mg/m^2 orally for 7 days, combined with doxorubicin (Adriamycin) 35 mg/m^2, both drugs given every 14 days for a total of five courses (CA × 5). Cyclophosphamide, vincristine and actinomycin (CVD) were then given for six courses. This was followed by local radiotherapy, in the case of expendable bone,

such as proximal fibula, distal four-fifths of the clavicle, body of scapula, iliac wing and ribs. Patients who underwent surgery and were left with microscopic or gross residual disease were given postoperative radiotherapy and were eligible for randomisation. Patients in whom surgery was not appropriate received either tailored field or whole field radiotherapy. This was given concomitantly with maintenance chemotherapy, which comprised cyclophosphamide 150 mg/m^2 combined with alternating doxorubicin 35 mg/m^2 and actinomycin D 1·5 mg/m^2. Chemotherapy was given for a total of 12 months.

Radiotherapy guidelines required a radiation course of 55·8 Gy given in 1·8 Gy daily fractions. Large irradiation fields, i.e. pelvic fields, could be delivered at 1·5 Gy daily fractions at the discretion of the radiation oncologist. Standard radiation treatment was defined as radiation to the whole bone, including the tumour, to a dose of 39·6 Gy followed by a boost to 55·8 Gy to the initial tumour plus a 2 cm margin. The tailored, involved field was the same as the field that was boosted in standard radiation, also to a total dose of 55·8 Gy. Patients who had involvement of a small bone, such as a vertebral body, where there would have been no difference between boost volume and whole bone volume, were not randomised but assigned to involved field radiation.

In 1986 randomisation was discontinued owing to low recruitment. This was apparently due to a high number of patients with secondaries or initial complete resection, and subsequently all patients received involved field radiotherapy.

Outcome measures included local control, event free survival (EFS) and overall survival.

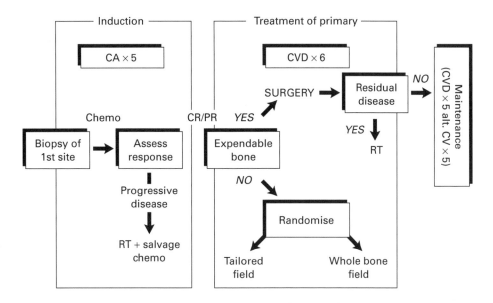

Figure 3.5 Protocol study design. Reprinted from Donaldson SS *et al*, *Int J Rad Oncol Biol Phys* (full reference p 68) with permission from Elsevier Science.

Outcome

One hundred and eighty-four patients were enrolled, of whom 178 were eligible. Six were excluded due to unconfirmed pathology. Primary sites comprised proximal extremity 30%, distal extremity 25%, pelvis 24% and other 21%.

All pathology was centrally reviewed, as were radiation planning fields. A major deviation in volume was defined as a field that missed a portion of the tumour, while a mild deviation was a field with less than a 2 cm margin. Major dose deviation was >10% variation, and a 6–10% deviation was dassed as mild. The influence of radiation deviations was analysed, although the percentage with minor or major deviations was not specified. Patients with major deviation, in either volume or dose, had a 5 year local control of only 16%, those with minor deviation 48%, while those treated appropriately had a 5 year local control rate of 80%. Of 141 patients with

localised disease, 104 non-surgical patients were eligible for randomisation or assigned to receive radiotherapy as local treatment.

Five year survival and EFS for this group was 52% and 41% respectively. Ninety-four patients actually received radiotherapy, the others are lost to follow up, refused radiotherapy or had progressive disease. Forty patients were ultimately randomised to receive either standard field (SF), i.e. whole bone, or involved field (IF) radiotherapy, with 20 in each group. The remaining patients were electively given involved field radiotherapy but these included 11 in whom the standard and involved fields would have been equivalent and who were therefore not eligible for randomisation (Figure 3.6).

Patients randomised to standard field had a 5 year local control rate of 53% ± 15% compared to 53% ± 14% for those receiving involved field treatment. Overall 5 year EFS in randomised

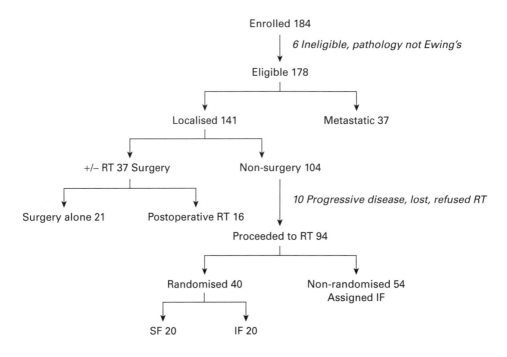

Figure 3.6 Flow chart showing patient distribution for all patients by extent of disease and treatment. Reprinted from Donaldson SS *et al*, *Int J Rad Oncol Biol Phys* (full reference p 68) with permission from Elsevier Science.

patients was 37% for whole bone, versus 39% for involved field.

Toxicity

No difference was documented in acute toxicity and follow up was too short to document any difference in late effects.

Conclusion

The conclusion was that there is no advantage to whole bone irradiation.

Study 5

Shamberger RC, LaQuaglia MP, Krailo MD, Miser JS, Pritchard DJ, Gebhardt MC, Healey JH, Tarbell NJ, Fryer CJH, Meyers PA, Grier HC.
Ewing sarcoma of the rib: results of an Intergroup study with analysis of outcome by timing of resection.
J Thorac Cardiovasc Surg 2000;**119**:1154–61.

This study was carried out by the Pediatric Oncology Group, CCG Intergroup between 1988 and 1992.

Objectives

The study addressed the value of intensified chemotherapy adding ifosfamide/etoposide to vincristine/doxorubicin/cyclophosphamide and actinomycin D (VACA).

This report considers only a subgroup within this large trial, namely those with rib primaries, and mainly addresses the issue of surgical timing.

Details of study

Patient eligibility for the Intergroup study comprised those under 30 years of age with Ewing's sarcoma, PNET or primitive sarcoma of bone and in whom treatment commenced less than 1 month from diagnosis.

Site of randomisation or randomisation details are not given. Patients were stratified by the presence of metastases. No predicted numbers or anticipated differences in the two chemotherapy groups are described.

Patients were randomised at study entry to receive standard chemotherapy with VACA or to receive experimental therapy consisting of these four drugs alternating with courses of ifosfamide and etoposide. Sizes of doses and schedules are not given in this publication, although the treatment was carried out around week 12.

For patients receiving radiotherapy alone, the initial treatment volume plus a 3 cm margin was treated with 45 Gy. This was followed by a reduction in treatment volume to the post-chemotherapy, pre-radiotherapy extent of tumour for an additional 10·8 Gy, resulting in a total dose of 55·8 Gy. Patients with residual tumour after surgery were irradiated, using the same dose volume guidelines in the case of gross residual disease, or 45 Gy with a 1 cm margin for microscopic residual disease.

The outcome measure of the study was event free survival (EFS).

Conclusion

Three hundred and ninety-three patients were entered in the overall study, with an EFS of 61%. Patients receiving VACA alone had a 54% 5 year EFS. The addition of etoposide/ifosfamide produced a 5 year EFS of 68%, hazard ratio 0·61, p = < 0·002. In the patients in this study with rib primaries alone the EFS was 64% versus 51%, hazard ratio 0·6, although not statistically significant. No details of toxicity in the chemotherapy arms were given.

Conclusions

The authors were more concerned with describing the timing of local surgery than the chemotherapy question and no specific analysis of the randomised group was presented. The full Intergroup study results have only been published in abstract form.

4

Wilms' tumour

Commentary – Dan Green

The treatment of Wilms' tumour has been the model for the multidisciplinary management of a paediatric solid tumour. Advances in anaesthesia, surgical techniques, radiation therapy equipment and planning and the demonstration that Wilms' tumour was responsive to several chemotherapeutic agents resulted in a transformation of the prognosis for children with this disease.

In this chapter the results of randomised clinical trials conducted by four groups are reviewed: the National Wilms' Tumour Study Group, the International Society of Paediatric Oncology, the United Kingdom Children's Cancer Study Group and the Brazilian Wilms' Tumour Study Group. The results of these trials form the basis for the management of children with Wilms' tumour throughout the world. The trials have had as a general objective defining the minimum necessary treatment for children with various stages and histologies of Wilms' tumour. The hypothesis has been that minimum necessary therapy would produce maximum survival rates with minimum late effects of therapy.

The trials conducted by the International Society of Paediatric Oncology (SIOP) had as a premise that treatment success was correlated with the presence or absence of residual intra-abdominal disease. They hypothesised that preoperative treatment would reduce the frequency of tumour rupture at the time of nephrectomy. This would lead to a lower frequency of post-nephrectomy abdominal radiation therapy in children with stages I—III Wilms' tumour. They demonstrated that pre-nephrectomy chemotherapy with vincristine and actinomycin D was as effective as abdominal radiation therapy in lowering the risk of tumour rupture. The most recent randomised trial conducted by SIOP demonstrated that 4 and 8 weeks of pre-nephrectomy chemotherapy were equivalent with respect to prevention of intraoperative tumour rupture and long term survival.

The trials conducted by the National Wilms' Tumour Study (NWTS) Group focused on minimising therapy for children treated with immediate nephrectomy. In their series of randomised trials, the Group demonstrated that abdominal irradiation was not necessary for children with stages I or II/favourable histology tumour. The addition of a third agent, doxorubicin, improved the outcome for those with stage III/favourable histology tumour randomised in NWTS–2, but a similar effect was not demonstrated in NWTS–3 when an intensified two drug regimen was compared to the three drug regimen. The most recent study of the NWTS Group demonstrated that single dose administration of actinomycin D and doxorubicin was as effective as the historical 5 and 3 day divided dose treatment courses.

The results of the SIOP and NWTSG studies are very difficult to compare due to the patient exclusions required by each study design. The SIOP studies exclude those with surgical emergencies (preoperative tumour rupture), a group that is at high risk of subsequent relapse. The number of patients excluded due to doubt in diagnosis, registration after nephrectomy or surgical emergency is 37–52%, the number of patients that were actually entered into the randomised trials. All of those considered to be surgical emergencies would have received post-nephrectomy abdominal radiation therapy. Thus the published figures regarding the percentage of children who receive post-nephrectomy abdominal radiation therapy are artifactually lowered due to the exclusion of those with preoperative tumour rupture from the randomised trials. Conversely, an increasing percentage of children registered on the NWTS Group protocols have not been eligible for randomisation because they received pre-nephrectomy chemotherapy. In general these children have large tumours, many of which may have been stage III. Thus the NWTS results may also underestimate the percentage of children who would require post-nephrectomy abdominal radiation therapy.

The role of doxorubicin in the management of children with favourable histology Wilms' tumour remains unclear. The intensity of the two-drug treatment regimen has an effect on the relapse free survival rate observed among those with stage II or III favourable histology disease. An anthracycline was added to the treatment regimen for SIOP patients with stage II N0 disease, based on the results of SIOP-6, but it is unclear from the most recent published results if there is a difference in outcome between children treated with doxorubicin (German Pediatric Oncology Group) or epiadriamycin (remainder of SIOP institutions).

The goal of maximising survival while minimising toxicity has historically been dependent upon light microscopic interpretation of histological findings, such as surgical margins and tumour subtype. More recent work has suggested that variables such as loss of heterozygosity at 1p or 16q may predict outcome, independent of traditional staging criteria. This hypothesis is being tested in the current NWTS Group protocol, where therapy is not being randomised. Future trials will build upon this model, with therapy first randomised and ultimately stratified, based on a combination of surgical, pathological and biological prognostic factors.

Studies

Study 1

Lemerle J, Voute PA, Tournade MF, Delemarre JF, Jereb B, Ahstrom L, Flamant R, Gerard-Marchant R.

Preoperative versus postoperative radiotherapy, single versus multiple courses of actinomycin D in the treatment of Wilms' tumour. Preliminary results of a controlled clinical trial conducted by the International Society of Paediatric Oncology (SIOP).

Cancer 1976;**38**:647–54.

The study was carried out between 1971 and 1974 by the International Society of Paediatric Oncology (SIOP) Collaborative Group.

> ## Objectives
> * To evaluate the role of preoperative radiotherapy.
> * To compare two schedules of actino-mycin D.

Details of the study

Eligibility included patients aged from 1–15 years with unilateral non-metastatic Wilms' tumour. Excluded were patients deemed to have very large tumours, in whom initial surgery was felt to be impossible without undue risk. Patients were excluded from the chemotherapy trial if they had marked intolerance to the first course of actinomycin D and also those in whom postoperative treatment could not be initiated 3 weeks after nephrectomy.

The randomisation method is not given in detail, but patients were stratified at the time of the second randomisation, based on stage, the use of radiotherapy, age and centre. An estimated 200–270 patients were planned to be included, at an accrual rate of 50–60 per year. The predicted difference between arms was not specified.

The first randomisation took place after a clinical diagnosis was made on the basis of imaging alone. Arm A received preoperative radiotherapy (20 Gy in 15–18 fractions). Following surgery those with stage I received no radiation treatment, stage II and III received a further 30 Gy. Arm B had primary surgery. Post-operative stage I received 20 Gy, stage II 30 Gy + boost to tumour residue and stage III, 30 Gy + boost to residue ± 30 Gy to the whole abdomen in case of tumour rupture.

Second randomisation was to either a single dose of actinomycin D following surgery, versus 3-weekly actinomycin D for a total of 6 courses. (Figure 4.1).

The main outcome measures were relapse free survival, operative complications and treatment tolerance.

A total of 422 patients were registered, 44 were excluded as not having Wilms' tumour (of these 19 were neuroblastoma). Another 203 were excluded from randomisation due to age < 1 year or > 15 years, stage IV or V, prior treatment, late registration or other causes. Ultimately, 169 patients were eligible for radiotherapy trial randomisation of whom 90 received preoperative irradiation and 79 received postoperative irradiation. In these two groups 17 and 15 patients respectively were excluded after randomisation

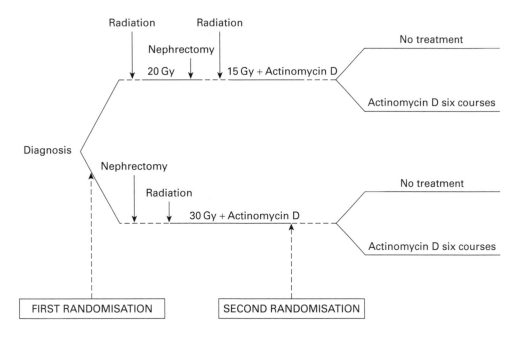

Figure 4.1 SIOP-I trial schedule. Copyright © 1976 American Cancer Society, Adapted and reprinted from Lemerle J *et al* (see p 74 for full reference) by permission of Wiley-Liss, Inc., a subsidiary of John Wiley & Sons, Inc.

because the tumour was not Wilms' or was stage IV. Therefore, a total of 137 were suitable for analysis.

Outcome

Stage distribution in arm A was as follows: stage I–31, stage II–33, stage III–9; there were 3 tumour ruptures at surgery. Arm B: stage I–14, stage II–28, stage III–22; there were 20 ruptures. The percentage of stage I tumours was significantly higher in arm A, $p < 0.025$, and there were significantly fewer ruptures in arm A, $p < 0.001$. Relapse free survival at 3 years was 52% for arm A, 44% for arm B and overall survival was 83% and 71% respectively–no significant difference.

In the actinomycin study, there were 161 eligible patients randomised, of whom 80 received a single dose. The RFS was 54% and overall survival, 82%. Eighty-one patients received repeated actinomycin, in whom relapse free survival was 58% and overall survival 86% – no significant difference.

The toxicities of the randomised arms with regard to other radiotherapy or chemotherapy were not given in detail.

Conclusion

It was concluded that preoperative radiotherapy reduced the tumour rupture rate at surgery but the administration of radiotherapy postoperatively diminished any potential outcome difference.

Study 2

Lemerle J, Voute PA, Tournade MF, Rodary C, Delemarre JF, Sarrazin D, Burgers JM, Sandstedt B, Mildenberger H, Carli M.
Effectiveness of preoperative chemotherapy in Wilms' tumour: results of an International Society of Paediatric Oncology (SIOP) clinical trial.
J Clin Oncol 1983;**1**:604–9.

The trial was carried out between 1977 and 1979 by the SIOP Group (SIOP-5).

Objectives

To determine the effectiveness of preoperative chemotherapy alone compared with chemotherapy plus radiotherapy.

Details of the study

Patients aged between 1 and 15 years with non-metastatic or bilateral tumours were eligible, the only exclusion being those with small polar tumours.

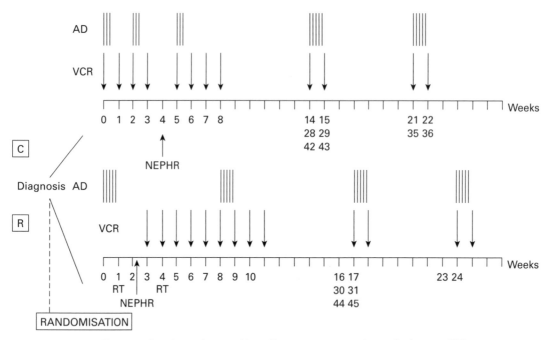

Preoperative chemotherapy (Arm C) versus preoperative radiotherapy (RT) 20 Gy plus actinomycin D 15 μg/kg/d (Arm R). In both arms, subsequent chemotherapy consisted of five courses of vincristine 1·5 mg/m² (VCR) plus actinomycin D (AD) at 6-week intervals

NEPHR: nephrectomy

Figure 4.2 SIOP-5 trial schedule

The randomisation methodology was not described and the predicted numbers required not detailed.

The trial consisted of randomising patients to receive either a combination of actinomycin D (AD) plus local radiotherapy prior to nephrectomy followed by 6 months of VA, or four doses of vincristine and two doses of actinomycin alone, prior to surgery, followed by VA plus local radiotherapy as appropriate. The patients with stage I disease post-surgery received no radiotherapy; stage II and III received 15 Gy postoperatively in the preoperative radiotherapy arm, or 30 Gy postoperatively in those receiving chemotherapy alone. The same total dose of chemotherapy was given postoperatively, although a slightly higher dose was given preoperatively where chemotherapy alone was given (Figure 4.2).

Major outcome measures were event free survival and overall survival.

Outcome

There were 397 eligible patients, of whom 233 were excluded. This was due to age < 1 or > 15 years (46), stage IV or V (56), small tumour (15), doubt in diagnosis (44), late registration (41) and other reasons (31). Ultimately 164 were randomised. Of these, 10 were excluded as not having Wilms' tumours.

With preoperative chemotherapy alone there was a clinical reduction in size in 84%. Tumour rupture occurred in 5 patients. After radiotherapy 88% showed tumour reduction and there were 7 ruptures after chemotherapy or radiotherapy. Stage distribution after chemotherapy or radiotherapy was similar: stage I, 43% and 52%; stage II, 36% and 32%; stage III, 21% and 16% respectively. A "major change" in pathological features (reflecting response) was seen in 53% of radiotherapy patients, compared to 17% after chemotherapy.

Event free survival at 4 years with chemotherapy alone was 76% and overall survival 89%, compared with 67% and 83% for radiotherapy.

Toxicity

Overall, there were four toxic deaths but it was not clearly specified in which arm this occurred.

Conclusion

It was concluded that preoperative chemotherapy was equivalent to radiotherapy.

Study 3

Tournade MF, Com-Nougue C, Voute PA, Lemerle J, de-Kraker J, Delemarre JF, Burgers M, Habrand JL, Moorman CG, Burger D.
Results of Sixth International Society of Paediatric Oncology Wilms' Tumour trial and study: a risk-adapted therapeutic approach in Wilms' tumour. *J Clin Oncol* 1993;**11**:1014–23.

The study was carried out between 1980 and 1987 by the International Collaborative SIOP Group (SIOP-6).

Objectives

This study addressed the issue of the duration of postoperative chemotherapy in stage I, the role of local radiotherapy in stage II node negative patients, and thirdly the role of doxorubicin (Adriamycin) in stage II node positive and stage III patients.

Details of the study

Eligible patients were 6 months to 15 years of age with stage I, II or III favourable histology. Patients could only have received vincristine and actinomycin preoperatively.

The method of randomisation is not defined and patients were stratified only on the basis of centre. Patients were randomised immediately after surgery before the initiation of continuing therapy. In stage I and stage II N0 these were de-escalation trials for chemotherapy and therefore designed as equivalence trials. For stage II N1 and stage III the design was of an efficacy trial. The same criteria were used for all trials: 2 years disease free survival (DFS), with type I error 5%.

For stage I patients, given the likelihood of complications due to chemotherapy and the 85% level of DFS at 2 years with the longer chemotherapy used previously, the short regimen would be considered to be equivalent if the 2 year DFS proved to be > 75%. A one-sided formulation to test the null hypothesis of inequivalence was applied, which stated that the difference in 2 year DFS between the long and short arm was > 10%.

The minimum number of patients required for a given power of 80% was at least 390. As this was not feasible within the time period, it was decided that the inclusion period would last 5 years and therefore the expected power would be approximately 45%.

For stage II N0, with the baseline DFS of 67%, too many patients would have been required to detect a difference of 10%. Therefore, again 5 year accrual was planned. The stopping rule was instituted whereby if the local recurrence increased from 5% to 15% this would be considered unacceptable. For stage II N1 patients and stage III patients a 5 year accrual would allow a 10% difference in 2 year DFS, with an error risk of 10%.

The protocol designed is outlined in Figure 4.3. The same preoperative chemotherapy comprising vincristine and actinomycin D over a 3 week period was followed by surgery. This consisted of radical nephrectomy, with examination and sampling of at least one hilar and one para-aortic node, as well as any suspicious regional lymph nodes. Patients were then stratified according to stage, lymph node involvement and histology.

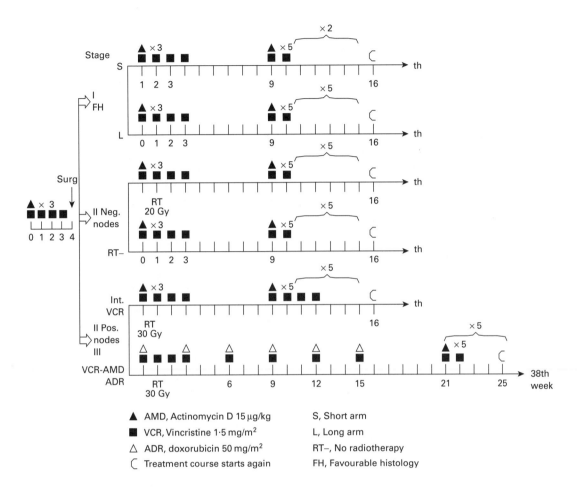

Figure 4.3 SIOP-6 Wilms' tumour protocol

Postoperative chemotherapy was started one week after surgery.

Radiation therapy, when given, had to be initiated within 2 weeks of surgery. The tumour bed was to be defined as the whole area of the kidney and the tumour according to the preoperative clinical and radiological extension criteria and based on the surgical and pathological reports. Total dose was 20 Gy in stage II N0 and 30 Gy in stage II N1 and III. A 5 Gy boost was permitted on areas of residual disease or in case of positive para-aortic lymph nodes.

The major outcome measure was 2 year disease free survival and 5 year overall survival.

Outcome

A total of 1095 patients were registered, of these 509 were assigned to the randomised trial group. Of the 586 who were found to be non-eligible, 421 were not included at initial registration due to age, stage or late registration. One hundred and sixty-two were excluded after nephrectomy due to other pathology or unfavourable histology. Fifty patients were taking part in the pilot study of SIOP-9. Patient accrual for stage I ended prematurely, whilst recruitment for stage II continued for a further period. A total of 442 patients with stage I–III disease were recruited in the initial period. In 7% tumour rupture occurred at the time of surgery. Of the 509 patients, 303 were stage I, 123 stage II N0, 83 stage II N1 and stage III. On central review, 47 patients were found to be misstaged (9% of the randomised tumours). Understaging mainly concerned stage II N0 patients. Fourteen patients were overstaged.

Histological review was carried out in 86% of the trial patients and 34 tumours that had unfavourable histology not identified by the local pathologist were redefined. Overall, the total rate of tumours with an unfavourable histology that were misclassified was 51%. Seventy-one patients were found to have a non-Wilms' tumour, 16 had benign disease and 22 a malignancy. Overall, benign disease represented 1·5 of the 1095 registered tumours.

Therapy compliance was reviewed by the Trial Committee, on the basis of recorded information regarding chemotherapy, irradiation, surgery and pathology. Complete evaluation was possible for all trial patients. Overall, 62% were treated strictly according to the protocols. Minor modifications involving a small reduction in dose or timing of radiotherapy were noted in 30%. Major deviations were noted in 8% (the precise definition of major deviation was not given). For chemotherapy a major deviation was a dose reduction to < 75% or the omission of one or more prescribed drugs, or delays of longer than one week in starting therapy.

For stage I patients the 2 year DFS rate was 92% in the short arm, versus 88% in the long arm, with a 5 year survival of 95% and 92% respectively. In stage II N0, abdominal recurrence occurred in 6 patients treated in the no-radiotherapy arm and as a consequence the trial was stopped in accordance with the stopping rule. Subsequently all stage II patients received local radiotherapy. The difference between the two regimens was less evident in terms of DFS. The number of events observed was higher in the radiotherapy arm, 18 versus 13, but 2 year DFS and 5 year survival were 72% versus 78% and 88% versus 85%. Statistical analysis concluded that there was equivalence between the radiation and non-radiation arms in terms of 2 year DFS, $p < 0.05$.

For node positive stage II and stage III patients the trial was also stopped prematurely but this was because of emerging results from the American NWTS trial, indicating an 80% event free survival at 5 years using a three-drug regimen. The 60% 2 year DFS rate obtained in SIOP-6 regardless of treatment was considered unsatisfactory. Despite this early closure, the DFS analysis shows a preference in favour of the doxorubicin-containing regimen, $p < 0.03$. Two year DFS and 5 year survival rates were 49% versus 74% and 77% versus 80%. The difference is not significant in terms of overall survival.

There was no significant difference in relapse sites in any treatment arm, although there was a suggestion of an increased rate of lung metastases in the radiation-plus and non-doxorubicin-containing regimen. It is possible that the higher rate of protocol modification in the radiation containing arm could have been responsible for this.

Conclusion

The study concluded that short postoperative chemotherapy is adequate for stage I favourable histology patients. For stage II N0 patients, it may be necessary to intensify chemotherapy to reduce the rate of local failure if radiotherapy is not given and the addition of doxorubicin is advantageous in patients with stage II node positive and stage III disease.

Study 4

De Camargo B, Franco EL.
A randomised clinical trial of single-dose versus fractionated-dose dactinomycin in the treatment of Wilms' tumour. Results after extended follow-up. Brazilian Wilms' Tumour Study Group. *Cancer* 1994;**73**:3081–86.

The study was carried out between 1986 and 1988 by the Brazilian Wilms' Tumour Study Group.

Objectives

The aim of the study was to evaluate the toxicity and efficacy of the more convenient single dose regimen of actinomycin D.

Details of the study

Eligible patients were those of any age with unilateral stage I–IV Wilms' tumour.

The method of randomisation was not described in detail and no predicted number of patients required was given. Patients did not appear to be stratified for any factor.

The main outcome measures were local and distant relapse rates, disease free survival and overall survival. The Cox's proportional hazards regression method was used to control for subset analysis bias.

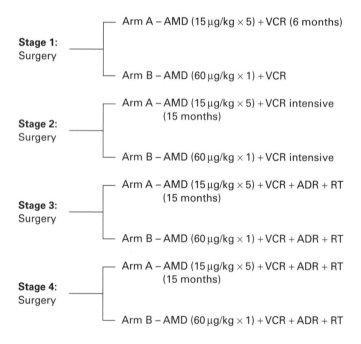

Figure 4.4 Treatment regimens according to disease stage. Copyright © 1994 American Cancer Society. Adapted and reprinted from De Camargo B *et al* (full reference above) by permission of Wiley-Liss, Inc., a subsidiary of John Wiley & Sons, Inc.

This was a prospective randomised study with three regimens as shown in Figure 4.4 and radiotherapy in stage III and IV. Chemotherapy comprised vincristine (VCR) and actinomycin D (AMD) or VCR/AMD and doxorubicin (ADR). The only variable was the dose and method of administration of actinomycin D. In arm A this was given as a fractionated dose of 15 µg/kg over 5 days and in arm B a single dose of 60 µg/kg. Courses of chemotherapy were given every 6 weeks.

Outcome

One hundred and ninety patients were registered, of whom 176 were confirmed with Wilms' tumour. One hundred and fifty-six patients were randomised. Physician decision or data entry problems were the main cause of non-randomisation. There were 33 major violations, which included the wrong chemotherapy, the wrong radiotherapy or non-completion of chemotherapy.

With arm A, at mean follow up of 38 months and median follow up of 47 months, there was an 80% 4 year relapse free survival and 84% overall survival. In arm B at mean and median follow up of 38 and 44 months respectively, the 4 year relapse free survival was 77% and overall survival 83%, i.e. no significant difference.

Toxicity

Little detail was given about the toxicity, although no clear difference appears to have been documented. Only a single toxicity was reported with regimen A, and hepatic toxicity was not observed in either arm. The 6 week gap between chemotherapies may account for the low toxicity observed in this study.

Conclusion

It was concluded that there was no significant difference between actinomycin D schedules, either in terms of efficacy or toxicity and the single dose was concluded to be more cost effective.

Study 5

D'Angio GJ, Evans AE, Breslow N, Beckwith B, Bishop H, Feigl P, Goodwin W, Leape LL, Sinks LF, Sutow W, Tefft M, Wolff J.
The treatment of Wilms' tumour. Results of the National Wilms Tumour Study.
Cancer 1976;**38**:633–46.

The study was carried out between 1969 and 1973 by the National Wilms' Tumour Study Group (NWTS-1).

Objectives

The study evaluates the role of radiotherapy in stage I patients, compares three chemotherapy regimens in group II and III (VCR alone, actinomycin alone or VA) and the role of preoperative vincristine in group IV patients.

Details of the study

Eligible patients were those of any age or stage of pathology.

Randomisation method was by telephone to the regional centre within two days of surgery for group I–III patients and group IV patients were randomised prior to surgery. Patients were stratified by age. The predicted number required or the differences to be detected were not detailed.

The primary outcome measures were relapse free survival and overall survival.

Details of treatment regimens are given in Figure 4.5.

For group I patients who received actinomycin D with or without radiotherapy the radiation therapy had to be started within 48 hours of surgery. The dose regimen was adjusted for age, ranging from 18 to 24 Gy for 18 months or less, up to 40 Gy for those over 40 months. The radiation field was designed to encompass the site of the kidney and associated tumour as visualised on a preoperative excretory urogram. Group I patients received actinomycin D (AMD) administered within 48 hours of diagnosis. Five daily injections were given at the time of surgery and at 6 weeks then 3, 6, 9, 12 and 15 months thereafter. Group II–IV patients who received vincristine (VCR) alone were given a dose at diagnosis and weekly for seven doses and thereafter at 3 monthly intervals for a period of 15 months. VA combined drugs in the same schedule, omitting the first VCR.

Outcome

Six hundred and six patients were registered, of whom 359 were randomised. Reasons for exclusion are given in detail, and included prior treatment, parental and institutional decisions. A diagnosis other than Wilms' tumour occurred in 30 patients. On central review, 16% of patients had been allocated to the wrong group.

Overall, there was good compliance with radiotherapy and chemotherapy. In only one patient was there a major deviation of radiotherapy due to a reduced dose, and there were eight chemotherapy deviations due to a reduced dose or delay.

For stage I patients < 2 years of age there was no difference between those given radiotherapy or actinomycin D alone, ith 2 year DFS of 90% and 88% respectively and overall survival of 97% and 94%. For those > 2 years of age the 2 year DFS

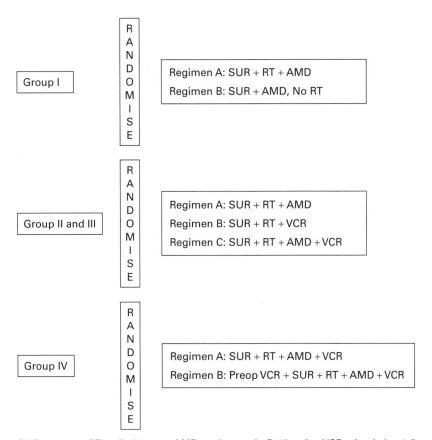

SUR, surgery; RT, radiotherapy; AMD, actinomycin D 15 μg/kg; VCR, vincristine 1·5 mg/m²

Figure 4.5 Treatment schemas of NWTS-1. Copyright © 1976 American Cancer Society. Adapted and reprinted from D'Angio GJ *et al* (full reference p 84) by permission of Wiley-Liss, Inc., a subsidiary of John Wiley & Sons, Inc.

appeared to be higher in those who had received local radiotherapy, being 77% versus 58% (p = 0·04), although overall survival was not different, at 97% versus 91%.

For stage II and III patients there was a significant advantage to the combination of vincristine and actinomycin D, with 2 year disease free survival of 81% for VA, versus 57% for actinomycin and 55% for vincristine alone. This was translated into an overall survival advantage with 86% for VA, versus 67% and 72% for actinomycin and vincristine respectively (p = 0·002).

In stage IV patients only 13 were included in each arm and the overall survival appeared to be superior in those who had immediate surgery without preoperative vincristine, 83% versus 29% (p = 0·02).

Conclusion

It was concluded that although in group I patients over 2 years of age the relapse rate appeared to be higher in the absence of radiotherapy, as the overall survival was no different this did not justify the late effects associated with radiation in this good outcome group.

The combination chemotherapy appeared to be more effective than either agent alone. The poor results with preoperative vincristine in group IV patients were unexplained, but the small number limited the strength of any conclusion.

Study 6

D'Angio GJ, Evans A, Breslow N, Beckwith B, Bishop H, Farewell V, Goodwin W, Leape L, Palmer N, Sinks L, Sutow W, Tefft M, Wolff J.
The treatment of Wilms' tumour. Results of the Second National Wilms Tumor Study.
Cancer 1981;**47**:2302–11.

The study was carried out between 1974 and 1978 by the National Wilms Tumor Study Group (NWTS-2). It considered the role of treatment duration in Group I, and the value of adding doxorubicin to vincristine and actinomycin in groups II–IV.

Details of the study

Eligible patients were those of any age or stage or pathology.

Randomisation method was not given in detail. Patients were stratified by institution, group and age. No predicted number of patients required or anticipated differences in outcome were given.

Treatment strategies are outlined in Figure 4.6. Group I patients did not receive any radiotherapy (RT) after surgery and all received actinomycin D (AMD) with vincristine (VCR) postoperatively and at 6 weeks, 3 months and 6 months. Actinomycin D dose was 15 µg/kg/day x 5 days and vincristine was given on days 7, 14, 21, 28 and 35 at 1·5 mgs/m^2. Patients were randomi-sed to receive either 6 months or 15 months VA treatment.

Group II–IV patients all received local radiotherapy, the dose to the tumour bed being age related, ranging from 18 Gy in those up to 18 months of age to 40 Gy for those above 40 months. Group IV patients initially received whole lung dose of 14 Gy but because of a 10%

incidence of pneumonitis this was reduced to 12 Gy. Other tumour sites received up to 30 Gy. Patients were randomised to receive two (VA) or three (AVA) drugs – doxorubicin (Adriamycin) 60 mg/m was given every 3 months for 4 doses.

Main outcome measures were relapse free survival (RFS) and overall survival.

Outcome

Of 755 patients registered, 513 were randomised. The reasons for non-inclusion and non-randomisation were given in detail and included 35 children who were determined to be inoperable by the local physician and received preoperative chemotherapy. Thirty- four tumours were bilateral and 15 patients received alternative chemotherapy. There were 12 cases of misdiagnosis.

Of the patients randomised, 22 switched chemotherapy regimens after central review resulted in a change of group. There were 31 major chemotherapy dose violations and 13 radiotherapy deviations.

For 188 group I patients there was no difference in outcome, with an overall 2 year RFS of 88%. There were 5/91 events in the short treatment arm versus 8/91 events in the long arm.

In groups II and III patients with favourable histology the addition of doxorubicin significantly improved outcome – 12/111 events versus 31/121 (p = < 0·004). Overall, group II–IV patients randomised to AVA had RFS at 2 years of 77% versus 62% (p = < 0·0004). For unfavourable histology patients there was no difference in RFS, although the overall survival appeared to be superior in the three-drug arm – 9/16 versus 4/19 (p = < 0·05). For favourable histology group IV patients alone, the RFS was 59% versus 43%,

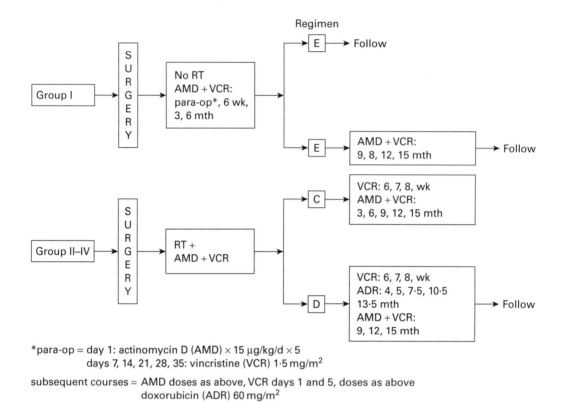

*para-op = day 1: actinomycin D (AMD) × 15 μg/kg/d × 5
days 7, 14, 21, 28, 35: vincristine (VCR) 1·5 mg/m²

subsequent courses = AMD doses as above, VCR days 1 and 5, doses as above
doxorubicin (ADR) 60 mg/m²

Figure 4.6 Treatment schemas of NWTS-2. Copyright © 1981 American Cancer Society. Adapted and reproduced from D'Angio GJ *et al* (full reference p 87) by permission of Wiley-Liss, Inc., a subsidiary of John Wiley & Sons, Inc.

again favouring the three-drug arm, although this was not statistically significant.

Toxicity

There was one toxic death in a group IV patient, who had received doxorubicin in addition to thoracic radiotherapy. The three-arm drug was predictably more myelosuppressive but there was no documented increase in other toxicity.

The authors mentioned that the outcome using the two-drug arm in the previous NWTS-1 study was superior for unexplained reasons. It is suggested perhaps the omission of actinomycin D on week 6 compared to NWTS-1 could have contributed to this difference.

Conclusion

The conclusions were that the short regimen is adequate for group I patients without the use of radiotherapy and that the addition of doxorubicin improves outcome in all other stages, particularly those with favourable histology.

Study 7

D'Angio GJ, Breslow N, Beckwith JB, Evans A, Baum H, deLorimier A, Fernbach D, Hrabovsky E, Jones B, Kelalis P.
Treatment of Wilms' tumour. Results of the Third National Wilms' Tumor Study.
Cancer 1989;**64**:349–60.

The study was carried out between 1979 and 1985 by the National Wilms Tumor Study Group (NWTS-3).

Objectives

The study addressed the issue of further shortening of the duration of treatment for stage I with favourable histology, the role of doxorubicin (Adriamycin) and local irradiation in stage II, the role of doxorubicin and the dose of radiotherapy in stage III, and finally the role of adding cyclophosphamide to AVA in stage IV and unfavourable histology.

Details of the study

Patients under the age of 16 years with any stage of pathology or histology were eligible.

Details of the randomisation method are not given. This was a factorial design, enabling the question regarding radiation and radiation dose, in addition to the role of doxorubicin, to be evaluated in the same patient group. Patients were stratified for histology and stage. No predictions of the numbers required or differences anticipated are given.

The outline of the study is given in Figure 4.7.

Stage I patients received a combination of vincristine and actinomycin D (VA) at a dose of 15 µg/kg/day x5 and 1·5 mg/m^2/week for 10 weeks. Patients were randomised to receive treatment for either 10 weeks or 26 weeks.

Stage II/III patients with favourable histology (FH) received the same initial 10 weeks but were randomised between VA with 5 day actinomycin D followed by 5 weekly injections of vincristine, repeated every 9 weeks, versus alternating actinomycin with two doses of vincristine and doxorubicin 20 mg/m^2/day on 3 consecutive day (AVA). Treatment duration was 65 weeks in both arms.

Stage IV patients with both favourable and unfavourable histology were randomised between the AVA regimen with or without cyclophosphamide 10 mg/kg/day IV on 3 consecutive days.

Stage II FH patients were randomised to receive or not receive 20 Gy local radiotherapy (RT) given not more than 10 days after nephrectomy. Stage III FH patients were randomised between 10 and 20 Gy. All stage IV patients received 12 Gy to the lung and mediastinum and FH patients with liver metastases received 20 Gy, UH received 30–40 Gy for metastases sites.

Close quality assurance monitoring took place, with deviations from timing and dosage of chemotherapy documented. All radiation therapy, machine calibrations, dose rates, physics and technical specifications were checked. All planning records and fields and doses used with imaging studies, operative and pathology reports were checked. Protocol deviations were defined as a delay in radiotherapy starting more

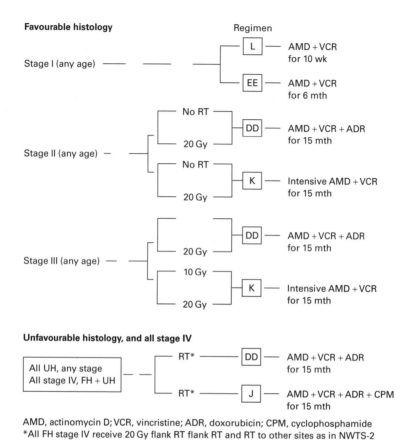

Figure 4.7 Treatment schemas of NWTS-3. Copyright © 1989 American Cancer Society. Adapted and reprinted from D'Angio GJ *et al* (full reference p 89) by permission of Wiley-Liss, Inc., a subsidiary of John Wiley & Sons, Inc.

than 10 days after nephrectomy, doses below the protocol stipulated level by more than 25% and failure to include all the tissues at risk as defined by the protocol. The Central Surgical Committee reviewed all operative and pathology reports.

Outcome

A total of 2496 patients were registered and of these 1489 were randomised. Three hundred and eight were non-eligible due to inoperability,

age and stage V. Five hundred and twenty-five eligible patients were treated with the protocol but not randomised and 174 eligible patients did not receive the protocol. Of the randomised patients, 24 were excluded. In 4 cases this was due to preoperative treatment, in 17 to stage IV disease which had been defined on the basis of CT scan alone. A further 26 children who had no follow up data of any kind were excluded from the survival and relapse free survival analysis. Ten per cent of patients switched regimen on review.

Relapse free survival and survival for the various study groups are both shown in Table 4.3. No significant difference is apparent relating to duration of treatment in stage I. The conclusions were less clear for the doxorubicin question. When stage II and III together are considered, there was no difference in outcome. Similarly, there was no difference for stage II alone. When stage III alone is considered, the relapse risk ratio for those receiving two versus three drugs was 1·6 (p = 0·07). There appeared to be fewer intra-abdominal relapses among those who receive doxorubicin, 4/134 versus 11/141, although this was not statistically significant. More than half the intra-abdominal relapses for stage III patients occurred among those given reduced irradiation of 10 Gy without doxorubicin. Relapse free survival and survival was no different in stage II patients who received no irradiation versus 20 Gy, or in stage III patients who received 10 Gy versus 20 Gy.

For high risk patients, namely the 279 patients with metastases at diagnosis, or tumours of unfavourable histology, the 4 year survival and RFS were 73% and 68% and the addition of cyclophosphamide did not improve outcome.

A separate analysis for unfavourable histology patients showed that the outlook for children with rhabdoid tumours was very poor whether or not cyclophosphamide was used, with only 25% alive at 4 years, contrasting with clear cell sarcoma, where the outcome was good, with 75% of patients alive at 4 years, irrespective of the chemotherapy given. For stage II, III and IV anaplastic tumours cyclophosphamide appeared to improve outcome, although the numbers are small – only 21 in the standard arm and 12 in the short arm. Four year survival was 37% versus 82% respectively. Combining log-rank scores for all anaplastic tumours, there were two relapses observed versus 6·7 expected for patients receiving four drugs (p = < 0·02).

Toxicity

Eighteen patients with stage IV disease developed radiological signs of pneumonitis; 3 with identified pneumocystis survived, 11 of the remaining 15 died. Although the addition of anthracycline was a specific question, there was no prospective documentation of cardiac function. Only "episodes of transient cardiotoxicity" were reported and these were seen more frequently in the doxorubicin-containing arm.

Conclusion

The conclusions from this study, which were brought forward into NWTS-4, were somewhat at odds with the published data. Although the short arm appeared to be equivalent for stage I patients, because "subset analyses, corrected for certain aberrations" resulted in a statistically significantly better survival for patients treated initially with 6 months rather than 10 weeks of chemotherapy, although the RFS rates were not different, it was decided to retain 6 months of treatment. Although the role of doxorubicin was not clearly demonstrated, the Committee favoured the use of the doxorubicin-containing regimen for stage III patients because this appeared to compensate for the lower dose of irradiation. Radiotherapy was concluded to play no role in stage II/FH patients.

The apparently beneficial effect of cyclophosphamide in stage II–IV anaplastic tumours was carried forward into the next study to obtain further data. The outline of NWTS-4 is given in Figure 4.8.

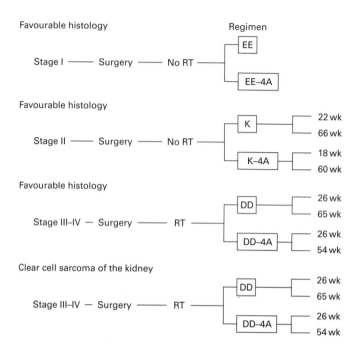

Figure 4.8 Treatment randomisation for NWTS-4. Copyright © 1989 American Cancer Society. Adapted and reprinted from D'Angio GJ *et al* (full reference p 91) by permission of Wiley-Liss, Inc., a subsidiary of John Wiley & Sons, Inc.

Study 8

Green DM, Breslow NE, Beckwith JB, Finklestin JZ, Grundy PE, Thomas PRM, Kim T, Schochat SJ, Haase GM, Ritchey ML, Kelalis PP, D'Angio GJ.
Comparison between single-dose and divided-dose administration of dactinomycin and doxorubicin for patients with Wilms' tumour: a report from the National Wilms' Tumor Study Group.
J Clin Oncol 1998;**16**:237–45.

This study was carried out by the National Wilms Tumour Study Group between 1986 and 1994 (NWTS-4).

Objectives
The study was designed to evaluate the efficacy, toxicity and cost of fractionated versus single dose of actinomycin D.

Details of the study
Eligibility included all those with Wilms' tumour under 16 years of age with untreated stage I–IV favourable histology, stage I anaplastic and stage I–IV clear cell sarcoma of the kidney.

Patients were treated by initial nephrectomy and lymph node biopsy. After surgical staging they were randomised within 5 days of surgery to receive a chemotherapy regimen that included actinomycin D, either as a single or divided dose. The initial dose of single fraction actinomycin D was 60 µg/kg but this was reduced to 45 µg/kg after early concern about hepatic toxicity.

Regimens were based on stage, as detailed in Figures 4.9, 4.10, 4.11. In summary, stage I patients received either 18 or 25 weeks of therapy with the frequency of actinomycin varying in addition to the schedule. For stage II, in addition to the schedule difference, the total number of doses differed: 8 in one treatment arm and 21 in the other. In stage III and patients with unfavourable histology, the number of doses of actinomycin D varied between study arms (10 v 6) as did the total number of doxorubicin doses (5 v 9), although the total dose was the same.

The study design was based on a two-sided test, with 95% power at the 0·05 level to detect a 2·5-fold reduction in the relapse rate, using the repeated dose schedule (pulse intensive) versus the standard regimen, or a 2-fold increase in relapse rate if the divided dose schedule was inferior.

Outcome
NWTS-4 registered 3335 patients, of whom 1756 were randomised. A further 1039 patients were treated on the same protocol but off study. Two hundred and seventy were not monitored. Of those randomised, 49 were excluded due to no pathological review or inadequate follow up and 69 due to anaplastic histology stage II–IV.

Five hundred and thirty-six low risk patients were randomised to standard and 528 to pulse intensive actinomycin D. In these patients the 2 year relapse free survival for the standard regimen was 91·4% (98·6% overall), and 91·3% RFS (97·9%) for the pulse intensive regimen. For the high risk patients, 284 received the standard regimen, with 90% RFS and 96% overall survival; 290 received pulse intensive therapy, with 87% RFS and 95·4% overall survival.

Toxicity
There was no significant difference in the haematological toxicity, nor at the 45 µg/kg dose level in the frequency of severe hepatic toxicity.

Week	0	1	2	3	4	5	6	7	8	9	10	11	12	13	14	15	16	17	18	19	20	21	22	23	24	25
Regimen																										
EE	A					A								A											A	
		V	V	V	V	V	V	V	V	V	V			V	V										V	V
EE–4A	A*			A*			A*			A*			A*			A*			A*							
		V	V	V	V	V	V	V	V	V	V		V*			V*			V*							

A, actinomycin D 15 µg/kg/d × 5 days IV; A*, actinomycin D 45 µg/kg IV; V, vincristine 1·5 mg/m² IV; V*, vincristine 2·0 mg/m² IV

Figure 4.9 Treatment randomisation for children with stage I/FH and stage I/anaplastic Wilms' tumour

Week

Regimen		0	1	2	3	4	5	6	7	8	9	10	11	12	13	14	15	16	17	18	19	20
K	A	A					A								A							
	V		V	V	V	V		V	V	V	V	V					V	V	V	V	V	V
K-4A	A*	A*						A*			A*			A*			A*			A*		
	V* / V		V	V	V	V	V	V	V	V	V			V*			V*			V*		

Week

		21	22	23	24	25	26	27	28	29	30	31	32	33	34	35	36	37	38	39	40	41	42	43	44	45	46	47
K	A		A									A									A							
	V			V	V	V	V	V	V	V	V		V	V	V	V	V	V	V			V	V	V	V	V	V	V
K-4A	A*				A*			A*			A*			A*			A*			A*			A*			A*		
	V*				V*			V*			V*			V*			V*			V*			V*			V*		

Week

		48	49	50	51	52	53	54	55	56	57	58	59	60	61	62	63	64	65
K	A		A									A							
	V			V	V	V	V	V	V	V	V		V	V	V	V	V	V	V
K-4A	A*				A*			A*			A*			A*			A*		
	V*				V*			V*			V*			V*			V*		

A, actinomycin D 15 μg/kg/d × 5 days IV; A*, actinomycin D 45 μg/kg/IV; V, vincristine 1·5 mg/m² IV; V*, vincristine, 2·0 mg/m² IV

Figure 4.10 Treatment randomisation for children with stage II/FH Wilms' tumour

Week 0–27

Regimen	0	1	2	3	4	5	6	7	8	9	10	11	12	13	14	15	16	17	18	19	20	21	22	23	24	25	26	27
DD	A						D							A						D							A	
DD		V	V	V	V	V	V	V	V	V	V	V	V	V	V												V	V
DD–4A	A*			D+			A*			D+			A*			D*			A*			D*			A*			D*
DD–4A		V*	V	V	V	V	V	V	V	V	V																	
	RT																											

Week 28–47

Regimen	28	29	30	31	32	33	34	35	36	37	38	39	40	41	42	43	44	45	46	47
DD					D							A						D		
DD												V	V							
DD–4A		A*				D*			A*			D*			A*			D*		
DD–4A		V*				V*			V*			V*			V*			V*		

Week 48–66

Regimen	48	49	50	51	52	53	54	55	56	57	58	59	60	61	62	63	64	65	66
DD					A						D							A	
DD						V	V											V	V
DD–4A		A*		D*		A*													
DD–4A		V*		V*		V*													

A, actinomycin D 15 μg/kg/d × 5 days IV; A*, actinomycin D 45 μg/kg IV; V, vincristine 1·5 mg/m² IV; V*, vincristine 2·0 mg/m² IV; D, doxorubicin 20 mg/m² d × 3 days IV; D*, doxorubicin 30 mg/m² IV; D+, doxorubicin 45 mg/m² IV; RT, abdominal irradiation

Figure 4.11 Treatment randomisation for children with stage III/FH and IV/FH Wilms' tumour and stages I to IV/clear cell sarcoma of the kidney

Conclusion

It was concluded that the divided dose schedule provides no therapeutic benefit, is no safer and has significant implications for cost effectiveness and patient convenience. It was recommended that the single pulse intensive regimen be adopted as standard therapy.

Study 9

Tournade MF, Com-Nougue C, de Kraker J, Ludwig R, Rey A, Burgers JMB, Sandstedt B, Godzinki J, Carli M, Potter R, Zucker JM.
Optimal duration of preoperative therapy in unilateral and nonmetastatic Wilms' tumour in children older than 6 months: results of the Ninth International Society of Pediatric Oncology Wilms' Tumour trial and study.
J Clin Oncol 2001;**19**:488–500.

The study was carried out between 1987 and 1991 by the SIOP Group (SIOP-9 trial).

Objectives

The purpose of this trial was to determine whether prolonged preoperative chemotherapy increased the proportion of stage I tumours, by comparing two regimens, one lasting 4 weeks and one lasting 8 weeks.

Details of the study

Eligibility criteria included patients aged 6 months to 16 years with untreated unilateral, non-metastatic tumours, where the clinical diagnosis appeared unequivocal and the child was fit to receive preoperative chemotherapy.

Randomisation was carried out at the Paris data centre. The method used is not stated. Patients were stratified by centre and balanced using randomised block permutation.

The baseline percentage of stage I patients was assumed to be 53%, on the basis of prior SIOP trials. It was predicted that 150 patients would be required in each arm to show a 15% increase in the number of stage I patients using the longer chemotherapy (80% power).

All patients following a clinical diagnosis of Wilms' tumour received a combination of vincristine and actinomycin D (VA). Patients were randomised only if they had responded to the initial 4 weeks chemotherapy. Surgery was carried out one week following completion of either 4 or 8 weeks chemotherapy and subsequent treatment depended on the surgical stage. Local radiotherapy (15 Gy favourable histology, 30 Gy unfavourable histology) was given to stage IIN, stage III and stage IINO unfavourable histology (Figure 4.12).

Because of an apparently high incidence of veno-occlusive disease, the schedule of actinomycin D was changed in April 1989 from single to split dose and two-thirds of the dose was given if the child was under 12 kg.

The main outcome measure was the percentage of stage I patients and tumour size following preoperative chemotherapy. Event free and overall survival were secondary endpoints.

Outcome

A total of 852 children were registered for the study, of whom 341 registered were not entered on the trial for a range of reasons, including age, doubt about diagnosis, surgical emergency and advanced stage. Five hundred and eleven patients received study chemotherapy but 129 were excluded from randomisation following 4 weeks preoperative chemotherapy. This was due to non-response, toxicity or refusal. Ultimately, 382 patients were randomised, 193 to 4 weeks and 189 to receive 8 weeks preoperative chemotherapy.

There was no difference in the rupture rate at time of surgery, 1% versus 3%, or in the 2 year

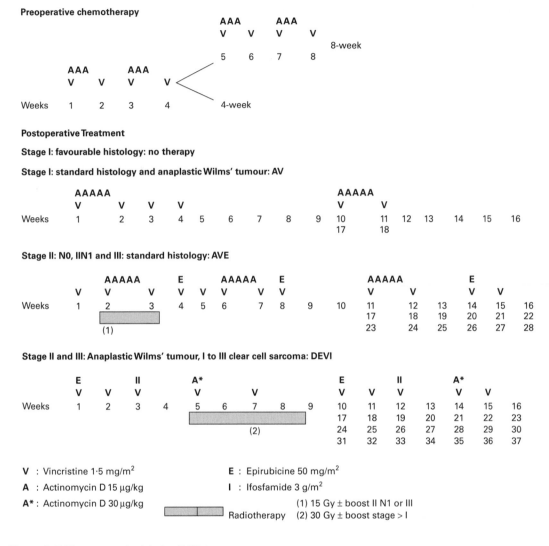

Figure 4.12 Treatment schedule for SIOP-9

event free survival, 92% versus 87%, and no difference in the site of failure between those receiving 4 or 8 weeks chemotherapy.

Volume assessment was available in 86% of patients, showing a > 50% reduction occurred in 52% of patients after four courses, and 64% of

patients were stage I at operation. Following an additional four courses of chemotherapy, a further reduction of 50% volume was seen in 33% of patients but the percentage of stage I was not further increased (62%). In both study arms 58% of patients received stage I postoperative therapy. Including non-randomised patients who received four courses of chemotherapy, there was no significant correlation between initial tumour reduction and event free survival.

Central pathology review showed an 82% agreement overall, with more discordance relating to unfavourable histology – 8/22 anaplastic and 8/16 clear cell sarcoma were discordant.

Toxicity

Toxicity was described in all patients receiving 4 weeks preoperative chemotherapy, with hepatic toxicity in 27%. Fifteen per cent developed veno-occlusive disease, 20% neutropenia, 17% gastrointestinal toxicity and 66% neurotoxicity. There was one death due to sepsis and liver dysfunction.

Conclusion

The conclusion was that there was no evidence of further downstaging by the addition of 4 weeks chemotherapy with vincristine and actinomycin D.

Study 10

Green DM, Beckwith JB, Breslow NE, Faria P, Maksness J, Finklestein JZ, Grundy P, Thomas PRM, Kim T, Shochat S, Haase G, Ritchey M, Kelalis P, D'Angio GJ.

Treatment of children with stages II to IV anaplastic Wilms' tumour: a report from the National Wilms' Tumor Study Group.

J Clin Oncol 1994;**12**:2126–31.

The study was carried out between 1979 and 1993 by the National Wilms Tumor Study Group.

Objective

This was a retrospective subgroup analysis of centrally reviewed anaplastic tumours in patients under the age of 16 years. It examined the influence of the addition of cyclophosphamide to a combination of vincristine, actinomycin D and doxorubicin (Adriamycin) in patients treated on NWTS-3 (Study 5 above) and NWTS-4 (Study 6 above).

Details of the study

On both studies the same chemotherapy regimens were used. Patients were randomised at presentation to receive either regimen DD with radiotherapy or regimen J, a similar protocol with the addition of cyclophosphamide at 10 mg/kg/day on three consecutive days every 6 weeks (Figure 4.13).

Details of the randomisation method are not given in the report.

For this study the definition of focal anaplasia was altered from an earlier quantitative definition, which included all cases in which less than 10% of microscopic fields contained anaplastic nuclear changes. This permitted the inclusion of cases in which anaplasia was widespread throughout the primary tumour, provided the affected cells were sparsely distributed. The new topographic definition required that anaplastic nuclear changes be strictly confined to a specified region of the primary tumour and absent from the surrounding portion of the lesions.

The outcome measure was relapse free survival (RFS) and overall survival.

Outcome

Seventy-two randomised patients were evaluated, 59 with diffuse anaplasia, and 13 with focal anaplasia. No information is given on patients with anaplastic pathology who were not included in the randomised study. Thirty-four received regimen DD and 38 regimen J.

The 4 year relapse free survival for regimen DD was 35%, overall survival 38%, and for regimen J 64%, overall survival 61%, p = < 0·03 and p = 0·04 respectively. For diffuse anaplasia, RFS for regimen DD was 27% versus regimen J 55%, for focal anaplasia (p < 0·02). Individual subgroup by stage contained small numbers, but a non-significant trend was clear for RFS: stage II, regimen DD 40% versus 72% for regimen J; stage III, 33% versus 58%; and stage IV, 0% versus 17%.

No details of any additive toxicity in the more intensive regimen are given.

Conclusion

The conclusion was that cyclophosphamide is of significant benefit with regard to outcome in anaplastic Wilms' tumour, particularly the diffuse subgroup.

Week 0–27

Regimen	0	1	2	3	4	5	6	7	8	9	10	11	12	13	14	15	16	17	18	19	20	21	22	23	24	25	26	27
DD–RT	A	V	V	V	V	V	D, V	V	V	V	V			A, V	V					D							A, V	V
		RT																										
J	A	V	V	V	V	V	D, V, C	V	V	V	V			A, V, C	V					D, V, C	V						A, V, C	V
		RT																										

Week 28–47

Regimen	28	29	30	31	32	33	34	35	36	37	38	39	40	41	42	43	44	45	46	47
DD–RT					D							A, V	V					D		
J					D, V, C	V						A, V, C	V					D, V, C	V	

Week 48–66

Regimen	48	49	50	51	52	53	54	55	56	57	58	59	60	61	62	63	64	65	66
DD–RT					A, V	V					D							A, V	V
J					A, V, C	V					D, V, C	V						A, V, C	V

A, Actinomycin D 15 μg/kg/d × 5 IV
D, Doxorubicin 20 mg/m^2/d × 3 IV
C, Cyclophosphamide 10 mg/kg/d × 3 IV

V, Vincristine 1·5 mg/m^2 IV
RT, Radiotherapy

Figure 4.13 Treatment schemas for children with anaplastic Wilms' tumour: regimen DD-RT and regimen J

Study 11

Green DM, Breslow NE, Beckwith JB, Finklestein JZ, Grundy P, Thomas PR, Kim T, Shochat S, Haase G, Ritchey M, Panayotis K, D'Angio GJ.
Effect of duration of treatment on treatment outcome and cost of treatment for Wilms' tumour: a report from the National Wilms' Tumour Study Group.
J Clin Oncol 1998;**16**:3744–751.

The study was carried out between 1986 and 1994 by the NWTS Group (NWTS-4).

Objectives

The study was designed to evaluate the efficacy, toxicity and cost of the administration of different regimens for the treatment of Wilms' tumour, which differed in schedule and duration (see Study 8).

Details of the study

Patients were aged under 16 years of age with Wilms' tumour but full eligibility requirements are not detailed. Patients with stage II–IV favourable histology and stage I–IV clear cell sarcoma were included. The randomisation method was based on a factorial design. The first randomisation was between single dose versus fractionated actinomycin D and the second between 6 or 15 months of chemotherapy. The first randomisation occurred within 5 days of nephrectomy and required neither final staging nor final histological information. Second randomisation was performed approximately 6 months after nephrectomy. The study was powered to detect an 80% increase in relapse rate in the short arm and 95% power, $\alpha = 0.05$.

The combinations of chemotherapy and the use of radiotherapy was stage dependent, but patients continued with the initial allocated schedule of actinomycin D.

The main outcome measures were relapse free survival (RFS) and overall survival (OS).

Outcome

Of 3230 patients registered, 1756 were randomised. Sixty-nine patients with anaplastic pathology were excluded from this analysis. Of 1687 randomised, 29 patients relapsed or died before the second randomisation, 665 patients had stage I favourable histology or anaplastic histology and were not randomised to receive additional therapy. The second randomisation was refused by patients or physicians in 88 cases. Forty patients had clear cell sarcoma stage I–V and are also not included in the analysis. The report describes the outcome of the 838 assessable patients randomised to the short or long treatments. The influence of actinomycin D schedule has been separately reported.

Patients were divided into low risk, i.e. stage II favourable histology, and high risk, stage III–IV favourable histology. One hundred and ninety low risk patients were randomised to the short arm and had a 4 year RFS of 84% and OS 96%. One hundred and eighty-seven low risk patients received the long arm therapy, with 4 year RFS of 88% and OS of 97% (not significant).

In the high risk group, 232 were randomised to the short arm, with 90% RFS, 94% OS, and 229 received the long arm therapy, with 89% RFS, 94% OS. There was no significant difference between the arms.

Conclusion

A complex analysis of cost concluded that the cost of treatment on the short arm, with the single dose actinomycin D, was approximately one-half that of those receiving the long arm with fractionated actinomycin D.

It was concluded that the addition of 9 months' chemotherapy was of no significant benefit with regard to outcome and had significant cost implications.

5

Neuroblastoma

Commentary – Katherine Matthay

Neuroblastoma, the most common extracranial tumour of childhood, remains a challenge among paediatric tumours, despite the astonishing advances seen in the outcome for children with leukaemia over the past 25 years. Fifty per cent of children with neuroblastoma present with high risk disease at diagnosis, with an expected survival below 40%, even with intensive multimodal therapy. In addition, late effects of treatment are particularly important in this tumour, where the peak age incidence is at 2 years. Thus, survivors will have many years for development of orthopaedic deformities, growth problems and second malignancies. Rapid testing of promising therapies and of means to diminish late effects in a randomised fashion has been difficult, due to the relative rarity of this tumour, with only approximately 650 new cases diagnosed yearly in the United States, for an incidence of 9.1 per million children age 0–15 years. This chapter evaluates six, randomised studies that have been completed in the past 15 years in Europe and the United States.

The important hypotheses to test in a randomised fashion for their possible contribution to an improvement of outcome in this disease are (1) increased dose intensity; (2) overcoming drug resistance using agents with new mechanisms of action; (3) local tumour control; (4) detecting and eliminating minimal residual disease; (5) how changes in therapy affect quality of life and late effects. The six randomised studies

summarised in this chapter have addressed the question of dose intensity using bone marrow support (Study 1 and 2); new non-cross-resistant chemotherapy for induction (Study 4 and 5); local control with radiation therapy in stage 3 neuroblastoma (Study 3); use of a differentiating agent for minimal residual disease (Study 1) and decreasing acute and late toxicity by changing the schedule of drug administration (Study 6).

Dose intensification to overcome resistance to therapy

The demonstration that hematopoiesis could be restored with autologous stem cells allowed the use of much higher doses of chemotherapy with autologous bone marrow support for treatment of solid tumours. The further advance showing that bone marrow tumour cells could be diminished or eliminated using immunomagnetic purging gave credence to the use of autologous marrow support in neuroblastoma, a tumour which is metastatic to bone marrow in 80% of children with high risk stage 4 disease. Early pilot studies showed that responses were seen in resistant patients after high dose melphalan and bone marrow reinfusion, and many subsequent single arm studies in the USA and Europe verified an apparent improvement in outcome for purged or non-purged autologous bone marrow transplantation (ABMT) compared retrospectively to results for chemotherapy[1–3].

Both cooperative paediatric groups in the US – the Pediatric Oncology Group (POG) and the Children's Cancer Group (CCG) – attempted statistical non-randomised comparisons of outcome for two concomitant groups of patients treated either with conventional doses of chemotherapy or myeloablative chemotherapy, total body irradiation and purged ABMT with mixed results[4,5]. On the basis of two POG studies, one a surgery plus conventional chemotherapy study (POG-8441) and the other an elective autologous transplant pilot protocol (POG-8340), there was no significant prognostic benefit of switching in remission from the chemotherapy protocol to the transplant protocol ($p = 0.91$). The analysis was based on 116 patients achieving a complete or partial remission, 32 of whom received transplants on the pilot protocol. The CCG examined the outcome of stage 4 patients under 1 year of age treated with identical induction chemotherapy on a CCG pilot protocol, who then either continued on the same chemotherapy ($n = 73$) for one year (CCG-321P2) or proceeded to CCG-321P3, with myeloablative chemotherapy, total body irradiation and purged ABMT ($n = 94$)[5]. The decision to use ABMT was non-random and depended on parental, investigator and institutional choice. The analysis was performed using Cox regression for censored failure-time data, treating time to ABMT as a time-varying covariate, and also by Kaplan Meier analysis comparing event free survival (EFS) from time of ABMT to EFS from 8 months after diagnosis for chemotherapy patients.

The advantage for ABMT versus chemotherapy was significant for the group as a whole, with respective 3 year EFS of 40% v 19%, different from the finding of Shuster et al[4]. The advantage for ABMT was greatest for certain very high risk subgroups, including those under 2 years of age at diagnosis, those with bone or bone marrow metastases, those with MYCN gene amplification, and those who had only a partial, rather than complete, response to the first four to six cycles of induction chemotherapy.

The European Neuroblastoma Study Group (ENSG) attempted the first randomized study, open 1983–85, using intensive therapy with autologous bone marrow support in neuroblastoma, very shortly after completion of the first pilot Phase II studies of high dose melphalan (Study 2). This study was actually a comparison of high dose melphalan compared to no further therapy, and showed a significant advantage in progression free survival for those patients with stage 4 disease over 1 year of age at diagnosis undergoing high dose therapy with bone marrow support. There are several problems, however, in application of these results. First, randomization was performed only for those patients achieving complete or good partial remission, and was not performed until approximately 10 months from diagnosis, after 10 cycles of chemotherapy. Of 84 eligible stage 4 patients, only 50 (59%) were randomised, for a variety of reasons ranging from toxic death to parental or physician preference. Thus, the applicability of these results is limited, because the group as a whole excludes the highest risk patients, including the 15% who are expected to progress early in the course of induction, and those who show a lesser response at the end of induction (perhaps another 20%), are not included in this study population. Secondly, bias may have been introduced by the high proportion of non-randomised patients. Overall survival curves are not shown, and the large difference in progression free survival (PFS) appears to diminish greatly after 2 years.

At the time of publication of these promising results, the CCG launched the first, large, randomised study comparing high dose chemoradiotherapy with purged ABMT to a new intensive non-myeloablative chemotherapy intensification (Study 1). This study differed from that of the ENSG by performing the randomisation much earlier in the course, after only two cycles of chemotherapy, at a time when 95% of the patients were still in the pool. The study was also much larger, with 190 patients in each randomised group. However, it still had the problem of refusal of randomisation, with a randomisation rate of 70%. Since ABMT was considered the experimental arm, patients who refused randomisation were assigned to the chemotherapy arm, but analysed separately. The results clearly showed a significant improvement for EFS for the patients randomly assigned to ABMT, both by an intent-to-treat analysis and also by treatment received.

As in the previous CCG non-randomised comparison, the highest risk patients, those with *MYCN* amplified tumours or those older than 2 years at diagnosis, had the most significant benefit. At the time of the analysis, with a median follow up of 43 months, there was no significant difference in survival. Further follow-up will be required to see if high dose therapy with hematopoietic support has truly made an impact on long term survival in this disease. The other notable finding from this randomised study was that there was no significant difference in the percentage of toxic deaths overall for patients randomised to the two arms, and the hospital days were identical, helping to validate the cost-effectiveness of this treatment. At present, many investigators are pursuing the strategy of trying to benefit from the further increase in dose

intensity obtainable with repetitive high dose myeloablative therapies with stem cell rescue, but a randomised study will be required to verify whether this approach truly improves EFS or survival[6,7]. Other groups are pursuing the use of further increase in chemotherapy dose intensity by eliminating total body irradiation, and instead using higher doses of chemotherapy and local irradiation[8].

Overcoming drug resistance with agents using new mechanisms of action

Since the limit of tissue tolerance has been nearly reached with current cytotoxic agents, even with hematopoietic support new approaches are required to overcome drug resistance, either by targeting therapy specifically to the tumour or by discovering agents that are non-cross resistant. The active cytotoxic agents added to the regular armamentarium of chemotherapy for neuroblastoma after 1985 have been the platinum compounds, ifosfamide and the inhibitors of topoisomerase, the epipodophyllotoxins (topoisomerase II inhibitors) and most recently the camptothecins (topoisomerase I inhibitors)[9–11]. Yet only one randomised study has been done to test the activity of these agents against the previous standard induction chemotherapy of doxorubicin and cyclophosphosphamide (Study 4).

This study compared the regimen which was the standard induction at that time when the study began, in 1981 (1050 mg/m^2 cyclophosphamide and doxorubicin, 35 mg/m^2), to the two newer agents with proven activity, teniposide (100 mg/m^2) and cisplatin (90 mg/m^2). There was no significant difference either in response rate or EFS, although the cisplatin regimen had an apparently slightly higher complete (CR) plus partial remission (PR) rate. The toxicity was not very different.

The value of this study was actually to show the tolerability and equivalent or better response with the newer agents. This, and other phase II studies using carboplatin with VP-16[12], led to the use of all four agents together in multiple induction regimens, with modestly improved overall response rates in cooperative studies in advanced neuroblastoma[13-16].

Further attempts to improve response rate were made in testing new agents in the context of an up-front phase II window (Study 5), rather than in relapsed patients, where resistance is known to develop to many agents. This study showed excellent and almost identical response rates (partial and minor response) of approximately 70% for ifosfamide, carboplatin and iproplatin, but an inferior response rate with epirubicin. The two platinum compounds were assigned in a randomised fashion, whereas the ifosfamide and epirubicin were given to sequential patients. The question of impact of the new drug on eventual outcome was not addressed in this study, although no deleterious effect of using a phase II window was demonstrated by comparing disease free or progression free survival in the group receiving the window therapy or not receiving it. However, as the 2 year PFS was only 40%, it is unknown whether further improvements in survival using combination therapy would result in the group receiving the single agent phase II window therapy for two courses to have a poorer outcome due to the possible more rapid development of drug resistance. In contrast, the European phase II window study of ifosfamide followed by conventional therapy, showed a lower survival and lower complete response rate for patients receiving the window therapy, despite good activity of the ifosfamide (44% response)[17].

The overall outcome for the two, randomised, continuation chemotherapy regimens has not yet been reported. An adjustment must be made to compare the response rate in the phase II window study reviewed here to previously reported results, since minor responses were included. If one only looks at those with partial response (there were no complete responses), then the response rates were ifosfamide 44%, identical to the up-front results in the European study[17], carboplatin 54%, iproplatin 35%, and epirubicin 17%. These response rates are generally higher than those in heavily pre-treated patients, as one would expect, but it is not clear that new information is gained, since traditional phase II testing also showed activity. The advantage of the phase II window approach is that it gives better information on quantitative response to the single agent in untreated patients, but these agents still then must be tested in a randomised fashion as part of a combination chemotherapy regimen to see if they improve overall response, or, more importantly, survival.

Local control

Recurrence in the local or regional area of primary disease is a component of relapse in a high proportion of children with high risk neuroblastoma, in rates ranging from 20 to 80% in reports that often include local radiotherapy and myeloablative therapy. There are both single arm studies and the randomised study reviewed here that demonstrate the benefit of local control measures for children with advanced but non-metastatic neuroblastoma[18-20], but the impact of local control in stage 4 disease has been mixed[21], possibly also due to problems with control of metastatic disease.

The study of Castleberry et al. (study 3) showed a benefit for the group of children with unresectable neuroblastoma who received radiotherapy. However, this group included both high risk and intermediate risk patients, since no biological markers were reported. There are problems in extrapolating the results of this randomised study, which took 8 years to complete, to current management, because of a now outdated chemotherapy regimen and the lack of biological risk factors. Because the protocol opened in 1981, this group only received cyclophosphamide and doxorubicin, without the benefit of platinum or etoposide. Furthermore, the group was heterogeneous in prognosis, since the only risk factors well known at the time were age and stage. It was shown in a subsequent CCG study that local control by surgery made a significant difference in EFS for high risk patients, but not those patients with stage 3 disease and favourable biology[19]. However, all patients on the CCG study were treated with four chemotherapy agents, and some of the high risk patients also had myeloablative therapy and ABMT.

Because of the POG study showing benefit from local radiation in incompletely resected tumours, all patients on the CCG study received local radiation for residual tumour. Therefore, no difference was shown in the CCG study for EFS of patients receiving radiation or those not receiving it, since those receiving the radiation were a higher risk group due to their residual disease.

Thus, although the study by Castleberry et al showed that radiotherapy in the dose of 24–30 Gy may make a contribution to EFS in locoregional neuroblastoma, it is unknown whether with more intensive chemotherapy the radiotherapy would have contributed to the EFS. The lessons to be extracted are that randomised studies that take more than 3–5 years to complete are likely to lose their usefulness because of changes in other factors, and that more information from treatment randomisation can be obtained in treating homogeneous risk groups.

Minimal residual disease

Even with intensive myeloablative therapy and hematopoietic stem cell support, relapse occurs in 50% of patients, including many who appear to be in complete remission at the time of consolidation. This suggests that microscopic viable disease is often present, which may not be entirely eradicated by myeloablative therapy, due to intrinsic resistance or anatomical problems with tumour cell hypoxia or uneven drug delivery. Approaches to this problem have suggested the use of non-cytotoxic therapy and therapy with a different mechanism of action such as immunological or differentiating agents. Study 1 showed that the addition of the differentiating agent 13-cis-retinoic acid, resulted in a significant increase in EFS when administered to patients post transplant, in a state of minimal residual disease. This study was based on previous data showing that 13-cis-retinoic acid caused differentiation and growth arrest of neuroblastoma in vitro[21], and anecdotal reports of responses in patients and one phase II study[22].

A phase 1 study of children with high risk neuroblastoma found that an intermittent schedule of high dose 13-cis-retinoic acid after bone marrow transplantation had minimal toxicity, achieved levels that were effective against neuroblastoma cell lines *in vitro* and resulted in the clearing of tumor cells in bone marrow, as determined by morphologic assessment, in 3 of 10 patients[23]. Thus, the second part of the CCG-3891 study examined the effect of treatment with 13-cis-retinoic acid after maximal reduction of the tumour with the use of chemotherapy, radiotherapy and surgery, with or without transplantation. There was a significant improvement in event free survival among children who were given 13-cis-retinoic acid, regardless of the type of prior consolidation therapy. The results suggested that 13-cis-retinoic acid is most effective in patients with minimal residual disease, because it did not appear to be effective in patients with proven residual disease who were non-randomly assigned to receive 13-cis-retinoic acid. The greatest effect of 13-cis-retinoic acid in patients with stage 4 neuroblastoma was found among those who had an initial complete response.

Minimal residual disease in bone marrow by immunocytology was shown, in the same CCG protocol, to adversely affect outcome. Patients with a quantitatively higher tumour content in bone marrow or blood at diagnosis and at the time of bone marrow harvest were shown to have a lower event free survival (EFS)[24]. This suggests that minimal residual disease in bone marrow may be either an important source of relapse, as also suggested by the gene marking study of Rill *et al*[25], or that it is a marker of general tumour resistance.

Recent studies using the polymerase chain reaction techniques for detection of minimal disease have also found that detection of circulating tumour cells at diagnosis or later also correlates with a worse outcome[26]. The CCG study used centralised quality controlled immunomagnetic purging of the autologous bone marrow. This had been used in other studies but not with the methodological improvements shown to eliminate 5 logs of tumour cells with immunocytologic testing before and after.

The contribution to event free survival of elimination of residual tumour from the bone marrow graft cannot be determined from this study, since purging was performed for all patients. The utility of purging deserves study as a randomised question in the future, given the increase in expense and cell requirement for purging versus the possible benefit by elimination of the minimal residual disease shown to be present in bone marrow and in peripheral blood stem cells using the sensitve RT-PCR technique for detection. The Children's Oncology Group protocol (opened February 2001) for high-risk neuroblastoma, A3973, is a randomized study of stem cell purging, as well as a prospective study of the impact of minimal residual disease by RT-PCR and immunocytology on event free survival.

Late effects

Study 6 reports the results for the French Society of Paediatric Oncology of an induction chemotherapy protocol, which included a randomized study of two methods of cisplatin administration. The goal of this randomization was to determine whether changing cisplatin from a one hour daily infusion for 5 days to a continuous 5 day infusion of the same total dose would diminish renal or ototoxicity.

A previous European pilot study had shown activity of the high dose cisplatin–etoposide regimen[27], but an associated high incidence of renal impairment, since 7 of 15 patients developed significant decreases in creatinine clearance. This is of concern both acutely during induction, then for later ability to tolerate a myeloablative chemotherapy, and long term, for development of late effects, including renal deficits or ototoxicity. Overall renal toxicity was lower in both treatment arms than expected, with only 8% of patients in the continuous infusion arm having a final creatinine clearance of < 90 ml/min/ $1.73m^2$, and 18% in the bolus arm, a difference that was not significant. Ototoxicity was also not significantly different on the two arms. Possibly, the toxicity was low due to the relatively low cumulative doses of cisplatin of 400 mg/m^2. It is stated in the article that response rates to the two regimens were equivalent, with an overall response rate (CR + VGPR + PR) of 74%. However, neither response nor survival data are given for the randomised regimens. It would have been useful to know if the late renal toxicity and ototoxicity were also similar, as many of these patients went on to receive carboplatin during consolidation.

Future important studies for toxicity and late effects in neuroblastoma should examine second malignancy, which has become increasingly prominent with the use of high doses of alkylating agents and epipodophyllotoxins during induction and consolidation, as well as radiation[28,29]. The genetic changes as well as the incidence could be compared on randomised treatment regimens. New studies to ameliorate the renal and ototoxicity of the very important platinum compounds could incorporate randomised addition of chemoprotectants.

Questions for future studies

The most important questions to address continue to be in the categories above, but with the emphasis on control of both local and late metastatic recurrence. Since dose intensity is close to the limits of tolerance, the emphasis should be either on ways to deliver dose intensity without increasing toxicity, or on agents with new mechanisms of action and on eradication of minimal residual disease. Increased dose intensity in the setting of myeloablative therapy might be accomplished by comparing a repetitive myeloablative consolidation to a single course. Adding agents with new mechanisms of action include comparing standard therapy to therapy with the addition of new immune modulators or new combinations of retinoids[30] or anti-angiogenic agents *et al* 2000;[31–33] in combination with chemotherapy. Treatment of minimal residual disease post myeloablative consolidation will be studied in a randomised fashion both in the ENSG and the COG studies testing the addition of anti-GD2 monoclonal antibody to 13-cis-retinoic acid. The COG study will also test, in a randomised fashion, the contribution of stem cell purging to elimination of minimal residual disease. Optimisation of the use of tumour radiation is also important, with a possible randomisation of [131] I-MIBG[34] versus external beam therapy, or a radiation dose question. Ways to decrease acute and late toxicity of treatment can also be tested in a randomised fashion, by the addition of chemoprotectants, schedule and dose alterations, and substitution of less toxic therapies. Only by timely, cooperative randomised studies will it be possible to verify the contribution of often costly and toxic new therapies to survival in this disease.

References

1 Matthay KK, Atkinson JB, Stram DO, Selch M, Reynolds CP, Seeger RC. Patterns of relapse after autologous purged bone marrow transplantation for neuroblastoma: a Childrens Cancer Group pilot study. *J Clin Oncol* 1993;**11**:2226–33.

2 Philip T, Bernard JL, Zucker JM, Pinkerton R, Lutz P, Bordigoni P, Plouvier E, Robert A, Carton R, Philippe N. *et al.* High-dose chemoradiotherapy with bone marrow transplantation as consolidation treatment in neuroblastoma: an unselected group of stage IV patients over 1 year of age. *J Clin Oncol* 1987;**5**:266–71.

3 Seeger RC, Reynolds CP. Treatment of high-risk solid tumors of childhood with intensive therapy and autologous bone marrow transplantation. *Pediatr Clin North Am* 1991;**38**:393–424.

4 Shuster JJ, Cantor AB, McWilliams N, Pole JG, Castleberry RP, Marcus R, Pick T, Smith EI, Hayes FA. The prognostic significance of autologous bone marrow transplant in advanced neuroblastoma. *J Clin Oncol* 1991;**9**:1045–9.

5 Stram DO, Matthay KK, O'Leary M, Reynolds CP, Haase GM, Atkinson JB, Brodeur GM, Seeger RC. Consolidation chemoradiotherapy and autologous bone marrow transplantation versus continued chemotherapy for metastatic neuroblastoma: a report of two concurrent Children's Cancer Group studies. *J Clin Oncol* 1996;**14**:2417–26.

6 Frappaz D, Michon J, Coze C, Berger C, Plouvier E, Lasset C, Bernard JL, Stephan JL, Bouffet E, Buclon M, Combaret V, Fourquet A, Philip T, Zucker JM. LMCE3 treatment strategy: results in 99 consecutively diagnosed stage 4 neuroblastomas in children older than 1 year at diagnosis. *J Clin Oncol* 2000;**18**:468–76.

7 Grupp SA, Stern JW, Bunin N, Nancarrow C, Ross AA, Mogul M, Adams R, Grier HE, Gorlin JB, Shamberger R, Marcus K, Neuberg D, Weinstein HJ, Diller L. Tandem high-dose therapy in rapid sequence for children with high-risk neuroblastoma. *J Clin Oncol* 2000;**18**:2567–75.

8 Villablanca JG, Matthay KK, Swift PS, Harris RE, Ramsay NK, Brodeur GM, Sondel PM, Stram D, Reynolds CP, Seeger RC. Phase I trial of carboplatin, etoposide, melphalan and local irradiation (CEM-LI) with purged autologous bone marrow transplantation for children with high risk neuroblastoma. *Med Pediatr Oncol* 1999;**33**:170.

9 Saylors RL, 3rd, Stewart CF, Zamboni WC, Wall DA, Bell B, Stine KC, Vietti TJ. Phase I study of topotecan in combination with cyclophosphamide in pediatric patients with malignant solid tumors: a Pediatric Oncology Group Study. *J Clin Oncol* 1998;**16**:945–52.

10 Tubergen DG, Stewart CF, Pratt CB, Zamboni WC, Winick N, Santana VM, Dryer ZA, Kurtzberg J, Bell B, Grier H, Vietti TJ. Phase I trial and pharmacokinetic (PK) and pharmacodynamics (PD) study of topotecan using a five-day course in children with refractory solid tumors: a Pediatric Oncology Group study. *J Pediatr Hematol Oncol* 1996;**18**:352–61.

11 Vassal G, Terrier-Lacombe MJ, Bissery MC, Venuat AM, Gyergyay F, Benard J, Morizet J, Boland I, Ardouin P, Bressac-de-Paillerets B, Gouyette A. Therapeutic activity of CPT-11, a DNA-topoisomerase I inhibitor, against peripheral primitive neuroectodermal tumour and neuroblastoma xenografts. *Br J Cancer* 1996;**74**:537–45.

12 Frappaz D, Michon J, Hartmann O, Bouffet E, Lejars O, Rubie H, Gentet JC, Chastagner P, Sariban E, Brugiere L. *et al.* Etoposide and carboplatin in neuroblastoma: a French Society of Pediatric Oncology phase II study. *J Clin Oncol* 1992;**10**:1592–601.

13 Coze C, Hartmann O, Michon J, Frappaz D, Dusol F, Rubie H, Plouvier E, Leverger G, Bordigoni P, Baehar C, Beck D, Mechinaud F, Bergeron C, Plantaz D, Otten J, Zucker JM, Philip T, Bernard JL. NB87 induction protocol for stage 4 neuroblastoma in children over 1 year of age: a report from the French Society of Pediatric Oncology. *J Clin Oncol* 1997;**15**:3433–40.

14 Matthay KK, Villablanca JG, Seeger RC, Stram DO, Harris RE, Ramsay NK, Swift P, Shimada H, Black CT, Brodeur GM, Gerbing RB, Reynolds CP. Treatment of high-risk neuroblastoma with intensive chemotherapy, radiotherapy, autologous bone marrow transplantation, and 13-cis-retinoic acid. Children's Cancer Group. *N Engl J Med* 1999;**341**:1165–73.

15 Pearson AD, Craft AW, Pinkerton CR, Meller ST, Reid MM. High-dose rapid schedule chemotherapy for disseminated neuroblastoma. *Eur J Cancer* 1992;**28A**: 1654–9.

16 Pinkerton CR, Blanc Vincent MP, Bergeron C, Fervers B, Philip T. Induction chemotherapy in metastatic neuroblastoma – does dose influence response? A critical review of published data standards, options and recommendations (SOR) project of the National Federation of French Cancer Centres (FNCLCC). *Eur J Cancer* 2000; **36**:1808–15.

17 Kellie SJ, De Kraker J, Lilleyman JS, Bowman, A, Pritchard J. Ifosfamide in previously untreated disseminated neuroblastoma. Results of Study 3A of the European Neuroblastoma Study Group. *Eur J Cancer Clin Oncol* 1998;**24**:903–8.

18 Haase GM, Atkinson JB, Stram DO, Lukens JN, Matthay KK. Surgical management and outcome of locoregional neuroblastoma: Comparison of the Children's Cancer Group and the International staging systems. *J Pediatr Surg* 1995;**30**:289–95.

19 Matthay KK, Perez C, Seeger RC, Brodeur GM, Shimada H, Atkinson JB, Black CT, Gerbing R. Haase GM, Stram DO, Swift P, Lukens JN. Successful treatment of stage III neuroblastoma based on prospective biologic staging: a Children's Cancer Group study. *J Clin Oncol* 1998;**16**: 1256–64.

20 Powis MR, Imeson JD, Holmes SJ. The effect of complete excision on stage III neuroblastoma: a report of the European Neuroblastoma Study Group. *J Pediatr Surg* 1996;**31**:516–9.

21 Reynolds CP, Kane DJ, Einhorn PA, Matthay KK, Crouse VL, Wilbur JR, Shurin SB, Seeger RC. Response of neuroblastoma to retinoic acid *in vitro* and *in vivo*. *Prog Clin Biol Res* 1991;**366**:203–11.

22 Finklestein JZ, Krailo MD, Lenarsky C, Ladisch S, Blair GK, Reynolds CP, Sitarz AL, Hammond GD. 13-cis-retinoic acid (NSC 122758) in the treatment of children with metastatic neuroblastoma unresponsive to conventional chemotherapy: report from the Children's Cancer Study Group. *Med Pediatr Oncol* 1992;**20**:307–11.

23 Villablanca JG, Khan AA, Avramis VI, Seeger RC, Matthay KK, Ramsay NK, Reynolds, CP. Phase I trial of 13-cis-retinoic acid in children with neuroblastoma following bone marrow transplantation. *J Clin Oncol* 1995;**13**:894–901.

24 Seeger RC, Reynolds CP, Gallego R, Stram DO, Gerbing RB, Matthay KK. Quantitative tumor cell content of bone marrow and blood as a predictor of outcome in stage IV neuroblastoma: a Children's Cancer Group Study. *J Clin Oncol* 2000;**18**:4067–76.

25 Rill DR, Santana VM, Roberts WM, Nilson T, Bowman LC, Krance RA, Heslop HE, Moen RC, Ihle JN, Brenner MK. Direct demonstration that autologous bone marrow transplantation for solid tumors can return a multiplicity of tumorigenic cells. *Blood* 1994;**84**:380–3.

26 Burchill SA, Lewis IJ, Abrams KR, Riley R, Imeson J, Pearson AD, Pinkerton R, Selby P. Circulating neuroblastoma cells detected by reverse transcriptase polymerase chain reaction for tyrosine hydroxylase mRNA are an independent poor prognostic indicator in stage 4 neuroblastoma in children over 1 year. *J Clin Oncol* 2001;**19**: 1795–801.

27 Hartmann O, Pinkerton CR, Philip T, Zucker JM, Breatnach F. Very-high-dose cisplatin and etoposide in children with untreated advanced neuroblastoma. *J Clin Oncol* 1988;**6**:44–50.

28 Donnelly LF, Rencken IO, Shardell K, Matthay KK, Miller CR, Vartanian RK, Gooding CA. Renal cell carcinoma after therapy for neuroblastoma. *AJR Am J Roentgenol* 1996;**167**:915–7.

29 Kushner BH, Cheung NK, Kramer K, Heller G, Jhanwar SC. Neuroblastoma and treatment-related myelodysplasia/ leukemia: the Memorial Sloan–Kettering experience and a literature review. *J Clin Oncol* 1998;**16**:3880–9.

30 Maurer BJ, Metelitsa LS, Seeger RC, Cabot MC, Reynolds CP. Increase of ceramide and induction of mixed apoptosis/necrosis by N-(4-hydroxyphenyl)-retinamide in neuroblastoma cell lines. *J Natl Cancer Inst* 1999;**91**:1138–46.

31 Erdreich-Epstein A, Shimada H, Groshen S, Liu M, Metelitsa LS, Kim KS, Stins MF, Seeger RC, Durden DL.

Integrins alpha(v)beta3 and alpha(v)beta5 are expressed by endothelium of high-risk neuroblastoma and their inhibition is associated with increased endogenous ceramide. *Cancer Res* 2000;**60**:712–21.

32 Katzenstein HM, Rademaker AW, Senger C, Salwen HR, Nguyen NN, Thorner PS, Litsas L, Cohn SL. Effectiveness of the angiogenesis inhibitor TNP-470 in reducing the growth of human neuroblastoma in nude mice inversely correlates with tumor burden. *Clin Cancer Res* 1999;**5**:4273–8.

33 Meitar D, Crawford SE, Rademaker AW, Cohn SL. Tumor angiogenesis correlates with metastatic disease, N-myc amplification, and poor outcome in human neuroblastoma. *J Clin Oncol* 1996;**14**:405–14.

34 Matthay KK, DeSantes K, Hasegawa B, Huberty J, Hattner RS, Ablin A, Reynolds CP, Seeger RC, Weinberg VK, Price D. Phase I dose escalation of 131I-metaiodobenzylguanidine with autologous bone marrow support in refractory neuroblastoma. *J Clin Oncol* 1998;**16**:229–36.

Studies

Study 1

Matthay K, Villablanca JG, Seeger RC, Stram DO, Harris RE, Ramsay NK, Swift P, Shimada H, Black CT, Brodeur GM, Gerbing RB, Reynolds CP. Treatment of high-risk neuroblastoma with intensive chemotherapy, radiotherapy, autologous bone marrow transplantation, and 13-Cis-retinoic acid.
N Engl J Med 1999;**341**:1165–73.

The study was carried out between 1991 and 1996 by the American Children's Cancer Group evaluated the role of high dose therapy and the differentiating agent 13-cis-retinoic acid.

Details of the study

Eligible patients were aged 1–18 years with stage IV pathology or <1 year with *NMYC* amplification, stage 3 poor risk patients on the basis of *NMYC* amplification, ferritin >143 ng/ml or unfavourable Shimada pathology.

The first randomisation was carried out just prior to cycle 3 of chemotherapy at week 8 for all patients with non-progressive disease. The second randomisation followed bone marrow transplant (BMT) or week 34 of the end of continuation (Figure 5.1). Details of the randomisation method are not given.

A permuted-block design was used for the random assignment of patients from two stratified groups, those with and those without metastatic disease, to receive transplantation or continuation chemotherapy. The second randomisation was similarly balanced with respect to the number of patients from each group of the first randomisation and non-randomised patients who were ineligible for transplantation.

Initial chemotherapy consisted of standard dose cisplatin 60 mg/m^2, doxorubicin 30 mg/m^2, etoposide 100 mg/m^2 ×2, cyclophosphamide 1 g/m^2 ×2 combination (see Figure 5.1). The patients received five cycles at 28 day intervals. They then received surgery plus local radiation to primary gross residual disease. Those randomised to receive high dose therapy were given carboplatin 1 g/m^2 combined with etoposide 640 mg/m^2 over 3 days with melphalan 210 mg over 2 days and total body irradiation 333 cGy × 3. Bone marrow was purged at a centralised purging centre, using immunomagnetic separation.

Patients randomised to continuing chemotherapy received cisplatin 160 mg/m^2, etoposide 500 mg/m^2 and doxorubicin 40 mg/m^2, all infused over 96 hours, combined with ifosfamide 2·5 g/m^2 × 4 doses. This was followed by prophylactic G-CSF. A total of three courses was given.

For the second randomisation patients received six courses of cis-retinoic acid 160 mg/m^2 per day orally in two divided doses for 14 consecutive days in a 28 day cycle or no further therapy.

The primary endpoint was event free survival (EFS) from time of randomisation. No details of the anticipated difference between the groups or the required predicted numbers are given.

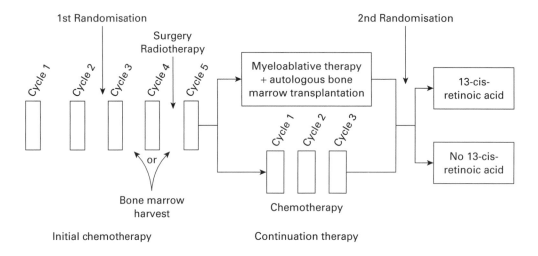

Figure 5.1 Treatment regimens. The conditioning regimen for autologous bone marrow transplantation consisted of carboplatin, etoposide, melphalan and total body irradiation. Adapted with permission, 2002 from Matthay K *et al, N Engl J Med* (full reference on p 115). Copyright © 1999 Massachusetts Medical Society.

Outcome

Five hundred and sixty patients were assessed for the study, of whom 539 were deemed eligible. Ineligibility included patients not of defined high risk, incorrect diagnoses, organ dysfunction and problems with local protocol review boards. Ultimately, 379 patients were randomised for high dose therapy and 258 were randomised for cis-retinoic acid. Overall, the treatment arms were well balanced for clinical features, except that 21% of stage 3 patients ended up in the non-randomised group, compared to 12% in the randomised group, i.e. more patients with lower stage disease refused randomisation.

One hundred and ninety patients were allocated to continuing chemotherapy, 189 to high dose therapy. One hundred and eighteen were non-randomly assigned to continuing chemotherapy. The remaining 42 patients never underwent randomisation, because of disease progression (16 patients), lack of parental consent (8), physician decision (4) and protocol deviations (11).

A total of 128 of 189 received BMT as per protocol, 150 of 190 received the full protocol chemotherapy. Overall, there was an 86% compliance if progressive disease is excluded.

Three hundred and nineteen patients completed induction and consolidation or BMT. One hundred and thirty patients were randomly allocated to cis-retinoic acid and 128 to no further treatment. Thirty-seven non-randomised patients were electively assigned to cis-retinoic acid due to residual disease and 24 declined randomisation. Overall, there was 98% compliance with the protocol of the second randomisation; two patients in the cis-retinoic group did not receive treatment according to protocol and four in the group assigned to no further treatment received cis-retinoic.

Outcome

Figures 5.2–5.4 summarise the outcome. For the whole group of 539 eligible patients the 3 year event free survival was 30% and overall survival

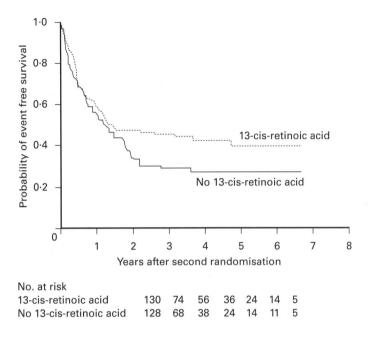

No. at risk
13-cis-retinoic acid	130	74	56	36	24	14	5
No 13-cis-retinoic acid	128	68	38	24	14	11	5

Figure 5.2 Probability of event free survival among patients assigned to receive 13-cis-retinoic acid or no further treatment. Follow-up began at the time of the second randomisation (34 weeks after diagnosis). The difference in survival between the two groups was significant at 3 years (p = 0·027). Adapted with permission, 2002 from Matthay K *et al, N Engl J Med* (full reference on p 115). Copyright © 1999 Massachusetts Medical Society.

45%; for the 379 randomised patients the 3 year EFS was 28%; in the 118 non-randomised patients who received chemotherapy alone it was 33%. In 189 patients randomised to bone marrow transplantation the 3 year EFS was 34%, compared with 22% in the 190 randomised to chemotherapy alone (p = < 0·03). Overall survival was 43% and 44% respectively (no significant difference). If only patients who actually received either BMT or continuing chemotherapy are analysed, the 3 year EFS is 43% and 27% respectively.

The 3 year EFS (from week 34) for patients receiving cis-retinoic was 46%, compared to 29% for those with no further treatment (p = < 0·03). Again, overall survival was not significantly

different, at 56% and 50% respectively. If the two study groups are combined, the best outcome was in the 50 patients who received both high dose therapy and cis-retinoic where 3 year EFS was 55% from the time of second randomisation. The worst outcome was in the 53 patients receiving standard chemotherapy alone, where 3 year EFS was 18%. In the subgroup non randomly assigned to chemotherapy and then included in the cis-retinoic randomisation, there again appeared to be benefit, although non-significant: 53% *v* 31% 3 year EFS (p = 0·13).

Overall, the event free survival for high dose therapy was greater in all prognostic subsets, which was evident on univariate analysis but particularly for those over 2 years of age

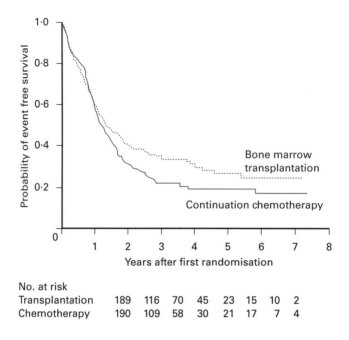

No. at risk
Transplantation	189	116	70	45	23	15	10	2
Chemotherapy	190	109	58	30	21	17	7	4

Figure 5.3 Probability of event free survival among patients assigned to bone marrow transplantation or continuation chemotherapy. Follow-up began at the time of the first randomisation (8 weeks after diagnosis). The difference in survival between the two groups was significant at 3 years ($p = 0.034$). Adapted with permission, 2002 from Matthay K *et al, N Engl J Med* (full reference on p 115). Copyright © 1999 Massachusetts Medical Society.

($p = < 0.01$) and those with MYCN amplification ($p = < 0.03$). Cis-retinoic acid was only of significant benefit for those in complete remission at the end of therapy, as opposed to those in partial remission.

If only stage 3 patients are considered, EFS for BMT was 30% versus 20% for chemotherapy alone, and for cis-retinoic 40% versus 25% for no further treatment.

Toxicity
The toxic mortality in the BMT group was 6% compared to 3% for chemotherapy alone. The incidence of grade 3 or 4 renal toxicity was 8% for chemotherapy versus 18% for BMT. There

was a 10% incidence of interstitial pneumonitis and 9% incidence of veno-occlusive disease with high dose therapy. Overall, the hospital stay duration did not differ: median 45 days for chemotherapy alone compared to 47 days for high dose therapy.

With cis-retinoic acid, 2% of patients had grade 3 or 4 significant skin toxicity and 2% had liver function test abnormalities.

Second malignancy occurred in two patients on study, one randomly assigned to transplantation and the other randomly assigned to continuation chemotherapy. One also occurred in a non-randomised chemotherapy patient.

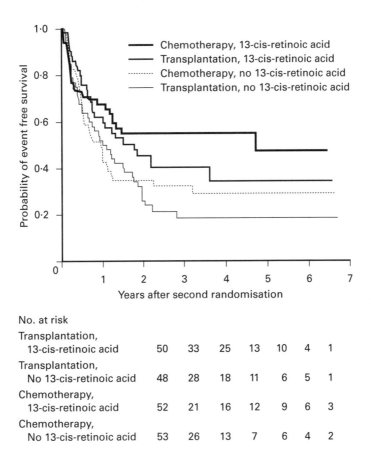

No. at risk

Transplantation, 13-cis-retinoic acid	50	33	25	13	10	4	1
Transplantation, No 13-cis-retinoic acid	48	28	18	11	6	5	1
Chemotherapy, 13-cis-retinoic acid	52	21	16	12	9	6	3
Chemotherapy, No 13-cis-retinoic acid	53	26	13	7	6	4	2

Figure 5.4 Probability of event free survival in the four randomised groups. Adapted with permission, 2002 from Matthay K *et al*, *N Engl J Med* (full reference on p 115). Copyright © 1999 Massachusetts Medical Society.

Conclusion

It was concluded that treatment with myeloablative therapy including total body irradiation followed by purged autologous bone marrow transplantation improved event free survival but not overall survival. In addition, treatment with cis-retinoic acid was beneficial for patients in complete remission, after either chemotherapy or high dose therapy.

Study 2

Pinkerton R, Pritchard J, de Kraker J, Jones D, Germond S, Love S.

ENSG 1 – Randomized study of high-dose melphalan in neuroblastoma.

In: Dickie K, Spitzer G, Jagannath S, *Autologous Bone Marrow Transplantation.* eds. Houston: University Texas Press, 1987.

The study was carried out between 1983 and 1985 by the European Neuroblastoma Study Group.

Objectives

The study addressed the issue whether the addition of high dose melphalan improved survival in patients with stage 3 and 4 neuroblastoma who were responding to initial induction chemotherapy.

Details of the study

Eligibility included all newly diagnosed patients with Evans' stage 3 or 4 disease aged over 6 months at diagnosis. In this report only the subgroup with stage 4 disease were described.

Patients received OPEC chemotherapy as induction, with cyclophosphamide at 600 mg/m^2, vincristine 1·5 mg/m^2, cisplatin 60 mg/m^2 and VM-26 150 mg/m^2. If the marrow was in complete remission after six courses patients proceeded to surgery and then received four further courses of OPEC. At this time, provided the patient was in complete remission (CR) or good partial remission (GPR), they were randomised to either 180 mg/m^2 of high dose melphalan followed by unpurged fresh autologous bone marrow, or no further treatment (Figure 5.5).

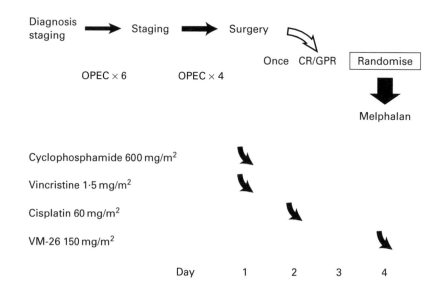

Figure 5.5 Treatment schema and OPEC chemotherapy regimen

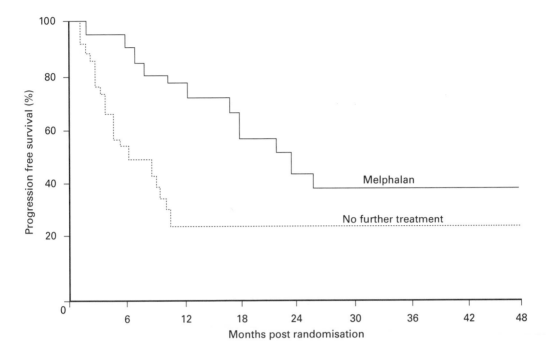

Figure 5.6 Actuarial disease progression free survival for the two randomised groups

No details of the randomisation method are given. There are also no details of the anticipated numbers predicted to be required nor the anticipated difference between groups.

The outcome measure was progression free survival and overall survival.

Outcome

One hundred and forty patients were registered. Of these 95 achieved CR or GPR with induction chemotherapy and surgery (68%) and of these 65 were randomised. Details for non-randomisation included medical reasons, physician preference, parental reluctance or death in remission (precise numbers not given). Thirty-two patients received high dose melphalan and 33 no further treatment. For stage 4 patients over 1 year of age, 24 were randomised to high dose melphalan. Two relapsed prior to high dose melphalan and there was one toxic death. Twelve of 24 patients were disease free at a median follow up of 32 months post ABMT.

Of 26 patients randomised to no further treatment, 8 were disease free. Median progression free survival was 23 months with melphalan, compared to 6 months with no further treatment (p = < 0·02) (Figure 5.6).

Conclusion

It was concluded that high dose melphalan prolonged progression free survival in stage 4 patients in complete remission after standard chemotherapy.

Study 3

Castleberry RP, Kun LE, Shuster JJ, Altshuler G, Smith IE, Nitschke R, Wharam M, McWilliams N, Joshi V, Hayes FA.
Radiotherapy improves the outlook for patients older than 1 year with Pediatric Oncology Group stage C neuroblastoma.
J Clin Oncol 1991;**9**:789–95.

This study was carried out between 1981 and 1989 by the Pediatric Oncology Group.

Objectives

The study addressed the role of local radiotherapy in patients with initially unresected stage C disease, i.e. those with complete or incomplete resection of primary tumour, with intracavitary lymph nodes not adhered to primary tumour, which were histologically positive.

Details of the study

Eligible patients were those 1–21 years of age with surgically proven node positivity and no prior chemotherapy or radiotherapy. The precise randomisation method is not given in detail.

It was predicted that 64 patients would be required to show a 50% reduction in local relapse for those receiving irradiation (single arm 80% power at 5% level), assuming that there was a 15% 2 year event free survival based on historical data.

After clinical staging all patients had surgery to the primary tumour. The aim of this was to the achieve maximum resection without vital organ damage, to search and sample non-adherent lymph nodes and to perform liver biopsy if the primary was in the abdomen. If the tumour was

too large for attempted resection, then it was assumed to be lymph node positive.

Patients received five courses of chemotherapy, with cyclophosphamide 150 mg/m^2 orally for 7 days and doxorubicin 35 mg/m^2 on day 8, given at 3-weekly intervals. Patients were randomised to receive local radiotherapy to the tumour plus regional lymph nodes. A dose of 24 Gy was given to those between 1 and 2 years of age and 30 Gy for those over 2 years of age. For abdominal primaries the field included the thoracic paravertebral and supraclavicular nodes, which were given 18–24 Gy depending on age. All patients had second-look surgery, except those with CT negative initial thoracic primaries. All patients achieving complete remission went on to receive alternating cyclophosphamide/doxorubicin with cisplatin 90 mg/m^2 and VM-26 100 mg/m^2, two courses of each.

Patients randomised to receive radiotherapy were treated within 3 weeks of initial surgery, concurrently with chemotherapy.

Outcome

Seventy-four patients were registered, of whom 8 were non-eligible due to diagnostic or staging errors and 4 were not randomised due to clinician decision. Twenty-nine received chemotherapy alone, 33 received chemotherapy plus radiotherapy. Five patients were non-evaluable due to protocol violations. Overall, the arms were balanced for clinical features.

There was a 46% complete response rate for chemotherapy alone, compared to 76% for chemotherapy plus radiotherapy (p = < 0·01). Nine of 28 patients randomised to chemotherapy remain disease free with a follow up off therapy of 1 to 52 months. Relapses occurred in both

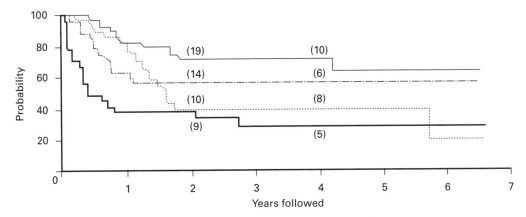

Figure 5.7 Event free survival (EFS) (p = 0·009) and overall survival (p = 0·008) for patients >1 year treated with chemotherapy (CT) alone *v.* identical chemotherapy plus radiotherapy (RT)

local (3) and metastatic (1) sites at 1 to 17 months after stopping treatment. In the combined therapy arm, 17 patients were disease-free at 1 to 77 months off treatment. Relapses were again seen at local sites alone (1), metastatic sites alone (2) or combined sites (2). All occurred within 2 months of stopping treatment. In the radiotherapy group, only patients having less than 50% resection of primary tumour at diagnosis developed recurrent disease.

The significant difference in survival remained when adjusted for Shimada classification. No biological studies were done (Figure 5.7).

Conclusion
It is concluded that local radiotherapy increases the initial complete response rate and reduces subsequent disease relapse.

Study 4

McWilliams NB, Hayes FA, Green AA, Smith EI, Nitschke R, Altshuler GA, Shuster JJ, Castleberry RP, Vietti TJ.
Cyclophosphamide/doxorubicin *v.* cisplatin/teniposide in the treatment of children older than 12 months of age with disseminated neuroblastoma: a Pediatric Oncology Group randomized phase II study.
Med Ped Oncol 1995;**24**:176–80.

The study was carried out between 1981 and 1984 by the Pediatric Oncology Group and compared two induction chemotherapy regimens in patients with stage 4 disease.

Details of the study

Eligible patients were over 1 year of age with POG stage D disease or Evans stage 4. Patients with dumbbell tumours were excluded from randomisation.

Patients were randomised at diagnosis to receive either cyclophosphamide 150 mg/m^2 PO × 7 + doxorubicin 35 mg/m^2 or cisplatin 90 mg/m^2 + VM-26 (teniposide) 100 mg/m^2 (or etoposide 200 mg/m^2 if allergic reaction). Both were given for a total of five courses prior to assessment of response.

No details of the precise randomisation method are given. Complete response rate and toxicity are compared by two-sided exact unconditional Z-test and event free survival by log-rank test. The predicted number or details required are not specified.

Outcome measures were remission rate, disease free survival and complete response post surgery to primary tumour.

Outcome

Of 157 patients registered, 4 were ineligible (reason not stated) and 13 patients with dumbbell tumours were excluded. The initial complete response (CR) rate to cyclophosphamide/doxorubicin was 13% compared to 22% for cisplatin/teniposide. CR rate following surgery was 27% versus 34% respectively. Overall, complete response and partial response including surgery was 59% versus 77% (p = 0·077). There was no difference in event free survival – 6% and 3% respectively at 5 years.

The cyclophosphamide/doxorubicin arm was significantly more myelosuppressive with a lower white cell count (p = < 0·02). The cisplatin/teniposide produced more nausea and vomiting (p + < 0·01) and more allergic reactions (p = 0·001).

Conclusion

It was concluded that the cisplatin/teniposide arm appeared to be an effective induction regimen, although overall outcome was very poor.

Study 5

Castleberry RP, Cantor AB, Green AA, Joshi V, Berkow RL, Buchanan GR, Leventhal B, Mahoney DH, Smith EI, Hayes FA.

Phase II investigational window using carboplatin, iproplatin, ifosfamide, and epirubicin in children with untreated disseminated neuroblastoma: a Pediatric Oncology Group study.

J Clin Oncol 1994;**12**:1616–20.

The study was carried out between 1987 and 1990 by the Pediatric Oncology Group. It was a randomised comparison of carboplatin with iproplatin as initial chemotherapy in metastatic neuroblastoma.

Details of the study

Eligible patients were those aged 1–21 years with POG stage D disease. Normal liver and renal function was required.

Patients were randomly assigned to receive carboplatin 560 mg/m^2 over 1 hour or iproplatin 325 mg/m^2 infused over 2 hours. In a separate group of patients, ifosfamide 2 g/m^2 daily × 4 was given and a sequential group received epirubicin 90 mg/m^2. The reason for allocation of patients to randomised or non-randomised therapy are not stated. With the carboplatin/ iproplatin study a second course was given 14–21 days later depending on count recovery.

No details of randomisation method are given nor of the predicted difference between arms and numbers required.

Following the accrual of an initial 25 cases within any of the single-agent stratum, the stratum was temporarily closed for analysis and a different stratum was opened. If five or more complete remissions and/or partial remissions were noted in the first 21 assessable patients treated with a particular drug, this stratum for that drug was again opened to accrue an additional 25 patients. If less than five CRs and/or PRs were noted in the first 21 patients analysed, the treatment arm was not opened for secondary accrual. This ensured that with 90% confidence the population CR/PR rate would be no less than 10% below the observed rate.

Following this window comparative study, patients proceeded to the phase III study (POG-8742) in which the efficacy and toxicity of two chemotherapy regimens were compared.

The major endpoint of the window study was the response to two courses of single agent therapy. Because it was anticipated there would be few, if any, complete responses after only two courses the number of objective responses, defined as PR plus minor response (MR), was used as a measure of efficacy.

Outcome

One hundred and seventy-nine patients were eligible. Six were excluded due to diagnostic error, early death or parental reluctance.

In the sequential study, 50 patients received ifosfamide, 23 received epirubicin. In the randomised arm 48 patients received carboplatin, 52 received iproplatin.

The patients in both arms were well balanced for primary site and nature of metastases. There were 26/48 partial responses with carboplatin, compared to 18/52 with iproplatin. The overall objective response rate PR + MR was 77% with carboplatin and 67% with iproplatin, i.e. no significant difference. In the sequential arm, the objective response rate was 70% with ifosfamide, 26% with epirubicin.

Ultimately, disease free survival did not differ in the subsequent phase III study for patients receiving, or not receiving, window chemotherapy.

Conclusion

Both iproplatin and carboplatin appear to be comparably active in metastatic neuroblastoma.

Study 6

Coze C, Hartmann O, Michon J, Frappaz D, Dusol F, Rubie H, Plouvier E, Leverger G, Bordigoni P, Cehar C, Beck D, Mechinaud F, Bergeron C, Plantaz D, Otten J, Zucker JM, Philip T, Bernard JL.
NB87 induction protocol for stage 4 neuroblastoma in children over 1 year of age: A report from the French Society of Pediatric Oncology.
J Clin Oncol 1997;**15**:3433–40.

The study was carried out between 1987 and 1992 by the French Paediatric Oncology Group. This was a single arm study assessing multi-agent chemotherapy but it included a randomised comparison of cisplatin scheduling.

Details of the study

Eligible patients were those over 1 year of age with INSS stage 4 disease.

No details of randomisation method are given. It was predicted that 44 patients would be needed in each randomised group to detect a reduction from 47% to 20% of decreased creatinine clearance. This was based on the incidence of renal dysfunction documented in the high dose cisplatin/etoposide phase II trial. This would have 80% power at 5% level.

Initial chemotherapy comprised (CADO) cyclophosphamide $1·5$ g/m^2, doxorubicin 60 mg/m^2, vincristine $1·5$ mg/m^2 × 2, alternating with (CVP) cisplatin 200 mg/m^2 divided over 5 days and etoposide 500 mg/m^2 over 5 days. Patients were randomised to receive the cisplatin either as a continuous infusion over 5 days or as a 1 hour bolus infusion.

In this trial there was also a randomisation question regarding the use of prophylactic G-CSF

and patients on this study were excluded from the cisplatin schedule randomisations.

Both groups had the same hyperhydration with added potassium chloride and the same post-hydration schedules were given.

Creatinine clearance was used to document renal function and audiometry was done before and after chemotherapy.

Outcome

Two hundred and eleven patients were registered onto the study. Nine were non-eligible due to prior chemotherapy or performance status, and 10 were excluded due to inadequate data collection. One hundred and eighty-three patients completed induction chemotherapy. Ninety-one patients were randomised on the schedule study: 43 received continuous infusion platinum and 48 bolus. They were well matched for age, sex, primary location, catecholamine increase, mIBG, marrow positivity and other secondary sites. Two patients who were given G-CSF were excluded for haematological evaluation. Three failed to complete the trial due to two early deaths and one progressive disease.

The GFR fell to below 90 ml/min/$1·73$ m^2 in 8% of those receiving continuous infusion cisplatin, compared to 18% with bolus infusion, (difference was not significant). Hearing was maintained at a Brock A level, i.e. none or <40 dB loss at any frequency in 81% of the continuous infusion and 86% of the bolus. Two patients in the bolus regimen had grade C ototoxicity, 3 had grade B; 6 in the continuous infusion had grade B ototoxicity (grade B = > 40 dB at 8000 Hz, grade C = > 40 dB at 6000 Hz). No patient had more severe hearing loss. The only significant difference between the two schedules was the degree of neutropenia after the first course of CVP, with 70% versus 43%, the higher incidence being in those who received continuous infusion (p < 0·02). This difference was not seen after the second course of CVP.

Conclusion

The incidence of both renal and ototoxicity appeared less than expected and at this high dose of cisplatin there appeared to be no significant difference between the two schedules.

Study 7

Kohler JA, Imeson J, Ellershaw C, Lie SO.
A randomized trial of 13-cis retinoic acid in children with advanced neuroblastoma after high-dose therapy.
Br J Cancer 2000;**83**:1124–7.

The study was carried out between 1989 and 1997 by the European Neuroblastoma Study Group.

Objectives

This trial was to establish whether 13-cis-retinoic acid used as continuation therapy after obtaining a good response to conventional chemotherapy could prolong disease free survival in children with advanced neuroblastoma.

Details of the study

Eligible patients comprised those with stage 3 or 4 disease of any age who had achieved complete response or very good partial response after induction and consolidation chemotherapy and surgery to the primary site.

Randomisation was carried out at the UKCCSG Data Centre. Method of randomisation, difference anticipated or numbers of patients needed are not given in detail. There was no stratification for risk factors.

This was a double blind placebo controlled trial. The dose of 0·75 mg/kg/day of cis-retinoic acid or masked placebo was given with milk or a fatty meal for a total of 4 years, or until disease recurrence. The primary endpoint was event free survival.

Outcome

One hundred and seventy-two patients were recruited on to the study. All received vincristine, carboplatin/cisplatin, etoposide and cyclophosphamide based regimens, with minor variations on the standard OPEC/OJEC regimen. Radiotherapy was not given routinely and high dose melphalan was recommended for children with stage 4 disease over the age of 1 year and stage 3 disease with MYCN amplification. Some patients received BCNU and VM-26 in addition to melphalan, and in a small number MIBG therapy was used.

High dose therapy was given to 126 patients. The median time to start cis-retinoic acid from diagnosis was 341 days. Eighty-eight patients were randomised to receive retinoic acid and 87 received placebo. Patients were well matched for age (under or over 1 year), complete response, very good partial response, UK centre versus non-UK centre, stage 3 disease and stage 4 disease.

Outcome

The 3 year event free survival for retinoic acid was 37% versus 42% for those on placebo. Adjusting for prognostic factors, such as age, abdominal primary and bone marrow metastases, did not change the lack of difference between the two arms. There was one death due to a second malignancy and one due to a cerebral haemorrhage following autologous bone marrow transplant.

Six patients relapsed before treatment started, within 2 months of randomisation. Four patients relapsed within 2 months of randomisation but had started treatment. A further 20 patients took treatment for less than 2 months from starting the first course, in 5 because of early relapse, and 15 were unable to take the capsules for a variety of reasons. Compliance with treatment assessed by parental reporting was a problem since the capsules were large and median age at randomisation was 3·5 years. Omitting all 30 patients, of whom 15 were taking retinoic acid and 15 placebo, there was still no difference in the outcome between the two randomised groups.

Toxicity

Treatment was discontinued because of presumed toxicity in 5 cases, one a recurrent skin problem and one bone pain, both on retinoic acid. Two children had eye symptoms, but were found to be on placebo. One who stopped medication because of slow blood count recovery was also on placebo.

Triglyceride and liver enzymes were monitored in 44 patients. They were normal in 35 and abnormal in 9.

Conclusion

It was concluded that this dose and schedule of retinoic acid did not significantly influence event free survival.

6

Hepatoblastoma and malignant germ-cell tumours

Commentary – Ross Pinkerton

Only a single randomised study has been published in full for both these tumour types. This reflects the perceived problem that it is very difficult, if not impossible, to run such trials in the rarer types of children's cancer. More recently, collaborative groups such as the CCG and SIOP have shown that if the question being addressed is perceived to be of sufficient importance and the infrastructure exists to support multicentre working, then these trials can be done.

Hepatoblastoma (HBL) and malignant germ cell tumours (MGCT) have a number of common features with regard to the questions that need to be addressed in their management. Both have subgroups in which the prognosis with current treatment strategies is good, namely localised HBL, where complete resection is feasible after non-intensive chemotherapy, and MGCT arising in the testis or ovary, where cure rate is high even with lung metastases. For these subgroups it is appropriate to determine whether chemotherapy with fewer early and late sequelae can maintain high cure rates. In contrast, those with non-localised HBL or extragonadal MGCT require more intensive treatment to try and improve outcome.

Hepatoblastoma

The CCG trial in HBL addressed the issue of whether doxorubicin with its attendant cardiotoxicity could be replaced by 5FU/vincristine. The conclusion appears to be that this is the case. Unfortunately, the size of the trial was rather small and it is difficult to separate out the different prognostic subgroups. The outcome in those with metastatic disease was poor in both groups and seems somewhat worse than that published in single arm studies by the German Society for Paediatric Oncology and Haematology and in the SIOPEL-1 study[1-4]. In SIOPEL-1 the small group of children with initially completely resected tumours had good outcome when given doxorubicin alone as adjuvant therapy. The SIOPEL-2 pilot study has suggested that cisplatin alone as pre-surgical therapy achieves tumour shrinkage and rates of operability comparable to cisplatin/doxorubicin (PLADO). The current randomised study SIOPEL-3 compares these two regimens in children with tumours that are localised to a single lobe, even if large. It is a matter of opinion whether the potential late sequelae of cisplatin alone i.e. hearing loss and nephrotoxicity, are necessarily more desirable than a comparatively low dose of doxorubicin, which given as a single agent can be infused over a 24 hour period with no concern about other acute morbidity such as oral mucositis. Future studies in this good prognosis group could compare the parent compound with either of the less toxic analogues – carboplatin and one of the liposomal anthracyclines.

In the poorer prognosis group the possible benefit from dose intensification is being addressed by the SIOP group in a single arm study of "super PLADO" in which carboplatin is combined with cisplatin and doxorubicin. Unfortunately, it was concluded that insufficient numbers could be recruited to carry out a randomised comparison with standard PLADO and this part of SIOPEL-2 can only be considered an extended pilot study from which no firm conclusion will be drawn.

To date, no useful biological prognostic marker has been identified on which to stratify treatment, other than the pattern of α-fetoprotein (αFP) decline, which has been shown to predict outcome.

Chemoembolisation has been recently used to try to improve resectability in tumours where standard approaches have failed. This technique should be evaluated further as failure to achieve complete resection remains the main cause of recurrent disease.

Malignant germ cell tumours

The introduction of cisplatin based treatment regimens in paediatric MGCT based on effectiveness in adults with testicular tumours had a dramatic effect on outcome[5-8], with outcome superior to the standard VAC protocol. It is less clear whether regimens with higher doses of both cyclophosphamide or ifosfamide and

doxorubicin would have achieved the same result. Subsequently PVB (cisplatin, vinblastine, bleomycin) or BEP (bleomycin, etoposide, cisplatin) regimens became part of standard protocols, although many groups continued to combine these drugs with VACA (vincristine, actinomycin D, doxorubicin, cyclophosphamide) based combinations.

The only randomised study in paediatric MGCT that has been completed is the CCG-8882/POG-9049 trial but this is available only in abstract form or subgroup analysis[9,10]. It did not take account of the good prognosis of those with gonadal tumours and evaluated dose escalation across all groups. This introduced the high dose cisplatin Einhorn regimen, which had been shown to have some efficacy in relapsed or refractory testicular teratoma. It was clear from earlier studies in metastatic neuroblastoma that this combination would have significant ototoxicity and renal toxicity, which one could argue would not be acceptable in children with already highly curable disease. The results of this study appear to show a small advantage to the high dose regimen but it is difficult to be clear in what specific subgroups the significant toxicity is justified.

The UKCCSG has taken the opposite approach and has introduced carboplatin in the JEB regimen to reduce cisplatin toxicity[11]. No alkylating agent or anthracycline is given. Although this has never been evaluated in a randomised trial, the results have been encouraging. It appears important that a relatively high dose of carboplatin (500–600 mg/m^2) is used, as poorer results have been reported by the French SFOP group using lower doses than the GFR formula base dose method achieves in the UK protocol.

Randomised trials in adults with good risk testicular teratoma have shown that cisplatin based chemotherapy provides a small but significant relapse free advantage. Some of these studies have again used a smaller dose of carboplatin than the UKCCSG. It would seem appropriate that the European and American groups consider a randomised trial to assess the role of carboplatin as there is no doubt about the significant hearing loss seen with cisplatin, particularly in this very young age group. There is also the possibility that cisplatin exacerbates bleomycin lung toxicity. The SIOP group has recently reached a consensus of risk grouping in MGCT which could be applied in such a study. For the poorer risk groups, such as those with extragonadal primaries and high αFP level, the addition of IVAd (ifosfamide, vincristine, doxorubicin) to PVB requires evaluation.

High dose chemotherapy with stem cell rescue has been introduced in relapse protocols following practice in adults. To date no adult study has shown significant benefit, although a number are under way. Whilst the number of children with relapsed MGCT is relatively small, the high number of failures following second line therapy means that in a combined international study this issue could be addressed.

References

1   Pritchard J, Brown J, Shafford E, Perilongo G, Brock P, Dicks-Mireaux C, Keeling J, Phillips A, Vos A, Plaschkes J. Cisplatin, doxorubicin and delayed surgery for childhood hepatoblastoma: a successful approach – results of the first prospective study of the International Society of Pediatric Oncology. *J Clin Oncol* 2000;**18**: 3819–28.

2   Perilongo G, Brown J, Shafford E, Brock P, DeCamargo B, Keeling JW, Vos A, Philips A, Pritchard J, Plaschkes J. Hepatoblastoma presenting with lung metastases: treatment results of the first cooperative, prospective study of the International Society of Paediatric Oncology on childhood liver tumours. *Cancer* 2000;**89**:1845–53.

3   Von Schweinitz D, Byrd DJ, Hecker H, Weinel P, Bode U, Burger D, Erttmann R, Harms D, Mildenberger H. Efficiency and toxicity of ifosfamide, cisplatin and doxorubicin in the treatment of childhood hepatoblastoma. Study Committee of the Cooperative Paediatric Liver Tumour Study HB89 of the German Society for Paediatric Oncology and Haematology. *Eur J Cancer* 1997;**33**:1243–9.

4   Shafford EA, Pritchard J. Hepatoblastoma – a bit of a success story? *Eur J Cancer* 1994;**30**:1050–1.

5   Pinkerton CR, Pritchard J, Spitz L. High complete response rate in children with advanced germ cell tumours using cisplatin-containing combination chemotherapy. *J Clin Oncol* 1986;**4**:194–9.

6   Ablin AR, Krailo MD, Ramsay NK, Malogolowkin MH, Isaacs H, Raney RB, Adkins J, Hays DM, Benjamin DR, Grosfeld JL et al. Results of treatment of malignant germ cell tumors in 93 children: a report from the Children's Cancer Study Group. *J Clin Oncol* 1991;**9**:1782–92.

7   Schneider DT, Calaminus G, Reinhard H, Gutjahr P, Kremens B, Harms D, Gobel U. Primary mediastinal germ cell tumors in children and adolescents: results of the German cooperative protocols MAKEI 83/86, 89 and 96. *J Clin Oncol* 2000;**18**:832–9.

8   Gobel U, Schneider DT, Calaminus G, Haas RJ, Schmidt P, Harms D. Germ-cell tumors in childhood and adolescence. GPOH MAKEI and the MAHO study groups. *Ann Oncol* 2000;**11**:263–71.

9   Rescorla F, Billmire D, Stolar C, Vinocur C, Colombani P, Cullen J, Giller R, Cushing B, Lauer S, Davis M, Hawkins E, Shuster J, Krailo M. The effect of cisplatin dose and surgical resection in children with malignant germ cell tumours at the sacrococcygeal region: a Paediatric Intergroup trial (POG 9049/CCG 8882). *J Pediatr Surg* 2001;**36**:12–17.

10 Billmire D, Vincur C, Rescorla F, Columbani P, Cushing B, Hawkins E, London WB, Giller R, Lauer S. Malignant mediastinal germ cell tumours: an Intergroup study. *J Pediatr Surg* 2001;**36**:18–24.

11 Mann JR, Raafat F, Robinson K, Imeson J, Gornall P, Sokal M, Gray E, McKeever P, Hale J, Bailey S, Oakhill A. The United Kingdom Children's Cancer Study Group's second germ cell tumour study: carboplatin, etoposide and bleomycin are effective treatment for children with malignant extracranial germ cell tumours, with acceptable toxicity. *J Clin Oncol* 2000;**18**:3809–818.

Studies

Study 1

Ortega JA, Douglass EC, Feusner JH, Reynolds M, Quinn JJ, Finegold MJ, Haas JE, King DR, Liu-Mares W, Sensel MG, Drailo MD. Randomized comparison of cisplatin/vincristine/fluorouracil and cisplatin/continuous infusion doxorubicin for treatment of pediatric hepatoblastoma: a report from the Children's Cancer Group and the Pediatric Oncology Group.
J Clin Oncol 2000;**18**:2665–75.

This study was carried out by the combined Pediatric Oncology Group and Children's Cancer Group (POG-8945, CCG-8881) between 1989 and 1992.

Objectives

The study was designed to determine whether the potentially more toxic combination of cisplatin/ doxorubicin was more effective than cisplatin/vincristine/5-FU in hepatic cancers. Data from hepatoblastoma only are presented here.

Details of the study

Eligibility included all those under 21 years with untreated hepatoblastoma or hepatocellular carcinoma. There was central pathology review. Normal creatinine clearance or GFR and normal cardiac function on echocardiogram or scan were required.

Patients were randomised immediately after surgery and staging and were stratified by stage. No other details of randomisation method are given.

Patients with stage I favourable histology, defined as pure fetal histology with minimal mitoses, were excluded from randomisation and electively given four doses of doxorubicin. It was calculated that 144 patients would need to be randomised to detect a 1·8-fold reduction in event risk between the two treatment arms, using a two-sided test with 80% power at the 0·05 level. This would require a 3 year accrual with an 18 month interim analysis that required a significant difference, p = 0·005, to close prematurely.

Stage I was complete resection with clear margins; stage II gross total resection with microscopic residue; stage III gross resection with nodal involvement or tumour spill or incomplete resection with gross residual intrahepatic disease; stage IV metastatic disease with either complete or incomplete resection.

Regimen A comprised cisplatin 90 mg/m^2 infused over 6 hours, vincristine 1·5 mg/m^2, and 5-FU 600 mg/m^2. Regimen B was also cisplatin 90 mg/m^2, with doxorubicin (Adriamycin) 60 mg/m^2 continuous infusion over 72 hours. All patients received four cycles of either regimen and then subsequent treatment depended on the response and surgical feasibility (see Figure 6.1).

Initial chemotherapy was delayed 2 weeks if more than 50% of the liver was resected. The cycles were given 3-weekly if the count had recovered to neutrophils ≥ 1000 cells/µl and

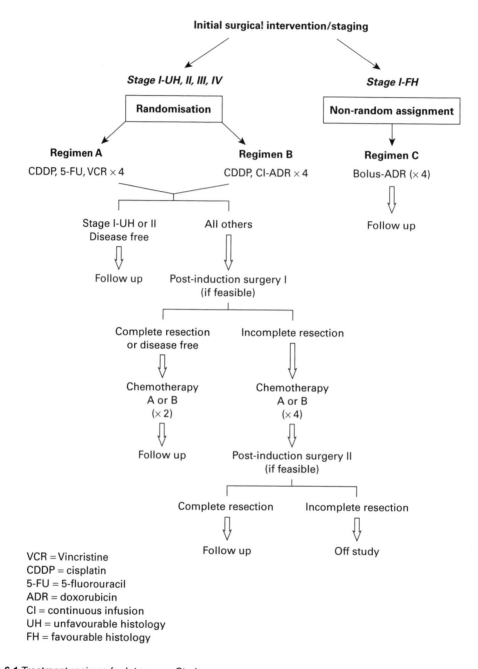

VCR = Vincristine
CDDP = cisplatin
5-FU = 5-fluorouracil
ADR = doxorubicin
CI = continuous infusion
UH = unfavourable histology
FH = favourable histology

Figure 6.1 Treatment regimen for Intergroup Study

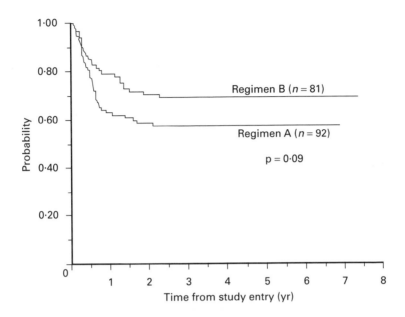

Figure 6.2 Event free survival for children with hepatoblastoma according to regimen

platelets ≥ 100 000 cells/μl. The doxorubicin dose was modified in relation to liver function tests, as was the dose of cisplatin in relation to GFR. Doses were also reduced if there was a delay in the time of chemotherapy.

The primary outcome measure was event free survival (EFS).

Outcome

Two hundred and forty-two patients were entered. One patient, who had stage I disease with unfavourable histology, was incorrectly given regimen C, i.e. doxorubicin alone, and was excluded. Ten patients were excluded owing to incorrect pathological diagnoses and 3 further patients were excluded due to local review board issues or prior chemotherapy. Two hundred and twenty-eight patients remained, of whom

182 had hepatoblastoma and 46 hepatocellular carcinoma; 9 received regimen C. Of the remaining 173 patients, 43 were classed as stage I unfavourable histology, 83 stage III and 40 stage IV. Ninety-two were randomised to regimen A and 81 to regimen B.

Five year EFS was 57% (± SD 5%), overall survival (OS) 69% (± 5%). For regimen B, EFS 69% (± 5%), OS 72% (± 5%), $p = 0.09$ (see Figure 6.2). Although no statistical difference was observed in EFS, the disease progression rate at 4 years was significantly higher for regimen A (39%) compared to regimen B (23%) ($p = 0.02$).

Toxicity

The toxicity for regimen B was significantly worse with regard to myelosuppression, stomatitis, cardiac toxicity and renal toxicity. Significantly more total parenteral nutrition was required and the hospital stay was longer (median 46 *v* 20 days). Rates of infection were, however, nodifferent. There were 3 toxic deaths on regimen A and 5 toxic deaths on regimen B.

Conclusion

Although the data indicate potential improved efficacy to the cisplatin/doxorubicin regimen, it was concluded that there was no advantage to this protocol when the enhanced toxicity was taken into consideration.

7

Medulloblastoma

Commentary – Joann Ater and Archie Bleyer

Medulloblastoma is one of the more common brain tumours in childhood, comprising about 20% of central nervous system tumours in children less than 21 years old. While it does occur in adults, the peak incidence is in early childhood. Despite the frequency, it is still a relatively rare tumour for performing clinical trials. Only approximately 300 cases of medulloblastoma are diagnosed in the United States each year.

In its narrowest definition, it is a highly malignant neoplasm that originates in the vermis of the cerebellum and roof of the IVth ventricle and because of its contiguity with the piaglia frequently enters the cerebrospinal fluid (CSF) and metastasises to all regions of the CSF space. In many clinical trials, the *supratentorial* primitive neuroectodermal tumor (PNET) has been included because of its similar microscopic appearance. Indeed, at one time Dr Rorke proposed that medulloblastoma and supratentorial PNET were the same tumour, just in different locations[1]. However, more information has evolved based on the cytogenetic abnormalities present in medulloblastoma and not present in supratentorial PNETs (gain of chromosome 17q)[2]. Hence, whether supratentorial PNETs are included in a trial, and if so whether or not a

randomised trial includes stratification of this subset, is important.

The treatment of medulloblastoma in children has clearly improved over the past 10–15 years, albeit many patients still succumb to the disease, and in most patients therapy-related morbidity is not acceptable. The advancement is due to multiple factors, including improvements in diagnostic imaging, biopsy techniques, pathology, surgery, anaesthesia, radiotherapy, chemotherapy and supportive care. Considerable diagnostic, prognostic and therapeutic information has been gained from phase II clinical trials and randomised phase III trials presented in this chapter.

Prognostic factors

Advancement in the care of children with medulloblastoma was also made with the identification of prognostic factors to help identify those patients who might best benefit from chemotherapy. In 1985 a group met in Niagara, NY and established criteria and definitions for response and relapse in children with brain tumours[3]. This group proposed using the Chang staging system for medulloblastoma, first proposed by Dr Chang is 1969. The Chang staging system utilised both T (tumour) staging, which quantified the size and extent of tumour at diagnosis, and

M (metastatic) staging, which identified extent of CNS and systemic metastases. White this system, those children with metastatic medulloblastoma (M1–4) or high T stage (T3 and T4) had a worse survival with radiotherapy.

Surgery

The role of surgery is undeniable, not only for therapeutic benefit but also in establishing the correct diagnosis and stage. Moreover, the beneficial effects of both radiotherapy and chemotherapy are largely dependent, when possible, on surgical debulking of disease to enable maximum benefit from the other treatment modality(ies). What seems remarkable is how long it took to demonstrate that prognosis after surgery is dependent on the degree of surgical resection, an observation that had been made years earlier in other types of brain tumours, particularly the gliomas. The difficulty in demonstrating the benefit of surgery on ultimate survival was probably due to the more difficult surgery in patients of younger age and in a location near the brain stem, and the propensity of CSF dissemination and a higher proportion of patients with metastases at diagnosis. Also, the conundrum of whether the improved prognosis is due to the extent of surgical resection *per se* or to the intrinsic nature of the tumour that makes it more resectable and is thereby independent of the operative intervention may apply more to medulloblastoma than to other brain tumours. None the less, the recent phase III trials provide at least circumstantial evidence that the completeness of the primary surgery is of benefit and should be accomplished without increasing the rate or intra- or postoperative mortality or unacceptable morbidity.

Radiotherapy

As early as 1926 Bailey and Cushing recognised that, following surgery alone, medulloblastoma was uniformly fatal within a year unless craniospinal radiation was applied postoperatively. Radiotherapy of the entire neuroaxis (craniospinal), as opposed to cranial alone, was recognised as important because of the contiguity of the site of origin of most medulloblastomas with the CSF space and the high propensity for meningeal dissemination, including the spinal compartment. In 1930, Bailey and Cushing reported that they were able to improve the median survival from 12 months with surgery alone, to 34 months with surgery followed by postoperative craniospinal radiation.

Further progress was made over the next two decades with improvements and refinements in radiotherapy equipment and techniques. Also it was found that there was a definite dose relationship between the radiation dose and the chance of curing the child. During the 1970s and early 1980s multiple radiotherapists reported over 70% 5 year survival rates for children with medulloblastoma with megavoltage radiation to > 54 Gy to the posterior fossa and 35 Gy to the brain and spine. The standard dose based on these related non-randomised studies became 35 Gy to the brain and spine with a boost to the entire posterior fossa resulting in a total of 54–55 Gy. The efficacy of this treatment with radiation mode has been reviewed in numerous single-institution studies with slightly variable results. However, these multiple studies reported similar 5 year survival rates ranging from 56% to 78% with cranial spinal radiation and posterior fossa boost to at least 54 Gy[4]. This improvement with radiation from 0 to 70% 5 year survival rate was so dramatic that no randomised study is necessary to prove the efficacy of radiotherapy.

The current issue is how to limit the amount of radiotherapy necessary and, if possible, identify subsets of patients, who will undoubtedly be relatively small in number, in whom radiotherapy is not necessary. The goal of the latter is paramount in very young children, in whom radiotherapy is not only more morbid but may of itself cause cancer[5]. From 50 years of study of nuclear bomb survivors, it is now known that the lifetime risk of cancer associated with radiation exposure is 10 times greater in children than it is in adults, and that this relative risk is similar at both low and high exposures of ionising radiotherapy[6].

Chemotherapy

Prior to 1985 there was no definitive evidence that chemotherapy could be of benefit in medulloblastoma, other than for the treatment of recurrence. The subsequent evidence for activity is irrefutable, but the overall contribution of chemotherapy to cure of children with medulloblastoma remains relatively modest compared to the strides that were made before 1980 with application of improvements in radiotherapy and surgery. Documentation of the value of chemotherapy for recurrent medulloblastoma was accumulated over many years, from the outcome of small groups of patients with recurrent disease.

Friedman and Oakes summarised the active agents in medulloblastoma in all studies prior to 1987 in a review[7]. These studies of recurrent disease revealed that there were a number of active agents that could produce responses. Prior to the CT scan and MRI era, judgement of

response was more difficult. In addition, response criteria were not uniform throughout these studies. Some recorded objective shrinkage of tumour, while others were called a response if the patient improved clinically. Despite these flaws a number of agents that were identified as being useful are still utilised for medulloblastoma. These included cisplatin, cyclophosphamide, methotrexate, procarbazine, VP-16 and various combinations, including procarbazine, CCNU and vincristine (PCV); vincristine, methotrexate and BCNU; nitrogen mustard, vincristine, procarbazine and prednisone (MOPP); "8-in-1" chemotherapy; and vincristine and cyclophosphamide. However, clinical trials were required over the next several years to identify the benefit of adjuvant chemotherapy for medulloblastoma. Most of the studies summarised in this chapter were formulated from this effort.

Randomised clinical trials

The first randomised trial in medulloblastoma was conducted by the Southwest Oncology Study Group and is described under Study 9 in this chapter. In this study van Eys et al evaluated the efficacy of the addition of vincristine (intravenous) and intrathecal hydrocortisone and methotrexate compared to radiation therapy alone. The doses of radiation given were 50 Gy to the primary site and 35 Gy whole brain and spine. Those patients under 3 years of age received 45 Gy to the posterior fossa. There were 63 patients entered. Fourteen were excluded because of either an incorrect diagnosis or incomplete follow-up data. Of the 44 evaluable patients, nine had inadequate data or refused to be randomised. Of the remaining 34 children, 8 of the 16 who received chemotherapy died, and

5 of the 18 who did not receive chemotherapy died, therefore showing no benefit to this chemotherapy. There were 2 toxic deaths and it was identified that the risk of administering intrathecal methotrexate in children with potential for meningeal disease – as further defined in other reports, methotrexate, IT/IV – especially following craniospinal radiation, has some risk of developing leukoencephalopathy. This risk was defined to be proportional to the number of inciting modalities used (radiotherapy + IV methotrexate + IT methotrexate worse than two of these, and any pair worse than a single modality), the total dose of the modalities, and if radiotherapy is used, the sequence or the modalities relative to the radiotherapy (worse if radiotherapy preceded the chemotherapy)[8–11]. However, based on the randomised results of the study, there was no benefit to delivering the chemotherapy. Possibly, the toxic death and small number of patients obscured the small benefit of vincristine.

The next randomised trials were conducted simultaneously by cooperative groups in Europe (International Society of Paediatric Oncology, SIOP) and the United States (Children's Cancer Group, CCG). Both randomised newly diagnosed patients between craniospinal radiation alone versus craniospinal radiation with chemotherapy and hence were adjuvant chemotherapy trials. The CCG study, Study 4 in this chapter, was performed from 1975 to 1981 and during the latter years of the trial was joined by the Radiation Therapy Oncology Group, RTOG. In this trial, vincristine, prednisone and CCNU constituted the adjuvant chemotherapy. The patients were randomised following surgery and, unlike previous studies, both M stage and T stage were identified for these patients and the randomisation was stratified by these factors. Radiation

doses were similar in previous studies. Of 233 patients with medulloblastoma, 179 were randomised, 88 to chemotherapy and radiotherapy and 91 to radiotherapy alone. Based on the prospective goal of the study the difference was not significant. Five year event free survival was 57% for chemotherapy and 52% for the control group. However, subset analysis showed that patients with a worse prognosis, based on M stage and T stage, had a statistically better outcome. Patients with M1, M2, M3, T3 and T4 disease had a 46% 5 year event free survival on chemotherapy regimen in contrast to no survivors on the radiotherapy arm ($p > 0.06$). The reciprocal observation, of course, showed no benefit of the chemotherapy for patients with no evidence for metastases (M0) and small tumors (T1, T2).

The SIOP trial (Study 1) was a randomised study carried out between 1975 and 1979. This study evaluated the role of chemotherapy added to the standard cranial spinal radiation. The eligibility allowed patients under 16 years of age with medulloblastoma and anaplastic ependymoma, either infratentorial or supratentorial. The staging requirements were based on T staging and assessment of preoperative tumour volume and extension as well as brainstem involvement. The M staging was apparently an exclusion criterion if metastatic disease was detected, but it was unclear how many patients actually had metastatic work ups that by current standards would have included lumbar puncture (LP), cerebrospinal fluid (CSF) examinations with cytology and myelography. During the time period of this study MRI was not yet available and accuracy of staging must be viewed with that in mind. Evaluating the extent of brainstem involvement is difficult even with contrast enhanced MRI and extremely difficult based on CT scans.

However, even with this limitation, the group is large enough that the randomisation should have been able to eliminate the bias in the final results related to the metastatic patients entered on this study incorrectly. However, the issue of accuracy of staging may have influenced the subgroup analysis.

Despite this concern, the differences observed in the control group ($n = 72$) versus the T3–4 ($n = 91$) disease group were extremely significant with 10 year event free survival 55% with chemotherapy, versus 25% with radiation alone ($p < 0.005$). Similarly for patients with incomplete resection, those who received chemotherapy had a 5 year EFS rate of 55% versus 36% for radiation alone ($p < 0.01$). As in the CCG study of similar time period (Study 4), those patients that would now be considered good or average risk with T1–2 disease and complete resection had no significant benefit from the CCNU and vincristine.

Despite the limitations and concerns, when this study is combined with others it appears to support the conclusion that chemotherapy is of benefit to children with medulloblastoma, especially those that have higher risk disease than average. This study's conclusion was reached for T stage, because M stage had to be M0 or was ineligible for this study. While a large number of patients were able to be recruited, the study closed prematurely due to the observation that there was a significance difference of survival at 2 years. Subsequently, the difference disappeared because the follow-up was inadequate to draw a conclusion about 5 year survival at that point.

The SIOP trial differed from the CCG trial in two basic ways. First, the chemotherapy was vincristine and CCNU and excluded prednisone. Second, the outcome of all patients entered, including the better prognosis patients, resulted in a statistically significant advantage for chemotherapy, at least in the initial reports. The trial showed a greater benefit in the worse prognosis patients, and a minimal benefit in the best prognosis patients, but the overall difference was greater than in the CCG–RTOG trial. This raised the question of whether prednisone was deleterious, since it was used in the trial with less of a beneficial outcome. It was subsequently shown that steroids might decrease the brain capillary permeability to chemotherapy agents, along with the general steroid effect of reducing cerebral oedema. Hence, in retrospect, the transatlantic difference in the simultaneous cooperative group trials may indeed have been due to adverse effects of the steroid.

A similar study (Study 6) was carried out by the Pediatric Oncology Group and reported in 1984. This early study was conducted in the current patients and randomised between MOPP chemotherapy versus the same regimen without nitrogen mustard (OPP) in children with recurrent brain tumours. The main outcome measure was clinical response. This was actually a randomised response study, and not a two-phase trial, therefore the results are not as conclusive. The numbers are very small and demonstrated 4 out of 9 patients with medulloblastoma had complete or partial response after MOPP, and 3 of 12 receiving OPP had partial response. It was concluded that MOPP produced more responses but with the very small numbers, this is hardly a justifiable conclusion.

A follow-up randomised study performed by the Pediatric Oncology Group tested MOPP adjuvant chemotherapy following radiation for newly diagnosed children with medulloblastoma. This is Study 3 in this chapter, reported by Kushner *et al* for the Pediatric Oncology Group, conducted between 1979 and 1986. This trial addressed the issue of adjuvant MOPP chemotherapy following radiation. The use of MOPP was supported by results from Study 6 comparing MOPP to OPP. Progression-free survival was the main outcome measure. Again, this early study did not apply stringent staging criteria and the M stage and other prognostic factors were not identified in these patients. After surgery patients were randomised between standard radiation and radiation plus chemotherapy. The radiation varied from 35 to 40 Gy to the cranial spinal access with the posterior fossa boost to 54 Gy, and the children were given lower doses. Over this 7 year period the study accrued only 78 patients, with 7 refusing randomisation. The 5 year event free survival was 68% with MOPP and 57% with radiation alone. However, despite this difference, the p value was only 0·18. Subgroup analysis was attempted only with the significant difference in the event free survival in children over 5 years old where the event free survival was 77% versus 52% for radiation alone (p = 0·05). There were similar differences for every subgroup, including extent of resection, T1–2 stage, and T3 stage with superior survival with MOPP. Again, the number of patients was really insufficient to reach a statistically significant conclusion and therefore, although there is a suggestion that MOPP may be useful in chemotherapy, the study does not definitively prove this.

Based on these early studies, Study 5 in this chapter, reported by Seltzer *et al* for the Children's Cancer Group, was conducted between 1986 and 1992. This study compared chemotherapy with an 8-in-1 regimen to adjuvant vincristine, CCNU and prednisone in medulloblastoma. Patients up to age 21 were eligible in high risk grouping and identified as M1–4 disease and T3B–T4. Again, the study required detailed investigations including post-operative myelograms, CTs or MRIs, CSF cytology and bone marrow evaluations.

Following surgery and staging all patients received radiotherapy. The vincristine, CCNU, prednisone regimen included weekly vincristine during radiation. The 8-in-1-chemotherapy arm included two cycles of chemotherapy prior to radiation and no vincristine during radiation. Radiotherapy doses were standard as reported in similar trials with 54 Gy to the posterior fossa and 36 Gy to the spine. The study included 155 medulloblastoma and 45 supratentorial PNET. Only patients considered high risk by M or T staging were allowed on the study. The results showed that progression free survival at 5 years was 53% for vincristine, CCNU and prednisone and 45% for the 8-in-1 regimen (p < 0·006). In addition, the 8-in-1 regimen was more toxic, with complications related to gastrointestinal, electrolytes and renal toxicity.

Following the results of this study, many have attempted to analyse the reasons for the significantly lower survival rate with the 8-in-1. Eight-in-1 chemotherapy includes vincristine, CCNU and prednisone given at similar dose intervals. It adds other chemotherapeutic agents to the regimen. The only differences between the two regimens other than the additional agents were that there was an approximate 6 week delay in beginning radiotherapy on the 8-in-1 arm and, additionally, possible delays in therapy because of toxicity. Also, one group did not receive weekly vincristine during radiation. Therefore, concern has been expressed that although the study provided other agents, these agents were not delivered in as dose intensive a manner as the more standard vincristine, CCNU. However, for high risk patients this study provides additional evidence that chemotherapy with vincristine, CCNU and prednisone is of benefit – not only compared to radiation alone, as shown in the previous study with subgroup analysis, but also when compared to another chemotherapy regimen.

SIOP also initiated a second randomised trial of chemotherapy in medulloblastoma, which is reported by Bailey *et al* and evaluated as Study 2 in this chapter. This study was carried out between 1984 and 1989 as collaboration between SIOP and the German Society of Paediatric Oncology. Whereas the SIOP-I study was a direct, uncomplicated clinical study design, this study attempted both to address the role of chemo-therapy as well as to evaluate the efficacy of radiation in low risk patients. Unlike the first study, the SIOP-II study attempted to divide the patients into two risk groups, again primarily utili-sing T staging. The low risk group was defined as those with total resection or only microscopic residual disease and neither brainstem involve-ment nor metastases. Again, however, the CSF cytology, CT and MRI imaging of the spine were not mandatory so the number of patients entered on the study without complete staging is unclear (refer to the detailed discussion of the study in this chapter).

There were many logistical difficulties in this study, some of which were directly related to the lack of complete staging that allowed "low risk" patients to be entered and randomised to lower dose cranial spinal radiation without complete end staging. In the low risk group only 132 of 229 had adequate imaging and proven negative CSF cytology. However, in the low risk group

event free survival was 55% for reduced dose radiation, 68% with standard dose radiation. Probably the most useful information derived from this study was the analysis of low and high risk grouped together with the therapy received. The most significant finding when adjusting for age and T staging was that there was a direct relation between radiation and chemotherapy. The negative effect on survival was associated with chemotherapy prior to radiation when the radiation dose was reduced. This was significant at $p < 0.005$. Both these facts suggested that the results were inferior when the radiation dose was reduced to 25 Gy to the cranial spinal axis, both with and without chemotherapy.

Although this study had many flaws, it raised concerns about reducing the dose of cranial spinal radiation in children with medullo-blastoma. This must, of course, be taken into context with the type of chemotherapy, which was of relatively low dose intensity. Despite these results, further studies have been imple-mented with different types of more aggressive chemotherapy to reduce the dose of cranial spinal radiation. This effort is due to the very real risk of long term deficits produced by the radia-tion to the cranial spinal axis. There have been a number of studies that indicate that 30–35 Gy to the whole brain can produce deficiencies, including growth hormone, thyroid deficiencies and, more significantly, intellectual deficit, espe-cially in children less than 7 years old.

The goal of most therapeutic trials in brain tumours is not only to cure the child, but also to provide a meaningful quality of life. This is of paramount concern. These concerns explain the continued study with the hope of providing therapy with reduced dose cranial spinal radiation. In fact, the recently completed study conducted by the Children's Oncology Group for average risk medulloblastoma included much more aggressive post-radiation chemotherapy given after 24 Gy to the cranial spinal axis. This same issue was explored in Study 7 in this chapter, reported by Deutsche *et al* for the combined Children's Cancer Group and Pediatric Oncology Group. This study was conducted from 1986 to 1990 and randomised good risk patients between full and reduced dose cranial radiation. Unlike the European studies, stringent staging was a requirement for study entry. This staging included myelography, MRI, CSF cytology, bone marrow examination and bone scan. The good risk group was required to have posterior fossa tumours that were T1–2 with more than 50% resection and less than 1·5 ml of residual tumour. They also could have no evidence of metastases. The difference of the relapse rate between the two arms of therapy was most significant when recurrences outside the posterior fossa were considered, with 7 out of 60 relapses in the low dose group versus 0 out of 34 in the full dose group (p < 0·004). Based on these results, the study was closed relatively early with a small number of patients entered. Follow up of the patients entered on this study was continued because the difference may become less significant as time passes.

The correct timing of radiotherapy and chemotherapy was investigated in Study 10, reported by Kortmann *et al* for the German GPOH group in 2000. This study conducted between 1991 and 1997 compared pre- and post-radiotherapy chemotherapy with chemotherapy given after radiotherapy. The chemotherapy used following radiotherapy was a regimen of CCNU, vincristine and cisplatin, previously reported by Packer *et al*[12]. The "sandwich" regimen did not improve survival for any group.

For average risk patients the 3 year progression free survival was 65% for the "sandwich" regimen and 78% for post-radiation chemotherapy (p < 0·03). For high risk patients, the pre-radiation chemotherapy also did not provide any benefit. This along with other single arm phase II studies, has shown that the survival in medulloblastoma was not improved with neoadjuvant or pre-radiation chemotherapy.

Important issues for future studies

Despite these randomised trials, several important questions concerning the best use of chemotherapy for treatment of medulloblastoma still need to be explored. And, as is usually the case in clinical trial outcomes, the results have also led to more questions being asked than were answered by the trials themselves. These include:

1   How can the promising newer imaging techniques of magnetic resonance imaging, helical CT, positron emission tomography and combinations thereof (e.g., CT–PET), be applied effectively or more effectively to evaluating the benefits, both quantitatively and qualitatively, and earlier, of chemotherapy?

2   Does reducing the dose of cranial–spinal irradiation with chemotherapy provide adequate survival rates and improve neuropsychological outcome, neuroendocrine outcome, physical and physiological growth, overall quality of life and survival?

3   Will a reduction in volume provided by conformal radiotherapy techniques be used to improve control of the tumour bed and simultaneously decrease the morbidity of normal tissue; to decrease late hearing loss without jeopardising tumor control; to enable on increase in the use of radiosensitising

chemotherapy that will offer better tumour control without increasing hearing loss and other adverse outcomes from local normal tissue effects?

4 Are there biological markers, such as c-trk, that can adequately predict a more favourable prognosis to allow treatment of some children with chemotherapy alone, especially young children?

5 How will genomics and protenomics alter the classification and treatment of medulloblastoma/PNET and related tumours? How will the gene array and multidimensional protein technologies revolutionise the field, as they most certainly will?

6 What is the role of other types of chemotherapy during radiotherapy?

7 Can disruption of the blood–brain barrier with osmotic or other techniques be successfully applied to the chemotherapy of medulloblastoma/PNET?

8 What is the optimal sequencing, combination and permutation of radiation therapy and chemotherapy?

9 Can neoadjuvant chemotherapy or radiotherapy, or both, be helpful to improve surgical resectability and postoperative function?

10 Will posterior fossa mutism and the related postoperative sequelae be understood and prevented?

11 Can intrathecal chemotherapy or biological agents provide prophylaxis to the cranial–spinal axis and replace some of the cranial–spinal radiation?

12 Will radioprotectors be clinically effective?

13 What targeted molecular therapies like the signal transduction inhibitor STI-571, which has dramatically altered the therapy of selected cancers, be discovered for the treatment of medulloblastoma/PNET and other brain tumours?

Overall, chemotherapy not only has a prominent, justified role in the treatment of medulloblastoma/PNET, but also there is every reason to believe that chemotherapy will be increasingly used, particularly in multimodal settings, over the coming decades.

References

1 Rorke LB. Experimental production of primitive neuro-ectodermal tumors and its relevance to human neuro-oncology. *Am J Pathol* 1994;**144**:444–8.

2 Russo C, Pellarin M, Tingby O, Bollen AW, Lamborn KR *et al*. Comparative genomic hybridization in patients with supratentorial and infratentorial primitive neuroectodermal tumors. *Cancer* 1999;**86**:331–9.

3 Zeltzer PM, Friedman HF, Norris DG, Ragab AH. Criteria and definitions for response and relapse in children with brain tumors. *Cancer* 1985;**56**:1824–1826.

4 Bloom HFG. Medulloblastoma in children: increasing survival rates and further prospects. *Int J Radiat Oncol Biol Phys* 1982;**8**:2023–7.

5 Pierce CA, Shimizu Y, Preston DL, Vaeth M, Mabuchi K. Studies of the mortality of atomic bomb survivors. Report 12, part I. Cancer:1950–90. *Radiat Res* 1996;**146**:1–27.

6 Brenner D, Elliston C, Hall E, Berdon W. Estimated risks of radiation-induced fatal cancer from pediatric CT. *Am J Roentgenol* 2001;**176**:289–96.

7 Friedmar HS, Oakes WJ. The chemotherapy of posterior fossa tumors in childhood. *J Neuro-Oncology* 1987;**5**:217–29.

8 Bleyer WA, Griffin TW. White matter necrosis, mineralizing microangiopathy, and intellectual abilities in survivors of childhood leukemia: associations with central nervous system irradiation and methotrexate therapy. In Gilbert HA, Kagen AR, eds. *Radiation damage to the nervous system*. New York: Raven Press, 1980, pp 115–74.

9 Bleyer WA. Neurologic sequelae of methotrexate and ionizing radiation. A new classification. *Cancer Treat Rep* 1981;**65**(Suppl 1):89–98.

10   Bleyer WA. Long-term adverse interactions between intrathecal and intravenous methotrexate and CNS irradiation. *Cancer Clin Trials* 1981;**4**(Suppl):33–4.

11   Bleyer WA. Chemoradiotherapy interactions in the central nervous system. *Med Pediat Oncol* 1998;Suppl 1:10–16.

12   Packer RJ, Sutton LN, Elterman R *et al*. Outcome of children with medulloblastoma treated with radiation, cisplatin, CCNU and vincristine chemotherapy. *J Neurosurg* 1994;**81**:690–8.

Studies

Study 1

Tait DM, Thornton Jones H, Bloom HJG, Lemerle V, Morris-Jones P.

Adjuvant chemotherapy for medulloblastoma: the first multi-centre control trial of the International Society of Paediatric Oncology (SIOP-I).

Eur J Cancer 1990;**26**:464–9.

The study was carried out between 1975 and 1979 by the SIOP Group (SIOP Study I).

Objectives
The study aimed to compare craniospinal radiation alone with radiation given simultaneously with vincristine and followed by a combination of vincristine and CCNU.

Details of the study

Patients under 16 with medulloblastoma or grade III or IV ependymoma were eligible. supra-and infratentorial tumours were included and patients were to have no detectable metastases. The latter was based on CSF examination, with or without myelography or CT scans. Radiation had to be given within one month of initial surgery.

The method of randomisation is not stated. Patients were stratified according to age, sex and extent of surgery. No details of anticipated number of patients or differences in outcome are provided.

Standard radiotherapy comprised 50–55 Gy to the primary tumour, with 35–45 Gy to the whole brain and 30–35 Gy to the spinal cord. Doses were reduced in children under 2 years of age.

They received 40–45 Gy to the posterior fossa with 30–35 Gy to the whole brian and 30 Gy to the cord.

In the chemotherapy arm, vincristine (VCR) was given weekly during the 8 weeks of radiotherapy, followed by a 4 week rest. CCNU and vincristine were given as a 3-weeks cycle every 6 weeks for a total of eight cycles (Figure 7.1)

Major outcome measures were overall survival and even free survival.

Outcome

A total of 286 patients with medulloblastoma were identified. Only patients who agreed to be randomised and were subsequently randomised are the subject of this report. No details about the overall patient population or reasons for refusal to be randomised are given.

Of the patients with medulloblastoma, 141 were randomised to receive adjuvant chemotherapy and 145 to receive radiotherapy alone. Twenty-six children were under the age of 2 years at the time of treatment. Chemotherapy details were available for review in 110 of 141 patients, as were radiotherapy details in 260 patients. Pathology was reviewed in 99% of cases: there were 286 medulloblastoma and 45 ependymoma. No case was excluded irrespective of the extent of protocol violation.

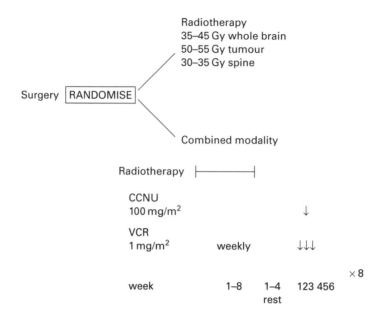

Figure 7.1 Study schema for SIOP 1. Reprinted from Tait DM *et al*, *Eur J Cancer* (full reference p 149) with permission from Elsevier Science.

At 2 years the event free survival was 71% in the chemotherapy arm, versus 53% in the radiotherapy alone (p = < 0·005). At subsequent follow ups there were more late relapses in the chemotherapy arm and as a result at 10 years EFS was 50% versus 46% (p = 0·07). Subgroup analysis suggested an advantage from chemotherapy. Of the 94 patients with brain stem involvement 48 were randomised to the chemotherapy arm and 46 to the control arm. At 10 years the EFS was 55% versus 25%, p = < 0·005. Similarly, the 91 patients with T3/T4 disease who received chemotherapy had better disease free survival than the 72 control patients (40% *v* 20%, *p* = < 0·002). For patients with incomplete resection the EFS with chemotherapy was 55% versus 36% for those with radiation alone, p = < 0·01. No difference was seen with chemotherapy for those without brian stem involvement, with T_1/T_2 disease of complete surgical resection.

Toxicity

There was one chemotherapy related death but this patient had received 2 years' maintenance chemotherapy rather than one. Two patients died of second malignancy but neither had received adjuvant chemotherapy.

Conclusion

A number of reservations were mentioned by the authors with regard to drawing firm conclusions from this study. The trial was closed before the anticipated accrual of 350 patients due to the large differences seen at 5 years, but follow up was probably too short. The multicentre international nature of the trial led to some problems with the staging of all patients. For example, of the 94 patients said to have brain stem involvement, 18 were

reported as having had total removal of tumour, which seems unlikely. Because of the duration of the study, towards the end recruitment fell off, in part because of the perception that the study chemotherapy was suboptimal compared to multiagent regimens.

Study 2

Bailey CC, Gneko A, Wellek S, Jones M, Round C, Brown J et al.

Prospective randomised trial of chemotherapy given before radiotherapy in childhood medulloblastoma. International Society of Paediatric Oncology (SIOP) and the (German) Society of Paediatric Oncology (GPO): SIOP-II.
Med Pediatr Oncol 1995;**25** 166–78.

The study was carried out between 1984 and 1989 by the SIOP and GOP groups.

Objectives

The study was designed to evaluate the possible benefit of adding vincristine, procarbazine and high dose methotrexate to radiotherapy and secondly to evaluate the efficacy of a reduced does of irradiation to whole neuraxis in low risk patients.

Details of the study

Patients were eligible if under 16 years of age and were divided into two risk groups. The high risk group were those with incomplete excision, brain stem involvement or metastases. It is unclear what method was used to define metastases, CSF cytology was recommended but was not mandatory and some, but not all, patients had CT or MR imaging.

The low risk group was defined as those with total resection or only microscopic residue and where there was neither brain stem involvement nor metastases.

Randomisation was done centrally by the GPO group in Mainz, using a minimising approach to avoid imbalance regarding age, sex and centre size.

Chemotherapy details are show in Figure 7.2 and consist of a "sandwich" regimen with pre-irradiation chemotherapy combining procarbazine, vincristine and methotrexate. A single course was given prior to radiotherapy and six further cycles at 42 day intervals, given after irradiation to all patients considered high risk. Radiotherapy was commenced within 28 days of surgery, or one week of the last dose of methotrexate: 35 Gy in 1·66 Gy fractions to the brain and spine with a boost of 20 Gy in 2·0 Gy fractions to the posterior fossa was compared with 25 Gy to the neuraxis and a 30 Gy boost. Some "variation" was allowed between centres, with dose schedules that were regarded as being biologically equivalent.

Patients with low risk could thus receive either no chemotherapy or pre-radiation chemotherapy, and one of two radiation schedules. High risk patients were randomised to receive pre-radiation chemotherapy or not, but all received standard dose irradiation and/or postoperative post-radiation chemotherapy.

It was calculated that 150 patients would need to be recruited per arm to detect an improvement in event free survival from 50% to 65% at 5 years, with 80% power at 5%. The level for the equivalence between the two doses of irradiation, $P_s - P_R$ was > 0·15 and a stopping rule was set at detecting a reduction in the EFS from 80% to 60% at one year.

Outcome

Four hundred and forty-six patients were registered. Of these, 60 were excluded by centres and 22 following randomisation. In 17 of these the diagnosis was incorrect. Three hundred and

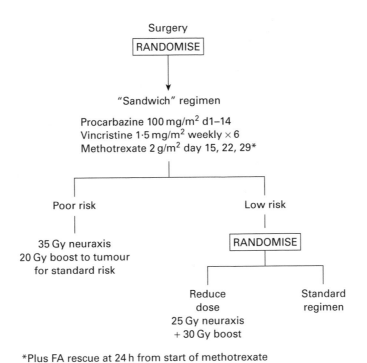

Surgery

RANDOMISE

"Sandwich" regimen

Procarbazine 100 mg/m^2 d1–14
Vincristine 1·5 mg/m^2 weekly × 6
Methotrexate 2 g/m^2 day 15, 22, 29*

Poor risk

35 Gy neuraxis
20 Gy boost to tumour
for standard risk

Low risk

RANDOMISE

Reduce
dose
25 Gy neuraxis
+ 30 Gy boost

Standard
regimen

*Plus FA rescue at 24 h from start of methotrexate

Figure 7.2 Study schema for SIOP II

sixty-four patients were analysed but 40 of these did not receive the treatment for which they were randomised. Overall event free survival was 58% for those receiving sandwich chemotherapy and 60% for those receiving radiation treatment alone. In the high risk groups this was 56% and 52% respectively. In the low risk group, only 132 of 229 had adequate imaging and 132 had proven negative CSF cytology. Of the 229 registered, 73 were not randomised. Of 74 patients receiving reduced dose radiotherapy event free survival was 55%, and of the 79 receiving standard dose the EFS a was 68% ($p = < 0.07$).

When the groups were combined, for those receiving standard dose radiotherapy (40 patients) the EFS was 60%; in those who received reduced dose irradiation treatment (36 patients) the EFS was 69%; in those receiving initial chemotherapy and standard dose irradiation treatment (38 patients) the EFS was 75%, whereas in those receiving chemotherapy and reduced irradiation (36 patients) the EFS was only 42%. Analysis of these data, adjusting for age, sex, centre size and TNM stage, showed a significant interaction between chemotherapy and radiotherapy ($p = < 0.005$), with a negative effect on survival associated by the insertion of chemotherapy prior to radiation where the radiation dose is reduced.

There were 12 non-tumour related deaths. Six were immediate postoperative deaths that occurred after randomisation had been carried out; 6 were treatment related – 1 methotrexate, 2 pneumonitis and 2 leukencephalopathy. One died of transfusion related AIDS.

Conclusion

As for SIOP-I, there was concern expressed by the authors about the quality of data and the central review showed a 30% discordance with regard to risk grouping and a 50% discordance regarding documentation of brain stem involvement. It was suggested that the dose of methotrexate was suboptimal and the folinic acid (FA) rescue given too early. Chemotherapy appea-red to be of no benefit to any subgroup and, moreover, appeared to have an adverse effect when given prior reduced dose radiation treatment.

Study 3

Krischer JP, Ragab AH, Kun L, Kim TH, Laurent JP, Boyett JM *et al.*
Nitrogen mustard, vincristine, procarbazine, and prednisone as adjuvant chemotherapy in the treatment of medulloblastoma.
J Neurosurg 1991;**74**:905–9.

The study was conducted between 1979 and 1986 by the Pediatric Oncology Group.

Objectives

The study addressed the question whether the addition of MOPP chemotherapy (mustine, vincristine, procarbazine and prednisolone) radiotherapy improved outcome when given after.

Details of the study

Patients aged 1–21 years were eligible. They had to have received no prior chemotherapy except corticosteroids and to have no evidence of metastases outside the central nervous system. The precise methods of spinal or CSF staging are unclear.

Randomisation method was not specified but was balanced by centre and patient age. Details of MOPP chemotherapy are given in Figure 7.3. Chemotherapy was given at 4-weekly intervals for a total of 12 courses, with a 25% reduction in dose if the white cell count fell below $3\cdot0 \times 10^9/1$.

Radiation dose to those over 3 years of age was 35–40 Gy, and less than 3 years 25–35·2 Gy (dose was increased 3 years into study). Boost to

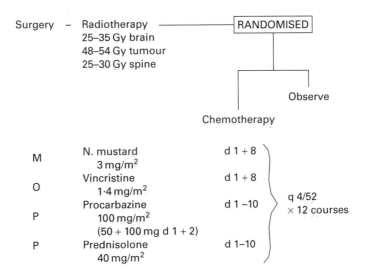

Figure 7.3 Study schema

posterior fossa consisted of 54–54·4 Gy in total, reduced to 48 Gy for patients under 3 years. Spinal irradiation consisted of 30 Gy, reduced to 25 Gy for patients less than 3 years.

Progression free survival was the main outcome measure. It was predicted that there would need to be 26 patients on each treatment arm to detect a 100% increase in the median time to progression, with 80% power at 5% significance level.

Outcome

Seventy-eight patients were eligible, of whom 7 refused randomisation.

Five year event free survival was at 68% for MOPP and 57% for radiation alone (p = 0·18). When subgroups such a race, sex extent of surgery and Change stage were separately analysed, event free survival appeared to favour irradiation plus MOPP, compared to irradiation alone, except for female patients (72% v 75% respectively) and in those under age 4 (51% v 67%). For children 5 years of age or older, event free survival was statistically superior with MOPP–EFS 77% v 52% (p = 0·05). For other subgroups the trend was in favour of MOPP (not statistically significant): for subtotal excision, 66% v 56%; total removal, 75% v 58%, Change $T_1 T_2$, 64% v 57%; T_3 72% v 61%.

Toxicity

There were no deaths associated with radiotherapy but one death occurred in the radiation alone arm from herpes zoster infection.

Conclusion

It was concluded that MOPP was beneficial in male patients over 5 years of age. The difference, however, was not apparent beyond 7 years follow up.

Study 4

Evans AE, Jerkin DT, Sposto R, Ortega JA, Wilson CB, Wara W *et al.*

Results of prospective randomised trial of radiation therapy with and without CCNU, vincristine, and prednisone.

J Neurosurg 1990;**72**:572–82.

The study was performed between 1975 and 1981 by the CCSG and the Radiation Therapy Oncology (RTOG) Group and evaluated the role of adding vincristine, prednisone and CCNU to standard surgery and radiotherapy.

Details of the study

Eligible patients were those aged 2–16 years with either medulloblastoma or infratentorial ependymomas with M_0 to M_3 disease. Method of spinal imaging was variable and documentation of CSF cytology was not mandatory.

Randomisation method is not specified but patients were stratified for T and M stage. Numbers required for a significant outcome measure are not specified.

The chemotherapy regimen is detailed in Figure 7.4. Vincristine (VCR) was given weekly for 8 weeks during radiotherapy (RT) and then eight 6-weekly cycles of post-radiation chemotherapy comprising vincristine, CCNU and prednisone (PDN).

The radiation dose was 35–40 Gy to the whole neuraxis, with 50–55 Gy to the tumour and 50 Gy to spinal metastases. Patients under 3 years of age received 5 Gy less. The extent of surgical removal was evaluated by the surgeon. There was no postoperative CT scanning.

Primary outcome measures were event free survival and overall survival.

Outcome

Three hundred and eleven patients were registered: 36 were not evaluable, 12 due to relapse or prior therapy, 10 due to supratentorial disease 10 due to incorrect pathology and 4 other reasons. One hundred and seventy-nine patients had medulloblastoma confirmed on central pathology review, plus 54 diagnosed on local pathology alone. Thirty-six patients with ependymoma were excluded from this analysis. Of the 233 patients with medulloblastoma, 179 were randomised, 88 to chemotherapy and radiotherapy, 91 to radiotherapy alone. A further 12 patients switched treatment after randomisation and 42 patients were electively treated without being randomised.

Of the 191 randomised, the 5 year event free survival (EFS) was 52% for radiation treatment alone and 57% with chemotherapy. For the whole group of 233 patients, both randomised and non-randomised, EFS for radiation alone was 50%, 59% for chemotherapy.

If T and M stage was considered, for M_0, T_1 and T_2, 26 had radiation plus chemotherapy and 41 radiation alone. There was no difference in 5 year EFS. By contrast, for patients with $M_1 - M_3$ or T_3/T_4 disease, 19 received chemotherapy and radiotherapy and 11 radiotherapy alone. There were no survivors in the radiotherapy alone arm, compared to 46% with chemotherapy (p = 0·006).

Toxicity

Chemotherapy was associated with four fatal infections.

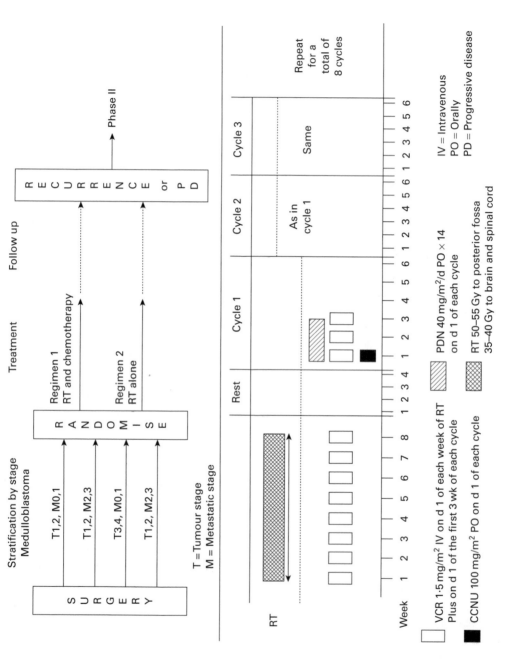

Figure 7.4 Study schema. Adapted and reproduced with permission from Evans AE *et al*, *J Neurosurg* (full reference p 157).

Conclusion

It was concluded that these data suggest a potential improvement for patients with advanced disease but not those with standard risk. Reservations were raised about the lack of standardisation in the initial staging and few had myelography or CSF, leading to a relatively small percentage of M_3 patients. When only randomised patients were considered in this subgroup all the numbers were smaller but there was still a significant difference in event free survival.

Study 5

Zeltzer PM, Boyett JM, Findlay JL, Albright L, Rorke LB, Milstein JM.

Metastasis stage, adjuvant treatment, and residual tumor are prognostic factors for medulloblastoma in children: conclusions from the Children's Cancer Group 921 randomised phase III study. *J Clin Oncol* 1999;**17**:832–45.

This study was performed between 1986 and 1992 by the CCG Group (CCG-921) and compared sandwich chemotherapy with the 8-in-1 regimen to adjuvant PCV in advanced medulloblastoma.

Details of the study

Patients between the age of 1·5 and 21 years were eligible. This high risk group was defined as having $M_1 - M_4$ and $T_{3b} - T_4$ (T_{3a} was included between 1986 and 1988). Patients with more than 1·5 ml of tumour residue following surgery on CT or MRI were also eligible. Detailed staging investigations were done and this was based on a combination of operative report, postoperative myelogram and CT or MRI, CSF cytology and bone marrow examination.

The randomisation method is not specified, nor where this was done. There was stratification by histology, site and T and M stage. It was calculated that a total of 204 patients would be required to detect an increase from 40% to 60% 4 year survival with 84% power.

The two chemotherapy regimens are detailed in Figure 7.5.

Following surgery, all patients received radiotherapy. They were randomly assigned to receive either weekly vincristine for 8 weeks during irradiation followed by eight cycles of VCP given every 6 weeks or two courses of 8-in-1 chemotherapy prior to radiotherapy, followed by eight courses of 8-in-1 at 6-weekly intervals. Overall, patients were well balanced for clinical features, however 24 patients in the PCV arm had M_3 disease, compared to 13 patients in the 8-in-1 arm.

Radiation doses were 54 Gy plus 36 Gy to the posterior fossa in patients over 3 years of age and 45 Gy plus 23·4 Gy in those between 105 and 209 years. The dose of 18 Gy was given to any spinal disease. There was central review of planning fields in all cases.

Main outcome measures were progression free survival and overall survival.

Outcome

A total of 212 patients were registered, of whom 9 were excluded due to inadequate data. Of the 203 remaining, 155 were registered as medulloblastoma and 48 as primitive neuroectodermal tumours. Pathology was reviewed centrally in 89% of cases After review, there were a total of 188 confirmed medulloblastomas, on whom survival analysis was based.

Progression free survival at 5 years was 63% ± 5% for PCV and 45% ± 5% for 8-in-1 chemotherapy (p = < 0.006).

Toxicity

The 8-in-1 regimen was more toxic with haematological complications, gastrointestinal, electrolyte and renal toxicity, and ototoxicity. Patients on 8-in-1 started radiotherapy on average 5 days later than planned.

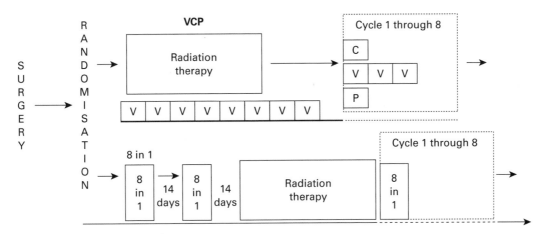

8-in-1 = Vincristine 1·5 mg/m^2
Methylprednisolone 300 mg/m^2 × 3
Lomustine (CCNU) 75 mg/m^2
Hydroxyurea 1·5 g/m^2
Procarbazine 75 mg/m^2
Cisplatin 60 mg/m^2
Cyclophosphamide 300 mg/m^2
Cytarabine 300 mg/m^2

PCV = Vincristine 1·5 mg/m^2 weekly during radiotherapy
then
Vincristine 1·5 mg/m^2 weekly × 3
Lomustine (CCNU) 100 mg/m^2
Prednisone 40 mg/m^2 × 14 days

Figure 7.5 Schema of Study CCG-921

Conclusion

It was concluded that the 8-in-1 chemo-therapy was inferior due either to the timing in relation to chemotherapy, i.e. the sandwich approach, with a delay in administering radiotherapy following surgery, or the reduced vincristine dose intensity compared to the PCV regimen.

Study 6

Cangir A, Ragab AH, Steuber P, Land VJ, Berry DH, Krischer JP.
Combination chemotherapy with vincristine (NSC-67574), procarbazine (NSC-77213), prednisone with or without nitrogen mustard (NSC-762) (MOPP v OPP) in children with recurrent brain tumours.
Med Pediatr Oncol 1984;**12**:1–3.

The study was carried out by the Pediatric Oncology Group and evaluated the role of mustine as part of combination chemotherapy in children with recurrent brain tumours. The trial date was not reported.

Details of the study

Patients under 18 years of age with a range of recurrent brain tumours were eligible. This was a randomised phase II study and randomisation was centralised in the POG office. The method of randomisation was not specified. Patients were stratified into the four major tumor groups, depending on histological type: medullobastoma, grade III and IV glioblastoma, ependymoma, and miscellaneous tumours. The Mantel–Haenszel statistic (log-rank) method was used to compare life tables of survival duration and median remission and survival comparisons were made using the Wilcoxon rank-sum test.

The main outcome measure was clinical response on CT scan.

Outcome

Fifty-four and 52 patients were randomised to MOPP (mustine 6 mg/m^2 days 1+8, vincristine 1·4 mg/m^2 d 1 + 8, procarbazine 50 mg/m^2 d 1, 100 mg/m^2 d 2–10, prednisone 40 mg/m^2 d 1–10 every 28 days) and OPP respectively. Thirty-one patients receiving MOPP and 14 patients receiving OPP were non-evaluable. This was due to a large percentage of early deaths and insufficient data. Overall, 4 of 9 patients with medulloblastoma had a complete or partial response after MOPP and 3 of 12 with medulloblastoma receiving OPP had a partial response. All patients on MOPP were reported to have myelosuppression with nausea and vomiting, and one life-threatening myelosuppression and two cases of pneumonia were reported in patients receiving MOPP but not among those receiving OPP. No clear details of these toxicities were presented.

Conclusion

It was concluded that the MOPP regimen produced more responses than the OPP regimen in patients with recurrent medulloblastoma. This conclusion was drawn despite the very small numbers and the absence of any statistical difference between the two groups.

Study 7

Deutsch M, Thomas PRM, Krischer J, Boyett JM, Albright L, Aronin P. *et al.*

Results of a prospective randomised trial comparing standard dose neuraxis irradiation with reduced neuraxis irradiation in patients with low-stage medulloblastoma.

Pediatr Neurosurg 1996;**24**:167–77.

The study was carried out between 1986 and 1990 by the combined Children's Cancer Group and Pediatric Oncology Group.

Objectives

The study addressed the issue whether reduced dose whole neuraxis irradiation could be safely given to good risk patients without adverse effect on recurrence rate and survival.

Details of the study

Patients between the ages of 3 and 21 were eligible. Stringent staging was necessary, including myelography, MRI, CSF examination, bone marrow examination and technetium bone scan. A good risk low stage subgroup was identified, comprising those with posterior fossa tumours with T_1/T_2 (T_{3a} was added in 1988), more than 50% resection, and <1·5 ml residue.

No details of randomisation methods are given. Stratification was by age alone.

It was predicted that 136 children would be recruited over 6·5 years and this would be sufficient to detect an increase in neuraxis relapse rate from 4% to 16% at 3 years, at the 10% level with 90% power. It would also detect an overall increase in recurrence rate, including primary site, from 23% to 33%.

In the control arm, a total of 36 Gy was given in 20 fractions at 180 cGy per day for 5 days per week, with an additional posterior fossa boost of 18 Gy in 10 fractions. Total posterior fossa dose was therefore 54 Gy. In the study arm, doses were reduced to 23·4 Gy in 13 fractions to whole neuraxis with a boost to the posterior fossa to achieve the same dose of 54 Gy. There was central review of all surgical details and radiotherapy, in addition to imaging.

The outcome measures were survival, progression free survival and isolated spinal relapses.

Outcome

One hundred and twenty-six patients were randomised. No details were given about the precise population base or randomisation refusal rate. Following randomisation, 32 patients were deemed to have been ineligible due to lack of postoperative contrast enhanced CT scan, > 1·5 ml residue, no myelography or evidence of brain stem involvement.

Patients' outcomes were analysed, both on the basis of the total group randomised ($n = 123$) and those deemed eligible after full review of eligibility ($n = 71$).

The overall relapse rate in the whole population was 5/63 (8%) for standard dose, versus 17/60 (28%) for reduced dose (p = < 0·002). For eligible patients only this was 2 out of 34 (6%) versus 2/37 (32%) (p = 0·02). If only recurrences outside the posterior fossa are considered in the whole patient group, there were 7/60 relapses versus 0/34 in the full dose group (p = 0·004). In the eligible group this was 4 versus none (p = 0·015).

On the basis of these findings accrual was discontinued in 1990 and with follow up there continued to be an excess in the number of total recurrences and neuraxis recurrences amongst patients treated with the reduce dose regimen.

Conclusion
It was concluded that in this good risk group dose reduction is not feasible and leads to a higher failure rate.

Comment
It is of note that there was a high ineligibility rate due to the stringent review and criteria, and numbers were relatively small once this was taken into account.

Study 8

Gerosa, M, DiStefano E, Carli M, Iraci G. Combined treatment of pediatric medulloblastoma. A review of an integrated program (two-arm chemotherapy trial).
Child's Brain 1980; **6**:262–73.

The study was carried out by the Padova Group and compared two different adjuvant chemotherapy strategies in surgically resected medulloblastoma. The date of the study is not stated.

Details of the study

Eligibility criteria were age 15 years or under and posterior fossa location medulloblastoma. No details of randomisation method or location are given. No details of anticipated difference in outcome or patient numbers are detailed.

Vincristine and cyclophosphamide were compared with vincristine combined with intrathecal (IT) methotrexate as adjuvant therapy. The vincristine dose was $1·5\,mg/m^2$, cyclophosphamide $600\,mg/m^2$, methotrexate $10\,mg/m^2$ IT Radiation dose was 55 Gy to the primary tumour with 40 Gy to the whole brain and 35 Gy to the spine. The overall dosage was reduced by 5–15 Gy in those under 3 years of age (Figure 7.6).

The primary outcome measure was event free survival.

Outcome

A total of 34 consecutively diagnosed patients were entered on the study, of whom 3 were lost to follow up and 2 excluded. Sixteen patients received cyclophosphamide/vincristine and 13 patients received vincristine/methotrexate. The mean interval to local recurrence was 30 months for the former and 27 months for the latter.

The local relapse rate with vincristine and cyclophosphamide alone was 69% and it was identical for the combination of vincristine with intrathecal methotrexate.

Conclusion

The conclusion was that neither regimen appeared to be particularly effective and there was no difference between the two regimens.

Comment

This was an early study with limited details regarding patient evaluation or methodology.

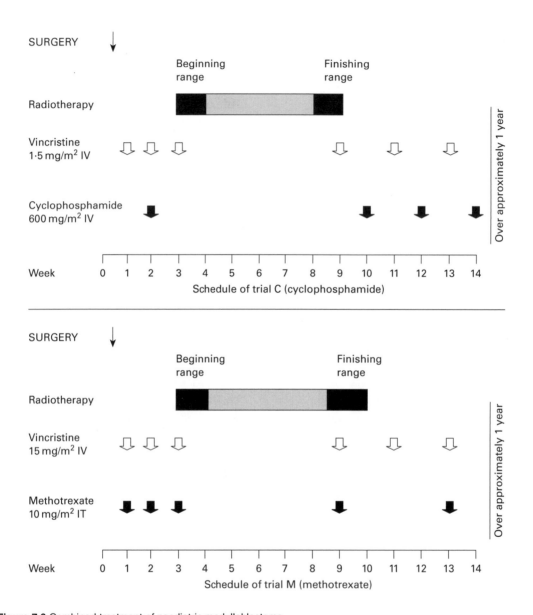

Figure 7.6 Combined treatment of paediatric medulloblastoma

Study 9

Van Eys J, Chen T, Moore T, Cheek W, Sexauer C, Starling K.
Adjuvant chemotherapy for medulloblastoma and ependymoma using IV vincristine, intrathecal methotrexate, and intrathecal hydrocortisone: a Southwest Oncology Study Group.
Cancer Treat Rep 1981;**65**:681–4.

The study was carried out by the Southwest Oncology Group. The date of the study is not stated.

Objectives

This was one of the first studies to address the issue of adjuvant chemotherapy and assess the use of intravenous vincristine and intrathecal methotrexate and hydrocortisone.

Details of the study

The eligibility criterion was biopsy proven diagnosis, either medulloblastoma or ependymoma.

No details of randomisation method or location are given. Patients were stratified by pathological type and also by the presence or absence of a ventriculoperitoneal or atrial shunt. No predicted differences in outcome or anticipated numbers are detailed.

Following trial details for initial surgery, radiotherapy commenced at around 10 days postoperatively. All patients received a total dose of 50 Gy to the primary site, with 35 Gy to the whole brain. Those under 3 years of age had a dose reduction to the posterior fossa of 45 Gy.

Vincristine 2 mg/m^2, hydrocortisone 15 mg/m^2 and methotrexate 15 mg/m^2 were initially commenced in combination 1 week following radiotherapy and then given weekly. This was found to be excessively myelosuppressive and therefore only vincristine was given for 4 weeks and the combination was then given monthly for a total of 1 year.

The main outcome measure was survival.

Outcome

Sixty-three patients were entered, of whom 2 were excluded due to incorrect diagnosis and 12 due to insufficient follow up data. Of 44 evaluable patients, 9 had inadequate data or refused to be randomised.

Of 34 children with medulloblastoma, 8 of 16 randomised to receive chemotherapy died, 5 of 18 who did not receive chemotherapy died. Median survivals were 128 days and > 134 days.

Toxicity

There were two toxic deaths in this group, one due to sepsis, and one due to unclear reasons.

Outcome

It was concluded that although this was a very small study, chemotherapy appeared to have no beneficial effect. The apparent adverse effect of chemotherapy was put down to the fact that these patients had closer surveillance and therefore relapse was noted earlier than in the radiotherapy alone arm.

Study 10

Kortmann R-D, Kuhl J, Timmermann B, Mittler U, Urban C, Budach V, Richter E, Willich N, Flentje M, Berthold F, Slavc I, Wolff J, Meisner C, Wiestler O, Sorensen N, Warmuth-Metz M, Bamberg M. Postoperative neoadjuvant chemotherapy before radiotherapy as compared to immediate radiotherapy followed by maintenance chemotherapy in the treatment of medulloblastoma in childhood: results of the German prospective randomised trial HIT '91.
Int J Rad Oncol Biol Phys 2000;**46**:269–79.

This study was carried out between 1991 and 1997 by the German GPOH group (HIT '91 trial).

Objectives

This study compared two chemotherapy strategies. The first a "sandwich" scheduling with chemotherapy before and after radiotherapy, the second less intensive chemotherapy given following radiotherapy.

Details of the study

The eligibility criteria a included patients between the age of 3 and 18 years. Study entry had to be within 4 weeks of surgery and no prior therapy apart from steroids was allowed.

Data was held centrally at Wuerzburg and quality control data in Tuebingen.

No details of the randomisation method are given, nor are there any details regarding predicted differences or numbers required. There was central pathological review and central review of all radiotherapy planning data.

Patients were randomised following initial surgery. Those who were to receive pre-radiotherapy chemotherapy were given a combination of ifosfamide 3 gs/m^2 ×3, and etoposide 150 mg/m^2 × 3 at around 2 weeks post-surgery. At weeks 5 and 6 high dose methotrexate 5 g/m^2 was given, and at week 7, cisplatin 40 mg/m^2 × 3 combined with cytarabine 400 mg/m^2 × 3 (see Figure 7.7).

Radiotherapy comprised a doses of 35·2 Gy in 22 fractions to the whole neuraxis, with a boost to 55·2 Gy to the primary site. Spinal metastases received a dose of 50 Gy. Those receiving initial radiotherapy were given weekly vincristine during radiotherapy and at 6 weeks following completion of irradiation a combination of oral CCNU 75 mg/m^2, cisplatin 70 mg/m^2 and vincristine 1·5 mg/m^2 was commenced. Vincristine was repeated on days 8 and 15 of each cycle. Cycles were repeated at 6-weekly intervals for a total of eight course.

The main outcome measures were PFS, overall survival and the toxicity of this NRO adjuvant chemotherapy aproach.

Outcome

One hundred and eighty-four patients were enrolled by 70 centres, of whom 137 were randomised, with 72 receiving arm 1, the "sandwich" regimen, and 65 arm 2, post-radiation chemotherapy. Forty-seven patients were not randomised due to parental refusal, but these are included in the subsequent analysis.

Of the randomised patients, 14% had M2/M3 disease and 60% had initial surgical complete excision.

Overall, 121 patients had full review of radiotherapy planning and a total of 23% were found

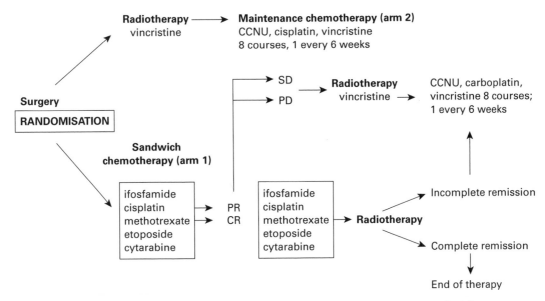

Radiotherapy: prescribed total dose and fractionation: 35·2 Gy craniospinal axis, 5 × 1·6 Gy/wk;
20·0 Gy posterior fossa, 5 × 2·0 Gy/wk

Figure 7.7 Treatment schedule of HIT '91 trial (CR, complete remission; PR, partial remission; PD, progressive disease; SD, stable disease). Reprinted from Kortmann R-D *et al*, *Int J Rad Oncol Biol Phys* (full reference p 168) with permission from Elsevier Science.

to contain errors. This included incomplete coverage of cribriform plate, middle cranial fossa and posterior fossa, or a gap between whole brain and craniospinal fields.

The response rate in the whole patient group with measurable disease entered into arm 1 was 13/23 patients with complete response. There were 5/12 complete responses in patients with M2/3 disease.

For the randomised study group only, the PFS was 66% ± 5% for those with no surgical residue, compared to 68% ± 9% for those with residue. In M2/3 disease PFS was 30% ± 15%. In those with M1 disease, treated with arm 1, i.e. sandwich

therapy, 3 year PFS was 65% ± 5%; in arm 2, post-radiation chemotherapy, it was 78% ± 6% (p = < 0·03). For those between 3 and 5·9 years of age, PFS was 60% versus 64% respectively, in contrast to those between 6 and 18 years of age where it was 62% versus 84%.

The relapse sites in the whole patient group were local 17%, other CNS sites 47% and combined 35%. There was only one extracranial recurrence in bone.

Toxicity
There were 2 toxic deaths – one septic death in arm 1 and one leukencephalopathy in arm 2 – in a patient given intrathecal therapy following irradiation contrary to protocol.

Conclusion

The conclusion is that although sandwich therapy is feasible, it does not appear to be of any benefit and may adversely affect outcome. Lower dose "maintenance" therapy appears to be superior, particularly in older children.

8
Glioma

Commentary – Joann Ater and Archie Bleyer

Gliomas constitute over 50% of central nervous system tumours in children, and most are low grade. Several clinical trials address the treatment of low grade glioma, but none of the randomised studies is yet complete. Hence this review will focus on treatment of high grade glioma.

The high grade glioma category of brain tumours includes anaplastic astrocytoma (AA), glioblastoma multiforme (GBM), high grade mixed glioma, anaplastic oligodendroglioma and high grade glioma not otherwise specified (NOS). They occur in any location in the central nervous system, but most commonly in the supratentorial cerebral hemispheres and brain stem. Less than 10% of gliomas that arise in or involve the optic pathway, hypothalamus and cerebellum are high grade. Most studies that address treatment of high grade glioma have either focused primarily on the supratentorial tumours or brain stem glioma. The supratentorial high grade glioma group comprises only 10% of brain tumours treated in children under the age of 21 and children with intrinsic pontine glioma make up another 8–10% of paediatric brain tumours. There are only approximately 150 cases in each group diagnosed annually in the United States. The reports cited in this chapter are specifically related to either supratentorial and cerebellar high grade gliomas or intrinsic pontine gliomas (brain stem glioma).

With the limitations imposed by small numbers, randomised clinical trials can only be performed within cooperative groups such as Children's Cancer Group (CCG) and the Pediatric Oncology Group (POG), that have now merged to form the Children's Oncology Group (COG). Indeed, all phase III studies included in this chapter are reports from these groups.

Other paediatric cooperative groups throughout the world are currently evaluating treatments of childhood high grade glioma with phase I and II studies, but have yet either to complete or report these trials. Some of these will be discussed as providing information for future randomised studies.

Surgery

The first element of treatment in high grade glioma is surgery. Surgery is performed to make the diagnosis, relieve symptoms of increased intracranial pressure and also, whenever possible, provide specific anti-tumour therapeutic benefit. While there is no prospective trial of the benefit of extent of resection on paediatric high grade gliomas, there is now evidence from the CCG that surgical removal of over 90% of the tumour is a favourable prognostic factor[1]. This group reports a significantly better 5-year progression free survival (PFS) for children who have greater than 90%

resection for both anaplastic astrocytoma (44% v 22%, p = 0·55) and glioblastoma multiforme (26% v 4%, p = 0·046). None the less, this trial does not ascertain whether this benefit is a surrogate for biology of the tumour and invasiveness, or simply a reflection that more aggressive removal will improve survival.

For most brain stem gliomas, surgery is not a useful treatment modality. Eighty-five to 90% of tumours that arise in the brain stem are diffuse, intrinsic pontine anaplastic astrocytoma or glioblastoma multiforme and 15% are focal low grade astrocytomas. The recognition of the relatively favourable focal low grade tumours is essential because of the relatively indolent course and distinctly different management. These tumours can be managed with surgery, observation and radiation or chemotherapy with progression, with good outcome. The focal brain stem gliomas are now excluded from clinical trials on intrinsic brain stem tumours, such as Study 2 in this chapter, reported by Mandell et al for the Pediatric Oncology Group (POG-9239). On the other hand, intrinsic pontine glioma is a diagnosis that is made by MRI criteria, has a very poor prognosis, and biopsy or surgery is usually of no benefit[2]. The risk of the biopsy and/or surgery seems to outweigh the benefit in the attempted resection.

In summary, from the evidence we now have it appears that, with one exception, high grade glioma should be completely resected whenever possible without inflicting life-threatening neurological deficit. The CCG trial indicates that this can improve survival, especially when given with other treatment. The exception is diffuse pontine glioma surgery in which the diagnosis rarely needs to be established with tissue confirmation and resection is neither of evidence-based benefit nor of sufficient safety.

Radiation therapy

The role of radiation dose and schedule in paediatric high grade glioma has been studied primarily in diffuse pontine glioma. There have been no randomised studies between surgery alone versus radiotherapy for high grade gliomas in children. However, there is evidence based on a number of adult studies that radiotherapy is of benefit in at least relieving symptoms and prolonging survival[3].

In the 1980s and early 1990s, there was initial interest in whether higher doses and different schedules of radiation fractionation may be beneficial in treatment of brain tumours. This approach was utilised in Study 2 by Mandell et al which investigated the issue of higher dose hyperfractionated radiation for brain stem gliomas. This study was based on numerous phase II studies from single institutions[4], CCG[5] and POG[6], that attempted to increase the dose of radiotherapy using a hyperfractionated (twice daily) treatment schedule to a variety of doses ranging from 64·5 to 78 Gy depending on the study. In retrospect, the early promising results may have included some patients with focal, more favourable tumour. The POG-9239 study (Study 2) randomised children with intrinsic pontine glioma between either the standard radiotherapy of 180 cGy daily to a total of 54 Gy or 117 cGy twice daily to 70·2 Gy. Both groups received concomitant cisplatinum. The median time to progression (MTP) is 6 months for 54 Gy and 5 months for 70·2 Gy. The survival at 2 years was 7% in both groups, showing no benefit for hyperfractionated radiation. In addition, these survival rates are the same as previous studies with radiation alone, showing no suggestion of benefit of the cisplatin as a radiation sensitiser. Finally, the hyperfractionated radiation was more toxic. Based on this study standard radiation is still the recommended treatment for intrinsic pontine glioma because of the benefit derived from temporary clinical improvement in most patients and tumour response in about 30%. These trials of radiation in brain stem glioma are important because when carefully done they demonstrated that hyperfractionation provided no objective benefit in prolonging survival beyond the benefit achieved with standard radiation. Numerous phase I and II studies are still ongoing to determine the effectiveness of chemotherapy and other radiation sensitisers for treatment of pontine glioma. These will be discussed below. As of now, despite numerous trials, there is no chemotherapy that appears to be of benefit in this disease.

In summary, the survival rates in brain stem gliomas are no better today than they were a quarter of a century ago, despite the trials and biological studies that have been conducted to date. This lack of progress is as dramatic as any failure in the discipline of paediatric oncology. To say that there is an urgent need for further laboratory and clinical studies in this type of glioma would be an understatement.

Chemotherapy

The role of chemotherapy has been the subject of most cooperative group studies in high grade glioma of children throughout the world. European groups, CCG and POG have focused on this issue. The results of randomised clinical trials related to the use of chemotherapy in supratentorial high grade glioma in childhood are difficult to interpret because of small numbers, changing neuropathological classification systems and discrepancy in diagnosis between neuropathology reviewers. These problems are most apparent in Study 3, a report by Sposto

et al for the CCG. Seventy-two children aged 2 to 21 years with high grade glioma were enrolled over a 5 year period between 1976 and 1981. This was the first randomised study in paediatric high grade glioma at a time when chemotherapy was not well accepted as a treatment for brain tumours in children. Therefore, only a small percentage of high grade gliomas diagnosed at CCG institutions were enrolled on this study. Thirteen patients were excluded for various appropriate reasons, leaving only 58 patients to be randomised between involved field radiation alone and involved field radiation with concurrent weekly vincristine followed by CCNU, vincristine and prednisone. The randomisation was not stratified by tumour type, and unfortunately the radiotherapy arm included 83% glioblastoma multiforme (GBM) and the radiotherapy and chemotherapy arm included 54% GBM. Overall event free survival at 5 years was 46% with chemotherapy versus 18% for radiotherapy alone ($p < 0.05$). For only the GBM patients, the 5 year EFS was 42% with chemotherapy versus 6% without ($p = 0.01$). These results appear to statistically prove that chemotherapy with CCNU, vincristine and prednisone is superior to radiation alone in paediatric high grade glioma.

The main concern is the small numbers of patients. When forced to statistically analyse studies with suboptimal numbers of patients, the results can often be indefinite and require further studies for confirmation. The second concern about this study is the pathology of these tumours. The survival rates on this study are much better than those reported in adult patients with similar treatment. One must conclude that either children have biologically different tumours that respond better to therapy than similar adult tumours, or perhaps subtypes of childhood low grade tumours were included erroneously. In reality it may have been a combination of both, as found in the review of the subsequent CCG-945 study (Study 1 in this chapter). (See further discussion below.)

Study 1 by Finlay *et al* reports the results of CCG-945, the study that followed Study 3 discussed above. This study logically seeks to build upon the finding that chemotherapy is of benefit to children with high grade glioma and to compare a then promising regimen "8-in-1" regimen to the CCNU, vincristine and prednisone regimen. The patients were randomised after surgery. Both groups received involved field radiation to 54 Gy. Weekly vincristine was given during radiation with PCV but not with the 8-in-1 regimen. In a 5 year period 185 patients were randomised, enabling further analysis of the effects of histology and extent of resection on progression free survival. The median survival of 14 months for both regimens is similar to results reported in adult patients with radiation and chemotherapy, with 5 year PFS 28% in AA, 16% in GBM and 64% for anaplastic ganglioglioma and anaplastic oligodendroglioma. These results show disappointingly lower survival rates than those achieved in the previous study, but are probably not statistically different.

This study suggests that the 8-in-1 regimen is not superior to PCV, but two design flaws compromise this conclusion. First, chemotherapy was not administered during radiotherapy on the 8-in-1 regimen and it was on the PCV regimen, so the conclusion remains tenuous. Had weekly vincristine also been given during radiotherapy on the 8-in-1 regimen the outcome may have been different. Secondly, the 8-in-1 regimen was administered for two cycles before radiation, thus delaying the start of the radiotherapy for at least 5 weeks.

The difference in survival compared to the previous study (CCG-943) led to renewed concern about the neuropathological diagnosis of the cases and discrepancy between reviewers. As noted, there was a large incidence of discordance for anaplastic astrocytoma and glioblastoma between reviewers. In 1998 Boyett *et al* reported a re-review of the cases enrolled on this study[7]. They found that when five expert neuropathologists reviewed 226 cases (98·3% of those enrolled on CCG-945), the five reviewers agreed on a specific diagnosis for only 25·2% of the cases. The consensus diagnosis confirmed high grade glioma in 136 patients (68·3%), while 75 (37·7%) of those entered on the study as high grade gliomas by institutional review were felt not to be high grade. When the 5 year PFS rates for each reviewer were compared for each tumour group to the institutional review, the survival of GBM and other high grade astrocytoma was relatively unchanged. However, the 5 year PFS rate for anaplastic astrocytoma dropped from 37% by institutional review to 18–27% for the reviewers. Since the reviewers were selected because they were experts in their field, the discrepancy was not due to incompetence or an inability to make the appropriate diagnosis. This discrepancy may be based on such items as insufficient tumour for review (the necessity for making a diagnosis with only one or two slides without immunohistochemistry). While the reviewers reportedly used a uniform system, the interpretations of the individual systems vary between neuropathologists. This variation is amplified when studies from different institutions using different neuropathologic classification systems are compared. Therefore, one must be particularly careful in overinterpreting the results of single institution studies in paediatric high grade glioma. Despite the difficulties, randomised multi-institutional studies that report both the institutional and reviewed diagnosis may provide the most reliable information for determining the treatment of childhood high grade glioma. Given these limitations, the papers and randomised studies published provide evidence-based information that can be useful in the treatment of children with high grade gliomas.

Clinical trials have shown that high grade gliomas in children can respond to a variety of chemotherapeutic agents. Study 4 by Kobrinsky *et al* for the CCG and Study 5 by Friedman *et al* for POG are essentially randomised phase II studies that evaluate response of tumour in recurrent patients. The Kobrinsky study had the hypothesis that mannitol could increase the efficacy of VP-16 by opening the blood–brain barrier in brain tumours. There were 15 low grade astrocytomas, 20 high grade gliomas, 22 brain stem gliomas and 42 PNETs entered on the study. The response rate on central review was 8% with mannitol and 13% without disproving the hypothesis. In addition, the response rate to VP-16 given with this intermittent dose schedule is low enough not to appear encouraging to pursue. Study 5 by Friedman *et al* randomised progressive or recurrent patients with brain tumours between carboplatin and iproplatin. The study was stratified by tumour histology to allow an assessment of response rate for each tumour type. For high grade glioma there was a 1/14 response with carboplatin and 0/12 for iproplatin and no responses in brain stem glioma. Based on this study carboplatin has a slightly higher response rate than iproplatin. These randomised phase II studies must be viewed in the same way as any other phase II study, in that they provide suggestive evidence of low levels of drug activity that would require further investigation in order to conclude that these drugs have any role in the treatment of children with newly diagnosed high grade glioma.

The efficacy of chemotherapy has been tested in both recurrent patients and pre-irradiation phase II window studies performed by the Pediatric Oncology Group, Children's Oncology Group and various other groups worldwide. The CCG and POG trials are complete but have not yet been reported in the literature. It is hoped that they will provide further evidence as to which types of chemotherapy would be most beneficial in high grade glioma. However, adult studies have shown that response rate alone is not sufficient to adequately choose the best chemotherapy. Therefore, they have taken the approach of evaluating both tumour response and also time to progression. The opinion is that while some agents provide a rapid response, the response is so short-lived that it is not significantly beneficial. On the other hand, some agents may produce a slower response, but one that is longer-lasting and consequently more beneficial to the patient. The adult North American Brain Tumour Consortium is now evaluating chemotherapy trials in high grade glioma using statistical methods that evaluate both response and time to progression.

Future studies

In an effort to improve efficacy of chemotherapy in childhood high grade gliomas investigators have utilised methods that include the following:

1   Neoadjuvant chemotherapy in a phase II window before radiation. This approach is based on the following premises: (1) reduction in the volume of the tumour enhances the efficacy of radiotherapy; (2) initiating multiple agent chemotherapy as soon as

possible reduces the advent of multidrug resistance which increases as a function of the time that the tumour is not treated with chemotherapy (Goldie Coldman hypothesis); (3) chemotherapy takes less to time to initiate than radiotherapy which requires referral to a radiotherapy unit, simulation, etc.; (4) chemotherapy is more able to more effectively penetrate the blood–brain barrier before radiation. The CCG and POG have completed studies utilising this approach which have been reported in abstract form only. POG randomised between BCNU and cisplatin versus cyclophosphamide and vincristine before radiation. In newly diagnosed patients with residual high grade glioma after surgery, CCG randomised pairs of agents for the phase II window (prior to radiotherapy). The pairs were etoposide (VP-16) and carboplatin, VP-16 and ifosfamide, and VP-16 and cyclophosphamide. Both studies are now closed and should be reported in the near future.

2   High dose chemotherapy with autologous bone marrow or stem cell rescue is currently under investigation by a number of groups as a method of increasing dose intensification. There is a notable lack of randomised phase III trials of this approach and it unlikely that any of the current trials will definitively demonstrate that high dose chemotherapy is a standard of treatment. Phase II studies have show that this method is not helpful with brain stem glioma or ependymoma, but it is still being pursued in supratentorial high grade glioma.

3   Dose scheduling and new agents are currently under investigation. The importance of route of administration and dose schedule for some agents has been identified. For example, while VP-16 appeared nearly inactive on the intermittent dosing schedule, subsequent studies utilising chronic low dose given daily have shown activity in low grade and high grade glioma and even brain stem glioma. New agents currently under investigation, such as irinotecan (CPT-11), are being investigated at different dose schedules. The phase II study of temozolomide in recurrent childhood brain tumours is now complete but not yet reported. As reported in abstract and preliminary studies in adults, this drug has activity in primarily anaplastic astrocytoma and possibly PNET. Because it is given orally and is well tolerated, it is likely to be incorporated into future studies evaluating different dose schedules and combined with other drugs. Adult groups are currently testing combinations with BCNU, CCNU, tamoxifen, thalidomide, cis-retinoic acid, carboplatin and others. Perhaps these studies will provide clues for future studies in childhood high grade glioma.

4   Blood–brain barrier disruption in the form of a bradykinin analogue that specifically opens the blood–brain barrier and not peripheral circulation (RMP-7) is under investigation in all types of brain tumours, including high grade glioma and brain stem glioma.

5   A new emphasis on chemotherapy during radiation as radiation sensitiser is now under investigation with a number of agents, including gadolinium-texaphyrin, topotecan, VP-16, temozolomide, and others.

6   Identification of new targets for therapy in laboratory-based studies and phase I clinical trials may provide evidence of new areas to pursue, including anti-angiogenesis agents, anti-invasiveness agents, and small molecule drugs such as tyrosine kinase inhibitors such as STI 571 (Gleevic).

It appears that currently in childhood high grade glioma there is no new treatment that appears promising enough to commit to a large phase III study that will take many years. Thus, most groups such as COG are continuing to pursue phase II studies. An exception is the putative value of high dose chemotherapy, but the lack of prospective, adequately designed phase III trials of this modality to date is disappointing.

Conclusions

Although the publications reviewed in this chapter may suggest otherwise, the treatment of paediatric high grade glioma continues to be a dilemma. The number of reported trials in childhood glioma is limited and their results are of insufficient power to provide unequivocal evidence-based outcomes for clear diagnostic, prognostic and therapeutic directions. In particular, they do not resolve the role of high dose chemotherapy in high grade glioma; the optimal radiotherapy volume, dose or fractionation; the best treatment in the youngest patients; when and how to manage the low grade astrocytomas; and how to follow patients for earliest sign of disease progression or recurrence. One of the reasons for this conundrum is that there are too few well-conducted trials. Compared to the number of clinical trials available for review in adult glioma, the number of trials in children is small. Despite the trials conducted to date, there is a compelling urgency to engage in clinical trials that will answer the questions that remain, many of which are generated by the very trials that were designed to settle some of these issues.

References

1   Wisoff JH, Boyett JM, Berger MS *et al*. Current neurosurgical management and the impact of extent of resection in the treatment of malignant gliomas of childhood. A report of the Children's Cancer Group trial CCG-945. *J Neurosurg* 1998;**89**:52–9.

2   Epstein F, McCleary EL. Intrinsic brain-stem tumours of childhood: surgical indications. *J Neurosurg* 1986;**64**: 11–15.

3   Levin VA. Neuro-oncology: an overview. *Arch Neurol* 1999;**56** (4):401–4.

4   Prados MD, Wara WM, Edwards MSB *et al*. The treatment of brain stem and thalamic gliomas with 78 Gy of hyperfractionated radiation therapy. *Int J Radiat Oncol Biol* 1995;**32**:85–91.

5   Packer RJ, Boyett JM, Zimmerman RA *et al*. Hyperfractionated radiotherapy [72 Gy] for children with brain stem gliomas. A Childrens Cancer Group phase I/II trial. *Cancer* 1993;**72**:1414–21.

6   Freeman CR, Krischer JP, Sanford RA *et al*. Final results of a study of escalating doses of hyperfractionated radiotherapy in brain stem tumours in children: a Paediatric Oncology Group Study. *Int J Radiat Oncol Biol Phys* 1993;**27**:197–206.

7   Boyett JM, Yates AJ, Gilles FH, Burger PC, Becker LE *et al*. When is a high grade astrocytoma (HGA) not a HGA? Results of 226 cases of anaplastic astrocytoma (AA), glioblastoma multiforme (GBM), and other HGA (OTH HGA) by five neuropathologists. *Proc ASCO* 1998; **17**:526a.

Studies

Study 1

Finlay JL, Boyett JM, Yates AJ, Wisoff JH, Milstein JM, Geyer JR, Bertolone SJ, McGuire P, Cherlow JM, Tefft M, Turski PA, Wara WM, Edwards M, Sutton LN, Berger MS, Epstein F, Ayers G, Allen JC, Packer RJ.
Randomised phase III trial in childhood high grade astrocytoma comparing vincristine, lomustine, and prednisone with the eight-drugs-in-1-day regimen.
J Clin Oncol 1995;**13**:112–23.

The study was carried out between 1985 and 1990 by the Children's Cancer Group (Study CCG-945).

Objectives

The aim was to determine whether pre- and postoperative 8-in-1 chemotherapy was superior to PCV as post-radiotherapy adjuvant treatment in high grade astrocytoma.

Details of the study

Eligible patients were required to have pathologically confirmed high grade astrocytoma outside the brain stem or spinal cord. Patients had to be less than 28 days from surgery unless pathological diagnosis had caused delay and no prior therapy was allowed. There was central pathology review but entry was based on the local pathology report. Histological types included were glioblastoma multiforme grade IV, anaplastic astrocytoma grade III, anaplastic ganglioglioma and anaplastic oligodendroglioma grade III.

The location and method of randomisation is not stated. It was planned to enter 60 patients in each arm, in order to show a 50% decrease in the estimated hazards ratio of 0·46% per year in the control group with 80% power and a two-sided test (= 0·1). To achieve the secondary objective, namely to study subgroups on pathological review with regard to prognostic factors, 172 patients were to be randomised, in order to have a 90% power to detect a 20% difference in 2 year progression free survival (40–60%) with a two-sided test (p = 0·05).

Study design involved standard treatment with local irradiation 54 Gy in 30 fractions at 1·8 Gy/fraction over 6 weeks with simultaneous weekly vincristine (eight doses), followed at week 10 by eight cycles of PCV chemotherapy with procarbazine, CCNU and vincristine, given every 6 weeks (Figure 8.1). Radiotherapy volume was the tumour on CT or MRI, including oedema, and adding a 2 cm margin. The experimental arm consisted of two courses of 8-in-1 chemotherapy given 2 weeks apart, followed by the same radiotherapy and subsequently eight courses of 8-in-1 chemotherapy given every 6 weeks.

Outcome

One hundred and eighty-five patients were randomised but it is unclear what number were eligible. Thirteen of those randomised were subsequently excluded, due to site (spinal cord) in 2, local repeat review of pathology in 7 or withdrawal in 4 of parental consent. Eighty-five

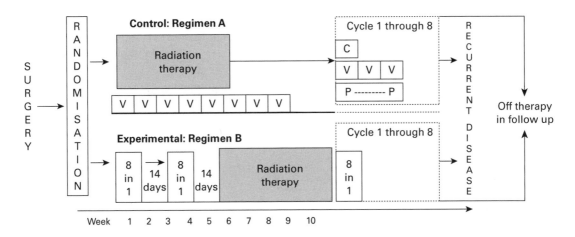

Figure 8.1 Schema for Children's Cancer Group Study CCG-945

patients received standard therapy with PCV and 87 the 8-in-1 chemotherapy (one patient given the treatment arm to which they were not randomised was analysed as randomised).

Age ranged from 21 months to 19 years, median 10 years. Resection greater than 90% varied by site, being achieved in only 7% of those with midline tumours, compared to 56% for the posterior fossa and 56% of those with hemisphere tumours. It was also lower in those with anaplastic astrocytoma, 34% versus 47% for glioblastoma multiforme.

Only one patient was noted to have spinal metastases on MR or myelography and 2 had positive cytology in the CSF.

Central pathology review revealed a high incidence of discordance. For anaplastic astrocytoma concordance was 63%, for glioblastoma multiforme 67%, but only 21% for other eligible tumour types. The radiotherapy planning volume

was reviewed in 77% of patients, in whom 30% had inadequate margins.

Overall, the 5 year progression free survival was 33%, 26% ± 8% with PCV and 33% ± 7% with 8-in-1. Median survival was 14 months in both arms. Five year PFS for anaplastic astrocytoma was 28%, 16% for GBM and 64% for other pathology. Ninety-seven per cent of failures were local.

Toxicity

Grade III or IV toxicity, predominantly neurotoxicity, was seen in 14% of those receiving PCV; 45% of these receiving the 8-in-1 chemotherapy had grade III or IV toxicity, predominantly myelosuppression. These were documented prior to radiotherapy. Following radiotherapy the degree of myelosuppression was comparable in the two arms.

Outcome

It is concluded that the more intensive 8-in-1 chemotherapy was of no significant benefit.

Comment

A subsequent paper gives further details of the tumour resection rates in the study arm of CCG-945: Wisoff JH, Boyett JM, Berger MS, Brant C, Li H, Yates AJ, McGuire-Cullen P, Turski PA, Sutton LN, Allen JC, Packer RJ, Finlay JL. Current neurosurgical management and the impact of the extent of resection in the treatment of malignant gliomas of childhood: a report of the Children's Cancer Groop trial CCG 945. *J Neurosurg* 1998;**89**:52–9.

Study 2

Mandell LR, Kadota R, Freeman C, Douglass EC, Fontanesi J, Cohen ME, Kovnar E, Burger P, Sanford RA, Kepner J, Friedman H, Kun LE.
There is no role for hyperfractionated radiotherapy in the management of children with newly diagnosed diffuse intrinsic brainstem tumours: results of a Pediatric Oncology Group phase III trial comparing conventional *v.* hyperfractionated radiotherapy.
Int J Rad Oncol Biol Phys 1999;**43**:959–64.

The study was carried out by the Pediatric Oncology Group between 1992 and 1996 (study POG-9239).

Objectives

The aim of the study was to assess the value of hyperfractionated radiotherapy in brain stem glioma.

Details of the study

Eligibility for the study required a clinical history of less than 6 months and at least two of the following clinical features: cranial nerve deficit, long tract signs or ataxia. Pathological confirmation was not required in all cases. A gadolinium enhanced MR had to show at least two-thirds of a lesion to be intrinsic to the pons.

Details of randomisation location or method are not given nor any prediction of the difference anticipated or numbers of patients required.

Radiotherapy started not more than 28 days from diagnosis. The study compared 180 cGy given in daily fractions to a total dose of 54 Gy, with 117 cGy fractions given twice a day to a total dose of 70·2 Gy. The radiation field included tumour volume plus a 2 cm margin.

Concurrent cisplatin was given as a continuous infusion over 120 hours on weeks 1, 3 and 5, combined with steroids. The exact dose is not given but prior dose finding studies suggest this was 100 mg/m^2.

Outcome

One hundred and thirty-two patients were entered on the study, of whom 67 received conventional radiotherapy and 65 hyperfractionated radiotherapy. Two patients were excluded due to diagnostic errors. The median ages were 78 months and 74 months respectively. A pathological diagnosis was obtained in 22 patients; 10 were anaplastic astrocytoma or glioblastoma multiforme.

Although 95% of patients had documented clinical improvement, the event free survival was short in both treatment arms. Three patients developed progressive disease during radiotherapy. Imaging reassessment 4 or 8 weeks after treatment in 108 evaluable patients showed a partial response in 18 patients with conventional radiotherapy, compared to 15 patients with hyperfractionated radiotherapy, stable disease in 25 versus 23 patients, and progressive disease in 13 versus 12 patients respectively. The median time to progression was 6 months (range 2–15) with conventional radiotherapy and 5 months (range 1–12) with hyperfractionated. Median time to death was 8 months in both arms of the study.

Overall survival at 1, 2 and 3 years with conventional treatment was 30%, 7% and 3%, compared to 27%, 7% and 4% with hyperfractionation.

No difference in toxicity was documented.

Conclusion
It is concluded that hyperfractionation did not appear to be of any benefit in this patient population.

Study 3

Sposto R, Ertel IJ, Jenkins RDT, Boesel CP, Venes JL, Ortega JA, Evans AE, Wara W, Hammond D.
The effectiveness of chemotherapy for treatment of high grade astrocytoma inchildren: results of a randomised trial.
J Neuro-Oncol 1989;**7**:165–77.

The study was performed between 1976 and 1981 by the Children's Cancer Group (Study CCG-943).

Objectives

This study evaluates the role of adding chemotherapy with vincristine, CCNU and prednisolone to standard radiotherapy in high grade astrocytoma.

Details of the study

Eligible patients were between 2 and 21 years of age with biopsy proven high grade astrocytoma (Kernohan grade II–IV). Brain stem and spinal cord tumours were excluded. Patients were grouped into those with anaplastic astrocytoma or glioblastoma multiforme. The latter was defined as one or more foci of necrosis in malignant astrocytes. There was central review of both pathology and radiotherapy planning fields.

Patients were randomised within 4 weeks of the time of surgery. The location and precise method of randomisation was not detailed. An adaptive procedure was used to balance for two major prognostic factors, namely extent of resection (total, partial or biopsy alone) and site (supratentorial and infratentorial).

The difference that was sought between the two study arms is not defined, nor is the number of patients required for the study.

The patients in both arms received standard radiotherapy 52·5 Gy in 28 fractions. Children between the ages of 2 and 3 years received reduced dose 45 Gy. The radiation field was to encompass all tumour plus a 4 cm margin. The lower surface of C2 was the field margin for cerebellar tumours. There was to be a minimum field of 100 ml.

Patients randomised to chemotherapy received weekly vincristine 1·5 mg/m^2 for 6 doses and, following a 4 week break after completion of radiation, were given 6-week cycles of vincristine on days 1, 8 and 15 (1·5 mg/m^2), CCNU on day 2, 100 mg/m^2, and prednisone days 1–14 (40 mg/m^2). Total duration of treatment was planned for 58 weeks.

At relapse, all patients were eligible for a phase II study of either procarbazine alone, in those who were previously treated with chemotherapy, or vincristine/CCNU in those who had received chemotherapy.

Major outcome measures were event free survival (EFS) and overall survival.

Outcome

Seventy-two patients were enrolled on the study. Thirteen were excluded: 3 had received prior therapy, in 6 there was an "incorrect pathological diagnosis", there was insufficient material for review in 2, 1 had a spinal tumour and 1 withdrew.

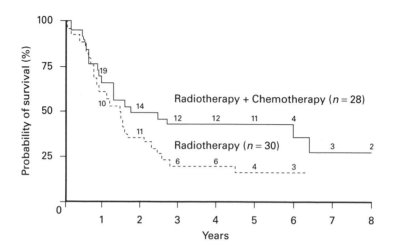

Figure 8.2 Survival (in years) by randomised treatment assignment

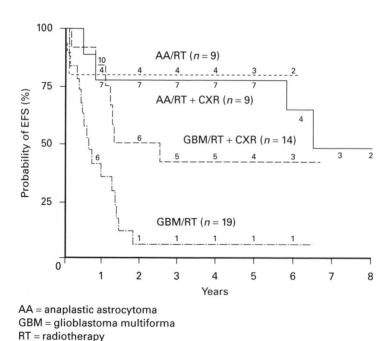

AA = anaplastic astrocytoma
GBM = glioblastoma multiforma
RT = radiotherapy
CXR = chemotherapy

Figure 8.3 Event free survival (in years) by pathology and randomised treatment assignment

Fifty-eight of 59 were randomised, 28 to radiotherapy plus chemotherapy and 30 to radiotherapy alone. Three patients randomised to radiation alone were given chemotherapy and were included in the analysis. Overall, the two arms were well balanced, except that a higher percentage of patients in the radiotherapy alone arm had glioblastoma (83% v 54%, p = <0·03).

Three patients died but there were no details of EFS. In the remaining population, the EFS at 5 years was 46% ± 10% in the combined therapy arm, versus 18 ± 7% for radiotherapy alone (p = <0·05). Overall survival at 5 years was 43% ± 9%, versus 17% ± 7% (p = 0·1) (Figure 8.2).

The difference was most marked for children with glioblastoma, where at 5 years 42% remained event free, versus 6% (p = 0·01) (Figure 8.3).

Eighty-two percent of the patients received radiotherapy, within 10% of the planned protocol. In 19 patients chemotherapy was delayed or drugs omitted. This was mainly due to infection. Of the 31 patients who were given chemotherapy, only 13 completed treatment. Of the 18 who failed to complete treatment, there were 10 with progressive disease and 4 refused further chemotherapy.

Conclusion
It was concluded that adjuvant chemotherapy may prolong event free and overall survival, particularly in glioblastoma multiforme. Unfortunately, the numbers in this study were too small to provide a reliable answer to the question posed.

Study 4

Kobrinksy NL, Packer RJ, Boyett JM, Stanley P, Shiminski-Maher T, Allen JC, Garvin JH, Stewart DJ, Finlay JL.

Etoposide with or without mannitol for the treatment of recurrent or primarily unresponsive brain tumours: a Children's Cancer Group Study, CCG-9881.

J Neuro-Oncol 1999;**45**:47–54.

The study was carried out by the Children's Cancer Group between 1988–1992 (Study CCG-9881).

Objectives

The aim of the study was to document the response in relapsed brain tumours to etoposide and the efficacy of mannitol when combined with this drug.

Details of the study

Eligible patients had recurrent or refractory brain tumours, and had received prior chemotherapy or radiotherapy. Disease types included medulloblastoma/PNET, grade I–IV astrocytoma and brain stem glioma. Patients were aged less than 21 years and at least 3 weeks had elapsed since prior treatment. They had a life expectancy of 12 months or over, creatinine clearance >50 ml/min/1·73m^2, bilirubin < 2·5 mg/dl, neutrophils, >1000/mm^3 and platelets >100 000/mm^3.

No details of the randomisation site or method used are given. No details are given of the predicted difference between the two arms or number of patients required. Patients were stratified by histological subtypes.

There was central review of response on imaging and a clinical scoring system was used that was based on steroid usage, signs and symptoms of raised intracranial pressure and neurological status.

Outcome

Ninety-nine patients were registered. The histological subtypes included 15 low grade astrocytomas, 20 high grade gliomas, 22 brain stem gliomas and 42 PNETs. Six patients were non-evaluable as they had complete surgical resection, and 6 had inadequate data. Of 87 patients, only 67 had evaluable imaging. Local review showed a total of 12 partial and no complete responses. This was reduced to 7 PR on central review of imaging. Overall response rate was 14% with local reporting and 10% after central review. Local reporting showed a 17% response rate with mannitol, compared to 10% without mannitol. On central review this was 8% with mannitol versus 13% without, i.e. no significant difference between the two arms. Survival with mannitol was 36 ± 7 months, without mannitol it was 28 ± 6 months. The clinical scoring system showed a poor correlation with radiological response and was not included in the analysis of response or outcome.

Conclusion

It was concluded that the overall response rate to single agent etoposide was low and mannitol did not significantly improve the efficacy of etoposide.

Study 5

Friedman HS, Krischer JP, Burger P, Oakes BW, Hockenberger B, Weiner MD, Falletta JM, Norris D, Ragab AH, Mahoney DH Jr, Whitehead MV, Kun LE.
Treatment of children with progressive or recurrent brain tumours with carboplatin or iproplatin: a Paediatric Oncology Group randomised phase II study.
J Clin Oncol 1992;**10**:249–56.

This study was carried out by the Pediatric Oncology Group between 1986 and 1990 (POG-8638).

Objectives
The aim of the study was to compare the activity of two non-nephrotoxic platinum analogues in relapsed brain tumours.

Details of the study

Eligibility included patients under 21 years of age with a range of intracranial malignancies. With the exception of brain stem glioma, this had to be histologically proven. A repeat biopsy was required if the relapse occurred more than 2 years from initial presentation. No more than one previous phase II study was allowed, neither was radiotherapy within 3 months, chemotherapy or increased dose of steroids within 6 weeks and no prior carboplatin or iproplatin. There had to be CT or MRI measurable disease, a predicted survival of at least 8 weeks and Karnofsky score >30. Other critieria were base line neutrophil count >1500/mm^3, platelets >100 000/mm^3 creatinine <1·2 mg/dl and bilirubin <1·5 mg/dl.

No details are given about the site of randomisation or the technique used. No predicted difference between the two groups is given or

Table 8.1 Response to therapy (PR/CR) in relation to histology

Histology	Carboplatin	Iproplatin
Low grade astocytoma	0/7	1/15
High grade astrocytoma	1/14	0/12
Medulloblastoma	1/15	1/14
Ependymoma	1/12	0/7
Brain stem glioma	0/14	0/14
Other	2/10	0/9

PR, partial remission; CR, complete remission.

anticipated numbers required. It is stated that randomisation was done mainly to document the comparative myelosuppression of the two agents. Patients were stratified by histology and prior cisplatin with regard to response analysis, and prior spinal irradiation with regard to toxicity.

Outcome

One hundred and seventy-one patients were enrolled. One with neuroblastoma was excluded, as were 30 who were non-assessable due to early, inadequate trial of chemotherapy, parental refusal or insufficient data.

The complete response/partial response rate with carboplatin was 9·5% ± 2·6% and with iproplatin, 6·3% ± 2·7%. No difference was seen in response rates in patients who had received cisplatin prior to carboplatin, whereas the response rate to iproplatin was higher in cisplatin naïve patients (20% versus 3% for those with prior therapy). Thirty-two per cent of patients had stable disease. Response by histological subtype for patients receiving carboplatin or iproplatin is shown in Table 8.1. Neutropenia was more marked with carboplatin – 20/83 v 4/88, $p = < 0.001$. No difference in thrombocytopenia and no difference in life-threatening sepsis was observed.

Conclusion

It was concluded that the drugs both had limited activity in this range of relapsed tumours and differed only with regard to toxic neutropenia.

9

Non-Hodgkin's lymphoma

Commentary – Tim Eden

It is difficult for the current practitioner to realise that before the mid 1970s the outcome for children with non-Hodgkin's lymphoma (unless they had truly localised disease treated with surgery and local radiation) was very poor. The use of pulsed chemotherapy with regimens such as CHOP yielded 5 year event free survival rates of 20% or less. The advent of truly intensive regimens for acute lymphoblastic leukaemia (ALL) protocols and their application to the non-Hodgkin's lymphomas (NHL) transformed the picture, not least the key study comparing the Sloan–Kettering intensive regimen LSA2-L2 with COMP (see Study 1 for details of regimens). Although Anderson *et al* reported the results in 1983, a dramatic change in survival was already evident in the late 1970s and spawned a series of other studies.

Identification by the CCSG group (Study 1, CCG-551) that patients with lymphoblastic disease fared better with the LSA2-L2 protocol whilst those with non-lymphoblastic disease fared better with COMP quite dramatically changed therapeutic approaches throughout the world. Suddenly there was a meaningful way in which to stratify treatment, although it is true to say that the argument as to how you should classify NHL and what constitutes adverse histological features has grumbled on to the present day (although in

paediatric practice there has been less dispute about classification and histology and less of an ability to write a book about the classification of classifications than has been the case in adult practice). The long term follow up from CCG-551 has confirmed the original finding.

Jenkin *et al.* reported in 1984 (Study 2) a follow up of the treatment of localised disease on CCG-551 showing no difference either in randomised or non-randomised patients between those who were treated either with COMP or LSA2-L2. Perhaps surprisingly in this series they had more deaths due to toxicity with COMP (3) than with LSA2-L2 (1), although 1 additional patient on the latter therapy developed a second malignancy. This report set the scene for attempts in localised disease to achieve comparable event free survival of 85–90% with least toxicity.

With the results of the CCG study looking favourable, at least at an early stage, the Pediatric Oncology Group (Study 3) conducted a randomised trial comparing LSA2-L2 with a regimen containing doxorubicin, vincristine, prednisolone, cyclophosphamide, intrathecal methotrexate and maintenance with the same drugs in addition to intravenous methotrexate and oral 6 mercaptopurine known as A-COP. This trial was for lymphoblastic lymphoma only and patients with stages I to III disease received 2 years of treatment and those with advanced disease, 3 years, more in line with the then current thinking on duration of therapy for ALL. Cranial irradiation was given in the first 2 years of the protocol and primary site radiation was given to patients with stage I and II disease and to residual sites at 4 weeks for those with stage III and IV disease with a variable radiation dose. There was a bias in the randomisation towards the A-COP protocol and only 85 patients were eligible for analysis. This A-COP protocol was much more intensive than COMP and gave comparable results to LSA2-L2. It is important to remember in both this and the original CCG-551 protocol that for stage IV disease event free survival was still very poor, the biggest advance being in stage III disease. But what would not be acceptable now was the use of adjuvant radiotherapy on top of such intensive chemotherapy. Of interest was the fact that patients with LSA2-L2 did not receive cranial irradiation, something that was generally ignored until almost two decades later, as was the truly remarkable event free survival of 93%, albeit from a small group of 15 patients with stage III disease treated on the intensive LSA2-L2 protocol.

The success of the LSA2-L2 protocol for lymphoblastic leukaemia had also led to a pilot study at Stanford Children's Hospital (Mott MG and Eden OB personal communication) which then resulted in the use of a modified LSA2-L2 protocol as the backbone of the UKCCSG T cell leukaemia/lymphoma study reported in Study 5. This study attempted to address in a limited number of centres whether adjuvant low dose irradiation, in particular 15 Gy delivered to the mediastinum, would carry any advantage over those treated with chemotherapy only. Forty-seven patients were randomised and the

study showed a highly significant benefit in favour of those receiving radiation (66% failure free survival for those who received radiation versus 18% who did not). This therapy was for T cell leukaemia and lymphoma but held up even if the leukaemic patients were excluded. Strangely the benefit for the radiotherapy appeared to be a reduction in frequency of spread to the bone marrow and/or CNS. This trial was run in parallel with a study by the remaining UKCCSG centres for all childhood non-Hodgkin's lymphoma which received a similar randomisation. Lymphoblastic disease treated either in the very intensive protocol or the standard protocol with or without irradiation was analysed. The benefit of local radiation was confirmed. The conclusion of the authors of those studies was that if more effective systemic chemotherapy had been given there would not be a requirement for irradiation, and of course that has proven true with more recent trial results, albeit in a non-randomised fashion.

Study 4 reported on a follow up study to CCG-551. Because of excess toxicity for those patients with localised disease receiving LSA2-L2 and given the fact that they appeared to have comparable outcome with COMP, after March 1979 patients with localised diseases were treated on CCG-551 with 18 months on COMP and after October 1979 there was a randomisation introduced to stop therapy at 6 or 18 months. The next study, which opened in 1982, continued the randomisation, although they did change one or two other items, particularly radiation doses and intrathecal therapy. It is always a pity if minor or apparently minor changes are made because one is never certain that they do not have an influence on the overall outcome and consequently it is wiser not to make ongoing small changes until a trial is concluded. As a result of an interim analysis in 1984, CCG actually removed lymphoblastic disease from this trial. Even with localised disease, such patients appeared to be faring adversely. The shortened therapy appeared to be adequate for all non-lymphoblastic patients, with a high event free and overall survival in excess of 90%. However, there were clearly defects in the trial apart from the minor changes that were brought about as the trial progressed, most notably a very low uptake for randomisation. Only 78 out of 115 patients/parents consented in CCG-551 and only 49 out of 99 in the subsequent CCG-501. It is always immensely difficult to get consent to trials with such a significant difference in length of treatment between arms of a trial. Details are not really included of the reasons for refusal. It would be interesting to note whether patients/parents or physicians opted for longer or shorter therapy since the standard arm had been 18 months previously.

Link *et al* reported in 1990 (Study 6) on their POG follow up study for children with localised NHL to address the question whether or not irradiation was required for such patients receiving a 6 week induction, 3 weeks of consolidation and 24 weeks of maintenance therapy. The irradiation was given during induction (27 Gy to the involved field, 15 Gy for abdominal tumours with a boost to the right lower quadrant and with any primary bone tumours receiving 37·5 Gy). This study showed comparable event free survival for those receiving chemotherapy alone and those receiving chemotherapy plus radiotherapy. This was the definitive study to confirm that for localised Murphy stage I and II lymphoma involved field irradiation was not required, particularly as it was associated with more severe toxicity. It also confirmed that 8 months of therapy was quite adequate for such tumours.

A further study reported by Link *et al* in 1997 (Study 10) tested whether a short 9 week regimen was adequate in patients with localised lymphoma. This study was conducted between 1983 and 1991 and was limited to Murphy stage I and II disease. The control arm was the same therapy given in their previous study for approximately 8 months. Randomisation was on a 2-to-1 basis to put more patients into the shorter therapy. The key finding was that for low stage disease with non-cleaved cell lymphoma and large cell lymphoma 9 weeks of therapy was found to be adequate. For lymphoblastic disease event free survival was poorer but overall salvage with further therapy appeared possible, yielding no significant overall survival difference between the two arms. The conclusion was clearly that for selected patients very short therapy based around a CHOP induction with a short duration of consolidation/maintenance including intrathecal therapy was quite adequate.

The Children's Cancer Study Group focused on lymphoblastic patients and reported (Study 8) on a study conducted between 1983 and 1990 (CCG-502 for lymphoblastic lymphoma) using the addition of daunorubicin and asparaginase to the basic COMP regimen, creating a protocol known as ADCOMP, and comparing that with the results of LSA2-L2. Both arms contained 18 months of therapy. Only patients with advanced disease had a more favourable outcome than previous reports, with an overall event free survival of 74% for LSA2-L2 and 64% for ADCOMP. Both arms were associated with toxic deaths but more on LSA2-L2 (3) compared with 1 on ADCOMP. There were 3 cases of secondary AML, all in the ADCOMP arm.

In 1987 the POG Group initiated a protocol (POG-8704) onto which they enrolled patients with advanced stage T cell lymphoma and leukaemia (Study 11). The important randomised question was whether patients would benefit from 12 weekly doses of high dose L-asparaginase (25 000 units per m^2 Im) during continuing therapy. There was perhaps a surprisingly significant benefit for the high dose asparaginase arm for those with ALL, and to a lesser degree those with non-Hodgkin's lymphoma. Of course, sadly the actual survival in the T-ALL group was poor at 30% (7 years) and around 50% for those with NHL. What was much more difficult to explain was an excess of second malignancies in the high dose asparaginase arm. This is an observation that still requires full clarification but has been seen in other non-randomised trials. Though lymphoblastic disease may be sensitive to a higher dose of asparaginase, it may carry with it this unusual and life threatening risk.

Some of the most successful studies, particularly in advanced stage B cell lymphoma and leukaemia, have been introduced by the French Paediatric Oncology Society in a series of studies some of which have not been randomised. The report by Patte referred to a study carried out between 1984 and 1987, building on their tremendously successful treatment for advanced stage B cell lymphomas (Study 7). This report refers only to patients with less than 25% bone marrow involvement and no CNS disease. Following cyto-reductive therapy with COP (two courses of CoPAdm and one course of CYM; for details see Table 9.1 in Study 7), patients were randomised between further CYM with either a short or long arm of maintenance. This was clearly another key study demonstrating that an intensive 4 month regimen was comparable to a longer 18 month course in advanced stage B cell NHL, which did not involve the CNS or more than 25% of blasts in the bone marrow. It laid the foundations for further subsequent reduction in therapy for other treatment groups.

Brecher *et al* reported in 1997 (Study 9) on a randomised trial from the Pediatric Oncology Group comparing a new "Total B" regimen which added doxorubicin along with fractionated cyclophosphamide to vincristine followed by cytosine and intravenous methotrexate in escalating dosages compared with a basic "best previous" regimen which consisted of cyclophosphamide, vincristine, prednisolone and methotrexate along with intrathecal therapy. Their more intensive protocol clearly demonstrated benefit in terms of event free survival.

In conclusion, in a small number of randomised trials since 1977 it has been confirmed that for non-Hodgkin's lymphoma: (1) therapy should be stratified by subtype; (2) lymphoblastic disease, whether it be low stage or more advanced, requires a different therapeutic approach and treatment more akin to that given to patients with acute lymphoblastic leukaemia; (3) localised non-lymphoblastic disease can be treated with short course pulsed therapy without adjuvant radiotherapy; (4) it is crucial to monitor for late sequelae, as exemplified by the excess of second malignancies in the long asparaginase arm of the POG-8704 protocol.

It is salutary to reflect upon the fact that it is only over the past decade or so that we have learnt that up to 15% of childhood NHL may consist of anaplastic large cell lymphomas and that we have only clearly been able to define them with the use of immunohistochemistry and molecular genetics (with the very characteristic KI-1 antigen positivity (CD30) and the presence of gene rearrangements involving the nucleolar phosphoprotein gene at 5q35 partnered with a range of protein kinase genes, commonly on chromosome 2 or 1). These patients appear to require rather different therapy but we are only now beginning to run the randomised trials to test for the truly optimal therapy for them. It is such a rare condition that international collaboration is clearly required. This has spurred an interest in running international trials also in lymphoblastic and non-lymphoblastic disease. Many of the answers to the questions that we have posed over the past 30 years could have been answered quicker if we had collaborated earlier and more enthusiastically. Only with large numbers in each trial, inclusion of all eligible patients, strict randomisation procedures and protocol compliance can results be trusted and applied more generally.

Studies (Review by A Davidson)

Study 1

Anderson JR, Wilson JF, Jenkin DT, Meadows AT, Kersey J, Chilc RR, Coccia P, Exelby P, Kushner J, Siegel S, Hammond GD.
Childhood non-Hodgkin's lymphoma. The results of a randomized therapeutic trial comparing a 4-drug regimen (COMP) with a 10-drug regimen (LSA2-L2).
N Engl J Med 1983;**308**:559–65.

This study was undertaken by the American Children's Cancer Study Group (CCSG) between 1977 and 1979 (CCG-551).

Objectives

The study compared two chemotherapy regimens and determined the influence of disease extent and histopathological subtype.

Details of the study

This was a multi-institutional prospective randomised trial. Initially, eligible patients were those aged less than 18 years with untreated, biopsy proven non-Hodgkin's lymphoma with no peripheral blood blasts and less than 25% blasts in the bone marrow, but after 5 months all patients with "undifferentiated" lymphoma regardless of peripheral blood blasts or bone marrow status were deemed eligible.

Staging investigations included clinical examination, bone marrow and CSF examination, chest X-ray, bone survey, intravenous pyelogram and radionuclide or CT scans of liver, spleen and bone. Localised disease was defined as a tumour limited anatomically either to a single extranodal site, with or without positive regional nodes, or to lymph nodes in one or two adjacent lymphatic regions. Grossly complete excision was required for tumours in the gastrointestinal system to be classed as localised. All other tumours (including mediastinal) were classified as non-localised.

The histopathological system of Rappaport was used and all specimens were reviewed by the study pathologist.

Randomisation was undertaken by phoning the Study Group's central office. Patients who met the eligibility criteria were assigned to one of the two treatments by means of an adaptive randomisation plan, to ensure a satisfactory balance of factors that were potentially important in the prognosis – namely, localised *v* nonlocalised, anatomic site, histology, bone marrow and CSF status and age above or under 13.

Interim analysis in 1979 showed no difference in outcome in those with localised disease treated on either regimen, but increased toxicity with LSA2-L2, and all patients with localised disease were thereafter assigned to COMP.

Predictions of expected difference or numbers required are not given in the study.

COMP (regimen 1) comprised induction therapy with 1·2 g/m^2 of cyclophosphamide, four doses of vincristine, intravenous methotrexate 300 mg/m^2 on day 12 and 4 weeks of oral prednisolone,

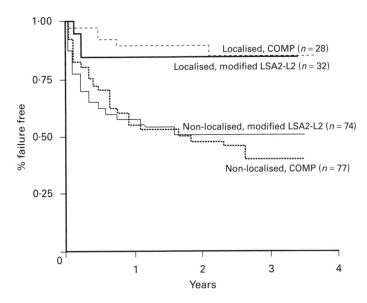

Figure 9.1 Failure free survival according to extent of disease at diagnosis and treatment regimen. Adapted with permission, 2002 from Anderson JR *et al*, *N Engl J Med* (full reference on p 194). Copyright © 1983 Massachusetts Medical Society.

with three doses of intrathecal methotrexate. Subsequent maintenance courses comprised 1 g/m² cyclophosphamide, with two doses of vincristine, 5 days prednisolone, one IT methotrexate and one IV methotrexate.

Modified LSA2-L2 (regimen 2) employed a similar induction regimen, but with the addition of daunorubicin at day 15/16. The major difference was in the addition of a consolidation phase, using cytarabine, 6-TG (thioguanine), asparaginase and carmustine, and more complex maintenance cycles, including cyclophosphamide, 6-TG, hydroxyurea, daunomycin, methotrexate, carmustine, cytarabine, vincristine and two doses of IT methotrexate.

Both regimens lasted for 18 months.

The same schedule of radiation was used in all patients. The objective was to irradiate all tissue volumes that were the sites of bulk disease (> 3 cm). Localised disease confined to lymph nodes was irradiated to 30 Gy with a 3 cm margin. Bulk disease (e.g. whole abdomen) was irradiated to 20 Gy. Radiation treatment was initiated during induction. Central nervous system radiation was used only for patients with CNS disease at presentation or in those suffering a CNS relapse within 6 months of commencing treatment.

The primary outcome measure was failure free survival (FFS). Adverse events comprised no response by the end of induction, a relapse of any kind and death. The product limit method was used to estimate the distribution of failure free survival and of overall survival. The statistical

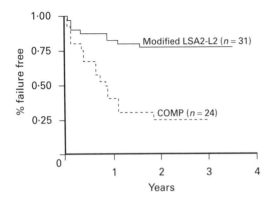

Figure 9.2 Failure free survival according to treatment regimen in patients with non-localised disease and lymphoblastic lymphoma only. Adapted with permission, 2002 from Anderson JR *et al, N Engl J Med* (full reference on p 194). Copyright © 1983 Massachuzetts Medical Society.

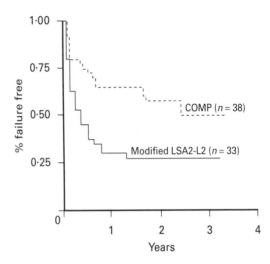

Figure 9.3 Failure free survival according to treatment regimen in patients with non-localised disease and non-lymphoblastic lymphoma only. Adapted with permission, 2002 (as with Figure 9.2)

significance of observed difference in FFS was assessed with the log-rank test.

Outcome

Two hundred and thirty-four eligible patients entered the study, of whom 23 were not randomised but treated according to an assigned regimen, including the 11 patients with localised disease who were assigned to COMP treatment after the interim analysis. These 11 were not included in the comparison of treatment regimens. Specimens from 25 patients were not reviewed by the study pathologist, and were not analysed in the comparisons of treatment regimens within histopathological groups. Median follow up for patients who had not had any adverse events was 28 months.

About one-third of patients had localised disease, and 34% were classified as lymphoblastic,

51% as undifferentiated Burkitt or non-Burkitt lymphoma, and 14% as histiocytic.

Sixty patients with localised disease were randomly assigned to treatment: 28 received COMP, 32 received modified LSA2-L2. Two year failure free survival was 89% and 84% respectively (p > 0·50) (Figure 9.1).

One hundred and fifty-one patients with non-localised disease were randomly assigned to a treatment group: 77 received COMP and 74 modified LSA2-L2. Overall results did not differ according to regimen, with 24 month FFS being 47% and 50% respectively (p > 0·50).

Significant differences were found only when treatments were compared within histopathological subgroups in patients with non-localised disease. Patients with lymphoblastic lymphoma had a significantly higher FFS at 24 months when treated with LSA2-L2 (76%) than when treated with COMP (26%) (p = 0·0002) (Figure 9.2). However, the opposite was true with non-lymphoblastic disease (including histiocytic as well as undifferentiated). FFS at 24 months for non-lymphoblastic disease was 57% for those treated with COMP compared with 28% for those treated with LSA2-L2 (p = 0·008) (Figure 9.3).

Further analyses of this group according to whether or not patients with non-localised disease had CNS or bone marrow involvement seemed to show that patients with lymphoblastic disease benefited from treatment with LSA2-L2 regardless of whether or not there was CNS/BM involvement, although the number of patients in this category was very small. Seven patients with CNS/BM involvement treated with LSA2-L2 had FFS of 71%, compared to 6 patients treated with COMP who had FFS of 0% (p = 0·01). However, COMP treatment benefited only those patients with non-lymphoblastic disease without CNS/BM involvement. For this group the FFS was 29% with LSA2-L2 ($n = 7$) and 33% with COMP ($n = 6$).

CNS relapse was rare and equally distributed between the two treatments.

Toxicity

There were 9 toxic deaths, equally distributed between the two regimens. Haematological toxicity was more common with LSA2-L2, although precise data were not presented.

Conclusion

It was concluded that for non-localised NHL LSA2-L2 was more effective than COMP for the lymphoblastic subtype and the opposite was the case for diffuse undifferentiated NHL. This was a "landmark" study demonstrating the importance of treating NHL according to histopathological subtype. However, follow up was relatively short, especially as late relapse is relatively more common in lymphoblastic disease compared with non-lymphoblastic disease.

Comment

A follow-up analysis of patients on CCG-551 was also reported:

Anderson JR, Jenkin DT, Wilson JF, Kjeldsberg CR, Spasto R, Chilcote RR, Coccia PF, Exelby PR, Siegel S, Meadows AT, Hammond GD. Long-term follow-up of patients treated with COMP or LSA$_2$L$_2$ therapy for childhood non-Hodgkin's lymphoma: a report of CCG-551 from the Children's Cancer Group. *J Clin Oncol* 1993;**11**:1024–32.

Event free survival of patients with localised disease was 84% at 5 years. No differences were noted between the two regimens. For disseminated disease, outcome was dependent on histological subtype. Patients with lymphoblastic lymphoma did better when treated with LSA$_2$L$_2$; 5 years EFS 64% *v* 35% for COMP. COMP produced better results for those with undifferentiated lymphoma: 5 year EFS 50% *v* 29%. In large cell lymphoma, results were similar: 5 year EFS of 52% for COMP, *v* 43% for LSA$_2$L$_2$.

Study 2

Jenkin RD, Anderson JR, Chilcote RR, Coccia PF, Exelby PR, Kersey JH, Kushner JH, Meadows AT, Siegel SE, Sposto R, Wilson JF, Hammond GD.
The treatment of localised non-Hodgkin's lymphoma in children: a report from the Children's Cancer Study Group.
J Clin Oncol 1984;**2**:88–99.

This was a collaborative group prospective randomised study which ran between 1977 and 1979.

Objectives

The study looked at the outcome of children with localised disease treated on CCG-551, and compared a 4 drug regimen (COMP) with the 10 drug LSA2-L2.

Details of the study

Eligible patients for CCG-551 were those aged less than 21 years with previously untreated non-Hodgkin's lymphoma, provided there were less than 25% blasts. Localised disease was defined as

1   Disease limited to a single extranodal site, with or without regional lymph node involvement.
2   Disease limited to one or two adjacent nodal regions.
3   Gastrointestinal disease was only defined as localised if a grossly complete surgical excision had been achieved.

Mediastinal disease was excluded, as were patients with Murphy stage II disease at more than two adjacent nodal sites, or those with disease at more than one extranodal site.

Central histology review was undertaken.

Randomisation was undertaken by phoning the study group's central office. A method of adaptive randomisation was employed to balance patient numbers with regard to localised versus non-localised disease, anatomical site of origin, institutional histological classification and age over or under 13 years. Following an interim analysis, randomisation for patients with localised disease was discontinued because of increased toxicity for those patients treated with LSA2-L2 regimen, and from March 1979 all patients with localised disease were treated with COMP.

Treatment was for 18 months on both regimens. Details were given in Study 1. Statistical predictions were not performed.

The primary outcome measure was relapse free survival.

Outcome

Of the total of 240 patients entered, 73 had localised disease. Follow up at the time of publication was 29–63 months, median 48 months.

Sixty patients were randomised. Two patients received COMP (investigators' choice) and 11 were electively given COMP after the protocol amendment discontinuing randomisation.

Overall event free survival by treatment regimen was 85% for COMP and 84% for LSA2-L2 (including non-randomised patients).

Outcome according to histology is shown in Figure 9.4.

The analysis of the subsets of patients for prognostic factors not fruitful. Overall analysis

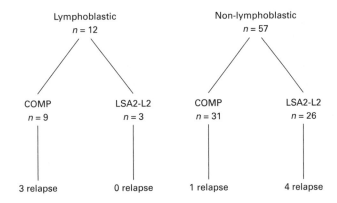

Figure 9.4

of relapse free survival rates by age, sex, site and treatment regimen gave no significant differences.

Toxicity

There were 4 toxic deaths, 3 with COMP and 1 with LSA2-L2. One patients who received LSA2-L2 developed a second malignancy.

Conclusion

It was concluded that the overall results were good and outcome did not appear to be influenced by the regimen used.

Study 3

Hvizdala EV, Berard C, Callihan T, Falleta J, Sabio H, Shuster JJ, Sullivan M, Wharam MD. Lymphoblastic lymphoma in children – a randomised trial comparing LSA2-L2 with the A-COP therapeutic regimen: a Pediatric Oncology Group Study.
J Clin Oncol 1988;**6**:26–33.

This study was undertaken by the Pediatric Oncology Group (POG) between the years of 1979 and 1983 (POG-7905).

Objectives

The study addressed the comparative efficacy of a 6 drug regimen, A-COP, with the 10 drug, modified LSA2-L2.

Details of the study

The study was conducted as a collaborative group multi-institutional prospective randomised trial.

The original design employed a stratification for histology, but did not plan for stratum specific analysis. However, following publication of the results of another study (CCG-551), this design was made obsolete, leading to a complete separation of the lymphoblastic and non-lymphoblastic patients. A second major change occurred when patients were retrospectively staged according to the Murphy system. For the first two years the randomisation was weighted 3:1 in favour of A-COP (regimen I), as the LSA2-L2 (regimen II) was identical to a previous study, but this was then discontinued.

Eligible patients were those aged less than 21 years with untreated biopsy proven lymphoblastic lymphoma. Specimens underwent central pathological review and were classified according to the system of Rappaport.

The randomisation method is not described and statistical predictions were not performed.

Both treatment regimens lasted 2 years for patients with stages I–III disease and 3 years for stage IV disease. The ACOP regimen comprised induction with doxorubicin, vincristine, prednisolone, cyclophosphamide, intrathecal methotrexate and maintenance with the same drugs, in addition to intravenous methotrexate and oral 6 mercaptopurine. Cranial radiation was only given to patients receiving A-COP. Primary site radiation was given in both regimens to stage I and II disease, and to residual sites at 4 weeks for those with stage III/IV disease. The dose for regimen I was 21 Gy compared with 30 Gy for regimen II.

The primary outcome measure was disease free survival.

Outcome

Eighty-five patients with histologically confirmed lymphoblastic lymphoma were entered. Eleven had localised (stage I and II) disease, 56 had stage III and 18 had stage IV. Fifty were randomised to A-COP and 35 to LSA2-L2. Nine patients were non-evaluable (failure to follow randomisation in 2, major protocol violation in 6, and inadequate data, in 1).

Overall DFS for A-COP was 53% (SE 8%) and 58% (SE 10%) for LSA2-L2 at 3 years. This was not statistically significant.

For stage IV disease, 3 year EFS was 14% and 12% respectively; in stage III, 93% and 54% (15/33 failures compared to 2/15; p = 0·055).

There was no increase in CNS relapse rates in the LSA2-L2 group who did not receive cranial radiation.

Toxicity

Induction toxicity was greater with regimen LSA2-L2, with 3 life threatening sepsis episodes compared to none with ACOP. Maintenance therapy toxicity was comparable, although there were 2 remission deaths due to infection on ACOP.

There were also 2 deaths from cardiotoxicity in the A-COP group.

Conclusion

It was concluded that, unlike COMP, the more intensive regimen A-COP was comparable to LSA2-L2 for lymphoblastic NHL. There appeared to be an advantage with LSA2-L2 for stage III disease, although numbers were too small to confirm this statistically.

Study 4

Meadows AT, Sposto R, Jenkin RD, Kersey JH, Chilcote RR, Siegel SE, Coccia PF, Rosenstock J, Pringle KC, Stolar CJ, Kadin ME, Hammond GD. Similar efficacy of 6 and 18 months of therapy with four drugs (COMP) for localized non-Hodgkin's lymphoma of children: a report from the Children's Cancer Study Group. *J Clin Oncol* 1989;**7**:92–9.

This study was undertaken between the years 1979 and 1986 by the Children's Cancer Study Group (CCSG).

Objectives

The study addressed the question whether a shortened duration of therapy (6 months) was sufficient for localised non-Hodgkin's lymphoma.

Details of the study

The study design entailed the randomisation of patients in two consecutive CCSG NHL studies, CCG-551 and CCG-501.

The CCG-551 study had originally randomised all NHL patients between COMP and LSA2-L2. Because of excess toxicity for patients with localised disease receiving LSA2-L2, from March 1979 all those with localised disease were allocated to 18 months of COMP. From October 1979 these patients were randomised between discontinuing therapy after 6 and 18 months therapy. The follow on study, CCG-501, opened in 1982, with slight modifications with respect to intrathecal and radiation doses but continuing randomisation between 6 and 18 months therapy with the same eligibility criteria. In 1984 a preliminary analysis suggested that those with lymphoblastic histology were doing less well and these were excluded from entry.

Eligible patients were those under the age of 21 years with localised disease, defined as no more than two lymph node regions on one side of the diaphragm, or a single primary site with or without regional node involvement. For abdominal disease, only those with a grossly complete excision were included. External review of the histology was undertaken and the classification was based on the system of Rappaport.

Patients were randomised after five cycles of maintenance therapy using an unstratified randomisation.

Primary endpoints were event free survival (EFS) and survival. Analysis of EFS was based only on patients accepting randomisation, whilst the analysis of overall survival included patients who electively continued or discontinued. Plots of survival and EFS were derived from the product-limit (Kaplan–Meier) estimate, and based on a one-sided log-rank test with 10% type I error. The power to detect a 10% decrease in EFS 2 years after randomisation was estimated to be > 75%. Statistical predications of numbers of patients required are not given in the study.

COMP treatment was detailed in Study 1. CCG-501 included minor modifications in the dosage and timing of intrathecal methotrexate doses and omitted IT chemotherapy for patients with localised abdominal disease. The radiation guidelines were modified, reducing the margin from 3 to 2 cm, and the dose to 15 Gy to the abdomen and 20 Gy to other areas.

Outcome

A total of 241 patients with localised NHL were registered. Nine were excluded on the basis of ineligibility: 3 were not localised, 3 were not classified as having NHL on pathological review and 3 who were diagnosed after 1984 with lymphoblastic histology were electively treated with LSA2-L2.

One hundred and thirty patients were registered on CCG-551, of whom 11 had an event before completing six cycles and 4 discontinued prior to completing six cycles at either parents' or physician's preference. Of 115 patients eligible for randomisation, 78 consented. For the CCG-501 study, 102 eligible patients were registered, of whom 2 had an event prior to completing six cycles, and 1 electively stopped treatment prior to completing 6 months' therapy. Of 99 eligible for randomisation, 49 consented.

Of the total randomised patients ($n = 127$), 12 had lymphoblastic histology and 115 non-lymphoblastic.

For the patients with non-lymphoblastic histology, 104 of the 115 patients followed the assigned length of treatment and results were presented for these patients (rather than on an intention to treat basis). There was no difference in EFS for those randomised to receive 6 months' treatment (EFS 95%) compared with those randomised to 18 months' treatment (EFS 98%).

Overall survival from diagnosis for patients with NHL treated on CCG-551 (median follow-up 60 months) was 91%.

For patients with lymphoblastic histology, because of small numbers, it was not possible to compare the efficacy of the two different lengths of treatment. Overall survival from diagnosis for patients with lymphoblastic disease treated on CCG-551 was less than 70% (i.e. 11/15 patients alive).

No details of toxicity are given in the study.

Conclusion

It was concluded that 6 months of therapy for patients with non-lymphoblastic localised lymphoma is sufficient.

Study 5

Mott MG, Chessells JM, Willoughby ML, Mann JR, Morris-Jones PH, Malpas JS, Palmer MK.
Adjuvant low dose radiation in childhood T cell leukaemia/ lymphoma.
Br J Cancer 1984;**50**:457–62.

The study was carried out by the United Kingdom Children's Cancer Study Group (UKCCSG)

between 1977 and 1983. Six centres within the UKCCSG contributed patients to the study.

Objectives

This study determined whether 15 Gy mediastinal radiation was necessary in the treatment of T cell leukaemia/lymphoma.

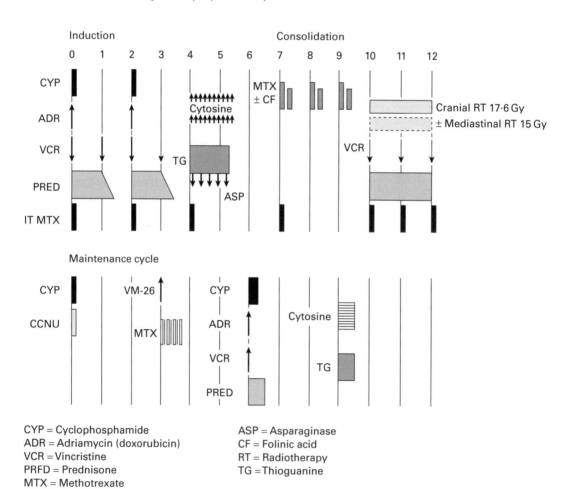

CYP = Cyclophosphamide
ADR = Adriamycin (doxorubicin)
VCR = Vincristine
PRFD = Prednisone
MTX = Methotrexate

ASP = Asparaginase
CF = Folinic acid
RT = Radiotherapy
TG = Thioguanine

Figure 9.5 Treatment schema: T cell protocol. Adapted and reprinted from Mott MG *et al, Br J Cancer* with permission from Nature Publishing Group (full reference above).

Details of the study

Eligible patients were those with localised or non-localised T cell lymphoma or T cell leukaemia with mediastinal disease.

It is not clear at what point patients were randomised to receive or not receive mediastinal radiation, but this appears to have been at the completion of successful induction treatment.

The chemotherapy was a complex multiagent regimen (Figure 9.5) including induction, consolidation and 2 years maintenance therapy.

All patients received cranial radiation therapy, 17·6 Gy. Patients were randomly assigned to receive 15 Gy to the mediastinum irrespective of whether there was a mediastinal mass at diagnosis.

The method of randomisation is not detailed and statistical predictions are not given.

Outcome measures were survival and failure free survival (FFS).

Outcome

Eighty-two patients were entered on the study, of whom 57 had more than 25% lymphoblasts in the bone marrow and or peripheral blood blasts and were classified as having T leukaemia. Twenty-five were designated as having T lymphoma.

There were 27 patients who presented with a mediastinal mass.

The overall FFS for patients with T leukaemia was 27%. FFS for patients with T lymphoma treated was 40%.

Forty-seven of 52 successfully completed induction and were randomised to receive or not

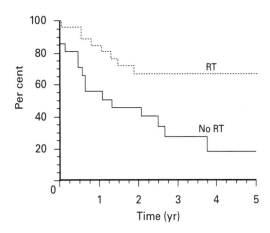

Figure 9.6 Failure free survival for T lymphoma patients randomised ± mediastinal radiation (RT). Adapted and reprinted from Mott MG *et al, Br J Cancer* with permission from Nature Publishing Group (full reference p 204).

receive mediastinal radiation. There was a highly significant difference in favour of those randomised to receive radiation (FFS 66% *v* 18%, p = 0·01) (Figure 9.6).

The difference remained significant when patients with T leukaemia were included (FFS 51% *v* 21%, p = 0·01).

Conclusion

Review of the first adverse events showed that the major differences in the two arms of the trial were in the frequency of spread to the bone marrow and/or CNS, and in the late occurrence of relapse in the non-irradiated patients. There were three patients randomised to receive radiation before completion of induction who then had early adverse events, but even when these patients were excluded from the analysis the difference between the two arms of the trial remained significant. It is suggested by the authors that the benefit observed from radiation would not have been seen if given in conjunction with more effective systemic chemotherapy.

A second paper describes all 120 children with T and B NHL in the same study showing no difference for non-mediastinal primary disease.

Mott MG, Eden OB, Palmer MK. Adjuvant low dose radiation in Childhood non Hodgkin's lumphoma. *Br J Cancer* 1984;**50**: 463–9.

Study 6

Link MP, Donaldson SS, Costan WB, Shuster JJ, Murphy SB.
Results of treatment of childhood localized non-Hodgkin's lymphoma with combination chemotherapy with or without radiotherapy.
N Engl J Med 1990;**322**:1169–74.

This study was undertaken by the Pediatric Oncology Group (POG) between 1983 and 1987.

Objectives

The study addressed the question of whether or not irradiation of primary involved sites could be safely omitted from the treatment of children with localised NHL. Additionally, treatment duration was shorter than in previously described regimens.

Details of the study

This was a multicentre, prospective randomised trial. Eligibility criteria were previously untreated patients aged under 21 years with biopsy proven non-Hodgkin's lymphoma, categorised as either Murphy stage I or II. Histology was reviewed by a panel of pathologists. Staging investigations included clinical evaluation, FBC, bone marrow aspirate, CSF examination, chest *x* ray, bone scan and CT scan in children with head and neck tumours or intra-abdominal disease.

Randomisation was performed by phoning the statistical office of the POG.

It was calculated that in order to detect a 10% improvement in EFS after 2 years, assuming an accrual rate of 80 patients per year, a power of 80%, and a one-sided p value of 5%, 127 patients were required. Because of the rarity of the disease this number of patients was deemed to be unachievable within an acceptable time frame and therefore a reduced power for the study was accepted.

The primary endpoints were event free survival (EFS) and overall survival (OS). Adverse events were defined as failure to achieve remission, relapse, death or a second malignancy.

Treatment consisted of a four drug, 6 week induction, including vincristine, cyclophosphamide, doxorubicin and prednisolone, followed by a 6 week consolidation using the same drugs, and 24 weeks of maintenance with mercaptopurine and methotrexate. CNS treatment comprised three doses of intrathecal methotrexate during induction, with further doses during maintenance only for those with head and neck tumours. For those assigned to receive radiation treatment, this commenced during induction, and comprised 27 Gy to the involved field. Abdominal tumours received 15 Gy whole abdominal radiation with a boost to the right lower quadrant. Primary bone tumours were all treated with 37·5 Gy to the involved bone.

Outcome

The study registered 144 patients, of whom 7 were ineligible following review, 2 because the diagnosis of NHL could not be confirmed and 5 because the staging definitions of localised disease could not be satisfied. Seven patients had primary bone disease and were not randomised. An additional patient was not randomised in error, leaving 129 eligible randomised patients. Three patients who were assigned to received chemotherapy plus radiation but who did not comply, receiving chemotherapy alone, were analysed on the arm to which they were allocated.

Twenty-one patients had lymphoblastic disease, 72 had small non-cleaved cell and 27, large cell.

All patients achieved complete remission at the end of induction.

Projected EFS at 4 years was 87·9 ± 8·8% for patients receiving chemotherapy alone and 87·3 ± 9·4% for those receiving chemotherapy plus radiotherapy.

There were 7 treatment failures in each group. These were all relapses in the chemo-therapy group, but in the combined therapy group there were 5 relapses, 1 toxic death and 1 acute myeloid leukaemia. Five of the

21 patients with lymphoblastic disease suffered a relapse, compared with 6 of the 72 with small non-cleaved cell.

Toxicity
Haematological toxicity was more severe in the combined group (36% severe neutropenia) than in the chemotherapy group (15% severe neutropenia)

Conclusion
Involved field radiation therapy is unnecessary for localised Murphy's stage I/II lymphoma. A shorter duration of therapy seems to cure the majority of children.

Study 7

Patte C, Philip T, Rodary C, Zucker J-M, Behrendt H, Gentet J-C, Lamagnere J-P, Otten J, Dufillot D, Pein F, Caillou B, Lemerle J.
High survival rate in advanced-stage B-cell lymphomas and leukemias without CNS involvement with a short intensive polychemotherapy: results from the French Paediatric Oncology Society of a randomized trial of 216 children.
J Clin Oncol 1991;**9**:123–32.

The study was organised by the French Paediatric Oncology Society (SFOP) between 1984 and 1987.

Objectives
The study addressed the possibility of reducing the length of treatment with multiagent chemotherapy from 7 months to 4 months.

Details of the study

Eligibility included patients 17 years or younger, with B cell lymphoma, defined by surface immunoglobulin positivity in addition to B cell antigen positivity. In the absence of immunophenotyping, only Burkitt or diffuse small non-cleaved lymphoma or lymphoma arising in the bowel were included. "Advanced" disease comprised Murphy stage III and IV without CNS involvement. Patients with more than 25% bone marrow or CNS disease were eligible for a more intensive regimen, LMB 86. Patients with extensive nasopharyngeal or facial stage II tumours were also included. Pre-treatment specimens were reviewed by a panel of pathologists and cytologists. Bone marrow evaluation consisted of at least two iliac crest bone marrow aspirates.

Randomisation was performed centrally at the Institut Gustave-Roussy. Patients were randomised after completion of CYM1, i.e. the third intensive induction course, when in first complete remission. Two arms were balanced in blocks of four and were stratified to take into account both stage and institution (Figure 9.7).

A sequential stopping rule was planned in order to detect an increase in the 9 month relapse rate from 5% to 25% (α error 10%, β error 5%). The 18 month EFS for patients in complete remission after the third induction course and receiving the long treatment was estimated to be equal to 90% in the previous study (LMB 81). The null hypothesis of inequivalence to be tested was whether short treatment reduced by 15% or more the 18 month EFS. A sample size of 75 patients in each group was required (α 5%, β 15%). Two successive analyses were planned: the first when the last patient was included, and the final one 18 months later. The upper limit of a one-sided 95% confidence interval for the difference between the 15 month EFS rate was calculated using the nominal significance levels of 5% and 4·8% respectively for the first and second analysis, necessary to achieve a 5% overall significance level. If this observed confidence limit was less than 15%, one could assume the two arms were equivalent.

The outline chemotherapy is given in Table 9.1. along with the drug doses in each arm.

The primary outcome measure was event free survival at 18 months.

Outcome

Two hundred and sixteen patients were registered, aged 6 months to 17 years, median 5·5 years. One

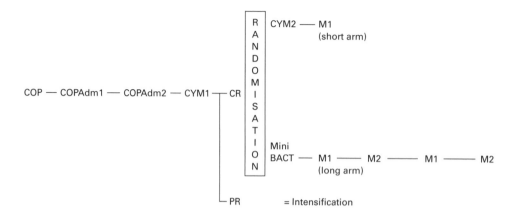

Figure 9.7 Schema of protocol LMB 84 (for abbreviations and details of chemotherapy see Table 9.1)

hundred and seventy-two patients were male. Sixty patients were of North African origin and 9 from other countries. Fifteen had stage II disease, 167 stage III and 34 stage IV, of whom 20 had more than 25% blasts in the bone marrow.

Two hundred and two patients achieved a complete remission, and of these 192 had received the planned initial treatment. In 3 cases CR was achieved with treatment modified due to toxicity, and 7 who were in PR at time of CYM1 achieved subsequent CR with intensified treatment. Fourteen patients failed to achieve CR and they all died. Of the 192 patients who received the planned protocol, 166 were randomised, 84 to the long arm and 82 to the short arm. Of the 26 not randomised, in 4 this was due to early toxic death and in 4 to early disease relapse. The variety of other reasons are also defined. Four African patients were lost to subsequent follow up.

In the randomised group, the overall survival and EFS at 18 months were 90 ± 4% and 89 ± 3% in the short arm and 89 ± 4% and 87 ± 4% respectively for the long arm. Numbers were insufficient to perform subgroup analysis on the basis of stage. For stage IV the EFS was not significantly different if there were less or more than 25% blasts in the bone marrow, 71% and 65% respectively. In the short study arm all 8 deaths occurred after a relapse, in the long arm 7 died after a relapse and 3 in first CR (one sepsis, one after sternal marrow puncture and one with EBV infection). The final analysis carried out in March 1989 showed the upper confidence limit of the observed difference between the 18 month EFS (87% and 89% respectively) for the long and short arm was 6%. This was, therefore, less than the 15% value fixed a priori. A comparison between the two proportions of failures (9 of 80 v 11 of 82 respectively for the short and long arm) according to the null hypothesis of inequivalence was significant (one-sided $p < 0.001$). The equivalence between the two arms was therefore concluded.

Conclusion

This study demonstrates that a short intensive 4 month regimen produces excellent event free survival in advanced B cell NHL and provided the basis for subsequent randomisations with further reduction of treatment intensity.

Table 9.1 LMB-84 chemotherapy regimens

COP	Cyclophosphamide 300 mg/m^2, vincristine 1·5 mg/m,^{2} prednisolone 2 mg/kg/d × 7, IT methotrexate/hydrocortisone
COPAdm 1	Cyclophosphamide 500 mg/m^2/d × 3, doxorubicin 60 mg/m^2, vincristine 1·5 mg/m^2, prednisolone 2 mg/kg/d × 7, IT methotrexate/hydrocortisone × 2, methotrexate 3 g/m^2 + folinic acid rescue
COPAdm 2	As for COPAdm1 but vincristine added on day 6 and cyclophosphamide dose increased to 1 g/m^2/d × 3
CYM	Methotrexate 3 g/m^2 + folinic acid rescue, cytarabine 100 mg/m^2 continuous infusion × 5 d, IT cytarabine/hydrocortisone
Mini BACT	CCNU 60 mg/m^2, cytarabine 100 mg/m^2/d × 5, 6 thioguanine 150 mg/m^2/d × 5 cyclophosphamide 500 mg/m^2/d × 3
M1	Vincristine 1·5 mg/m^2, methotrexate 3 g/m^2 + folinic acid rescue, prednisolone 2 mg/kg × 5, cyclophosphamide 500 mg/m^2/ d × 2, IT methotrexate/hydrocortisone
M2	CCNU 60 mg/m^2, cytarabine 100 mg/m^2/d × 4 subcutaneously, 6 thioguanine 150 mg/m^2/d × 4, IT cytarabine/hydrocortisone

Study 8

Tubergen DG, Krailo MD, Meadows AT, Rosenstock J, Kadin M, Morse M, King D, Steinherz PG, Kersey JH.

Comparison of treatment regimens for pediatric lymphoblastic non-Hodgkin's lymphoma: a Children's Cancer Study Group study.

J Clin Oncol 1995;**13**:1368–76;

The study ran between the years of 1983 and 1990 was undertaken by the Children's Cancer Study Group (CCSG), and was a collaborative group prospective randomised study (CCG-502).

Objectives

This study determined whether in lymphoblastic lymphoma the addition of daunorubicin and asparaginase to the basic COMP regimen (ADCOMP), would improve or at least equal the results achieved with modified LSA2-L2, but with lower toxicity.

Details of the study

The study was open to newly diagnosed patients with lymphoblastic NHL aged less than 22 years with 25% or less lymphoblasts in bone marrow aspirate. Marrow involvement up to 5% was defined as M1, whilst marrow involvement of 5–25% was defined as M2. Central review of histology was undertaken. A diagnosis of lymphoblastic histology was made when there was a monotonous population of medium sized cells, with sparse cytoplasm, irregular, often convoluted nuclear membrane, fine delicate chromatin and small nucleoli. Immunophenotyping was performed if there was sufficient material.

Randomisation was performed separately for each of five groups defined by presentation:

1 Localised disease.
2 Disseminated disease without mediastinal involvement with M1 bone marrow.
3 Disseminated disease without mediastinal involvement with M2 marrow.
4 Disseminated disease with mediastinal disease with M1 marrow.
5 Disseminated disease with mediastinal disease with M2 marrow.

Localised disease was defined as:

1 Completely grossly resected gastrointestinal disease.
2 Waldeyer's ring with/without cervical and or supraclavicular disease.
3 Single extralymphatic site with/without regional node involvement.
4 Nodal disease limited to a single or two adjacent lymphatic regions.
5 Exclusions – mediastinal, bone, bone marrow, CNS involvement.

The study was designed to accrue sufficient patients to detect a twofold decrease in the failure rate associated with LSA2-L2 as compared with the ADCOMP regimen with probability 0·80 when using a two-sided log-rank test at the 0·05 level of significance.

Treatment details of modified LSA2-L2 were given in Study 1 (Anderson *et al*).

ADCOMP added daunorubicin at day 16 to the basic COMP induction, and 9 doses of asparaginase also commencing at day 16. "Maintenance" COMP cycles added daunorubicin at 30 mg/m². Both regimens lasted for a minimum of 18 months and included radiation therapy to areas of bulk disease greater than 3 cm diameter either in the mediastinum or elsewhere, beginning on day 5 of induction therapy.

The primary outcome measure was event free survival (EFS). The duration of EFS was from entry on to the study to disease progression, death in remission, occurrence of a second neoplasm, or last contact. Plots of estimated survivor functions were constructed using the method of Kaplan–Meier, and treatment comparisons made using the stratified log-rank test. Analyses were performed according to intent to treat.

Outcome

Three hundred and seven patients were entered, of whom 26 were excluded. In 19 this was following histopathological review. Six patients were not randomised and one who was not entered had more than 25% lymphoblasts in the bone marrow. Twenty-eight patients had localised disease. One hundred and forty-four specimens had immunophenotyping performed locally, showing a T cell phenotype in 79%, B cell in 5% and null cell in 17%.

The overall 5 year EFS was 74% for LSA2-L2 and 64% for ADCOMP (p = 0·17). When analysed according to the extent of disease groupings, there was no difference by treatment group, except in those with the most advanced disease, i.e. mediastinal disease and a M2 marrow, who had fewer relapses with LSA2-L2 (3/12) than on the ADCOMP therapy (8/11) (p = 0·026).

Toxicity

Toxicity was moderately severe on both regimens. There were 4 toxic deaths, 3 with LSA2-L2 and 1 with ADCOMP. There were 3 cases of AML, all in ADCOMP patients.

Conclusion

The addition of daunorubicin and asparaginase to COMP therapy for patients with lymphoblastic lymphoma did not result in a more effective treatment than LSA2-L2.

Study 9

Brecher ML, Schwenn MR, Coppes MJ, Bowman WP, Link MP, Costan WB, Shuster JJ, Murphy SB.

Fractionated cyclophosphamide and back to back high dose methotrexate and cytosine arabinoside improves outcome in patients with stage III high grade small non-cleaved cell lymphomas: a randomised trial of the Pediatric Oncology Group. *Med Ped Oncol* 1997;**29**:526–33.

This was a multicentre prospective randomised trial undertaken by the American Pediatric

Oncology Group (POG) between 1986 and 1991 (POG-8616.)

Objectives

The study addressed the question of whether the "Total B" regimen, which had been reported to give encouraging results in a single institution study, would prove superior when compared in a prospective randomised fashion against the group's previous best standard therapy, protocol 8106.

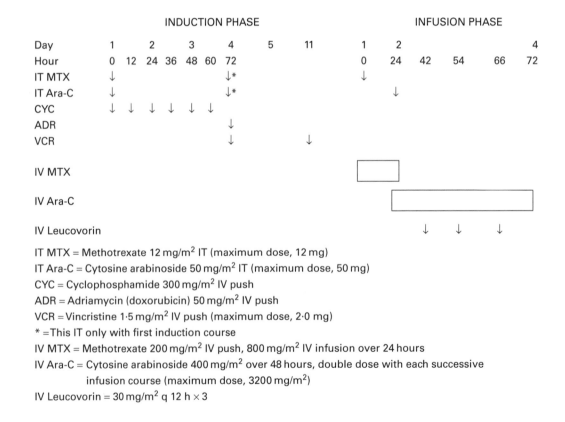

IT MTX = Methotrexate 12 mg/m^2 IT (maximum dose, 12 mg)
IT Ara-C = Cytosine arabinoside 50 mg/m^2 IT (maximum dose, 50 mg)
CYC = Cyclophosphamide 300 mg/m^2 IV push
ADR = Adriamycin (doxorubicin) 50 mg/m^2 IV push
VCR = Vincristine 1·5 mg/m^2 IV push (maximum dose, 2·0 mg)
* = This IT only with first induction course
IV MTX = Methotrexate 200 mg/m^2 IV push, 800 mg/m^2 IV infusion over 24 hours
IV Ara-C = Cytosine arabinoside 400 mg/m^2 over 48 hours, double dose with each successive
 infusion course (maximum dose, 3200 mg/m^2)
IV Leucovorin = 30 mg/m^2 q 12 h × 3

Figure 9.8 Regimen B chemotherapy

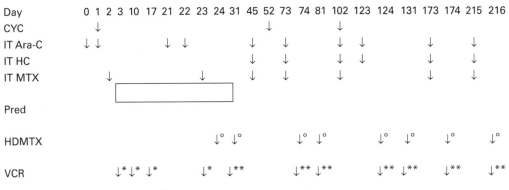

IT MTX = Methotrexate 15 mg/m² IT (maxmimum dose 15 mg)

IT HC = Hydrocortisone 30 mg/m² IT (no maximum dose)

IT Ara-C = Cytosine arabinoside 60 mg/m² IT (45 mg/m² during induction) (no maximum dose)

Pred = Prednisone 60 mg/m² PO (maximum 60 mg)

CYC = Cyclophosphamide 1200 mg/m² IV

*VCR = Vincristine 2 mg/m² IV (maximum dose 2 mg)

**VCR = Vincristine 1 mg/m² IV or 0·03 mg/kg

HDMTX = Methotrexate 200 mg/kg IV (given 1 hour after VCR)

° = Citrovorum factor 15 mg IV q 4 h × 9, beginning 4 h after HDMTX completed

Figure 9.9 Regimen A chemotherapy

Details of the study

Eligible patients were under the age of 21 years, with newly diagnosed diffuse, undifferentiated NHL, small non-cleaved cell (Burkitt or non-Burkitt), according to the Working Formulation, which was stage III according to the Murphy staging system. Staging investigations included clinical evaluation, FBC, bone marrow and CSF examination, and CT scan of involved areas.

Other than stating that all patients were randomised no further details are given in the study about randomisation methods.

Statistical predictions do not seem to have been performed prospectively. However, calculations were performed based on the number of eligible patients actually recruited, and it was calculated that based on a proportional hazards model, a

study of 123 eligible patients has a 80% power to detect a 20% improvement in EFS from 65% at p = 5%, one-sided. The power number is exact if failure is deemed impossible after 2 years, and higher if failure is possible.

Protocol 8106 (regimen A) employed cyclophosphamide, vincristine, prednisolone and methotrexate, with triple intrathecal chemotherapy throughout the 7 months of therapy, whereas "Total B" (regimen B) added doxorubicin, along with fractionated cyclophosphamide and vincristine, followed by cytosine and intravenous methotrexate, the doses of which escalated with subsequent courses (Figures 9.8 and 9.9). No patient received radiotherapy.

Intention to treat was utilised in all of the analyses, and event free survival (EFS) was the primary end

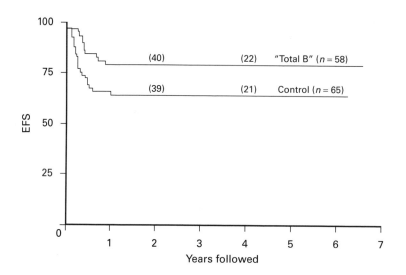

Figure 9.10 Event free survival (EFS) for patients treated on the control arm (regimen A) and total B therapy (regimen B). EFS was measured from time of initial therapy, utilising the log rank method

point measured from the time of initial therapy. Events were defined as induction death, progressive disease, relapse and death in remission or second malignancy.

Outcome

One hundred and thirty-four patients were registered, of whom 11 were excluded after central pathology review. Sixty-five patients were randomised to regimen A, 58 to regimen B. On regimen A 52/64 achieved complete response, compared to 55/58 on regimen B. The difference was statistically significant with a p value of 0·014. EFS was 64% for regimen A

compared to 79% for regimen B (p = 0·027) (Figure 9.10).

Toxicity

There were 2 induction deaths on each regimen, but haematological toxicity was more severe on regimen B.

Conclusion

The "Total B" therapy resulted in a significant improvement in EFS, which seemed mainly to result from a better initial complete response rate.

Study 10

Link MP, Shuster JJ, Donaldson SS, Berard CW, Murphy SB.
Treatment of children and young adults with early-stage non-Hodgkin's lymphoma.
N Engl J Med 1997;**337**:1259–66.

This was a Pediatric Oncology Group study undertaken between 1983 and 1991.

Objectives

The question addressed was whether a short 9 week regimen was adequate in patients with localised non-Hodgkin's lymphoma.

Details of the study

Eligible patients were those aged under 21 years with untreated biopsy proven NHL categorised as Murphy's stage I/II. The histopathological findings were classified according to the Working Formulation.

The study was designed to allow the inclusion of patients treated on a study undertaken between 1983 and 1987 in which all patients had received 8 months of chemotherapy, with a 6 week induction, 3 week consolidation and 24 week "maintenance" phase, but had been additionally randomised to receive or not receive radiation therapy. In the second trial, undertaken between

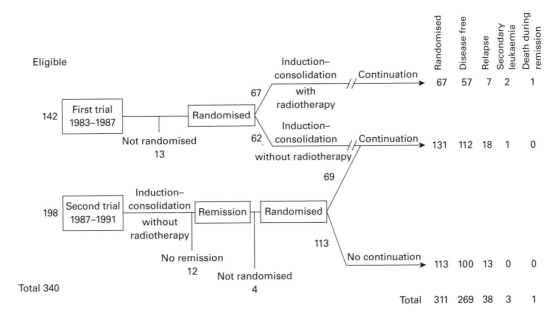

Figure 9.11 Design of two consecutive trials of therapy for patients with early stage non-Hodgkin's lymphoma, with the treatment assignments and outcomes shown for all 340 eligible patients. Adapted with permission, 2002 from Link MP *et al, N Engl J Med* (full reference above). Copyright © 1997 Massachusetts Medical Society.

Table 9.2 Treatment regimens for patients with early-stage non-Hodgkin's lymphoma

Therapy	Route of administration	Schedule			
Induction and consolidation therapy (9 weeks)					
Vincristine	Intravenous	1.5 mg/m^2 weekly for 7 weeks			
Doxorubicin	Intravenous	40 mg/m^2 on days 1, 22 and 43			
Cyclophosphamide	Intravenous	750 mg/m^2 on days 1, 22 and 43			
Prednisone	Oral	40 mg/m^2 daily on days 1–28 and 43–47			
Continuation therapy (24 weeks)					
Mercaptopurine	Oral	50 mg/m^2 daily			
Methotrexate	Oral	25 mg/m^2 weekly			
Central nervous system		Age adjusted doses given on days 1, 8, 22, 43 therapy* and 64 on induction–consolidation therapy and every 6 weeks during continuation therapy			
		1-yr-olds	2-yr-olds	3–8-yr-olds	> 9-yr-olds
Methotrexate	Intrathecal	8 mg	10 mg	12 mg	15 mg
Cytarabine	Intrathecal	16 mg	20 mg	24 mg	30 mg
Hydrocortisone	Intrathecal	8 mg	10 mg	12 mg	15 mg

*Intrathecal methotrexate alone (12 mg/m^2) was used in the first trial.

1987 and 1991, patients who were in complete remission after induction/consolidation were randomly allocated between 9 weeks of induction/consolidation treatment only *OR* 9 weeks of induction/consolidation *plus* 24 weeks of therapy (Figure 9.11).

Patients were allocated between the 9 week versus the 8 month therapy on a 2:1 basis.

Chemotherapy comprised standard CHOP, with 6 MP/methotrexate maintenance and intrathecal methotrexate, cytarabine and hydrocortisone (Table 9.2).

Because the study question was negative, a one-sided p value of 0.10 or less in favour of the 8 month therapy was taken as evidence of the efficacy of "maintenance" therapy. For a power of 90% to detect this difference it was calculated that an additional 183 patients were required as well as the patients accrued from the first study.

The primary outcome measures were event free survival, continuous complete remission and overall survival. Comparisons were made with the log-rank test and life tables constructed according to Kaplan–Meier.

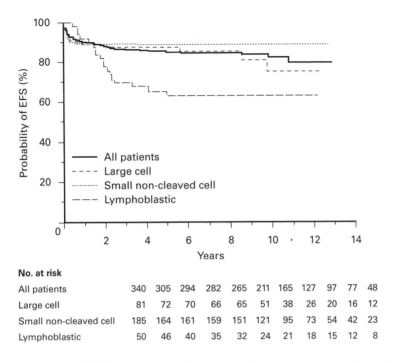

Figure 9.12 Event free survival (EFS) in relation to histology. Adapted with permission, 2002 from Link MP *et al*, *N Engl J Med* (full reference on p 217). Copyright © 1986 Massachusetts Medical Society.

Outcome

Three hundred and fifty-five patients entered the two studies. Fifteen were excluded: pathology unconfirmed in 7, non-localised disease in 8. In the first study 13/42 were not randomised, 7 of whom had primary lymphoma of bone. In the second trial 16/198 were not randomised: 4 declined and 12 failed to achieve complete remission. One hundred and thirteen patients were randomly assigned to the 9 week treatment arm and 69 to receive treatment for 8 months.

Sixty-two patients from the first study who had received 8 months of treatment and no radiotherapy were analysed with the latter group to produce a total of 131.

There were no differences in the projected 5 year rates of continuous complete remission: 89 ± 4% for those treated with 9 weeks of chemotherapy compared to 86 ± 4% for those treated with 8 months of chemotherapy. Details on those randomised are not given.

A total of 54 patients had adverse events: 12 did not achieve a complete remission (all from the second trial), 38 had recurrent disease, 1 died of sepsis and 3 had second malignancies.

Important differences were found when results were analysed according to histopathological subtype. Projected complete clinical remission rates for those with lymphoblastic disease was 63% compared with 89% for those with small

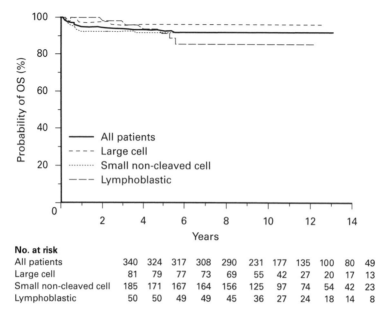

Figure 9.13 Overall survival (OS) in relation to histology. Adapted with permission, 2002 from Link MP *et al, N Engl J Med* (full reference on p 217). Copyright © 1986 Massachusetts Medical Society.

non-cleaved cell lymphoma. The failure rate was higher in those with lymphoblastic disease treated for 9 weeks (8/14) compared with those treated for 8 months (7/21) (p = 0·24). There was, however, no difference in overall survival between histological groups, suggesting that there is a high salvage rate with further therapy in relapsed lymphoblastic disease (Figures 9.12, 9.13).

Conclusion

It was concluded that 9 weeks' treatment is sufficient for localised Murphy's stage I/II small non-cleaved cell lymphoma and large cell lymphoma.

Study 11

Amylon MD, Shuster J, Pullen J, Berard C, Link MP, Wharam M, Katz J, Yu A, Laver J, Ravindranath Y, Kurtzberg J, Desai S, Camitta B, Murphy SB.

Intensive high-dose asparaginase consolidation improves survival for pediatric patients with T cell acute lymphoblastic leukemia and advanced stage lymphoblastic lymphoma: a Pediatric Oncology Group study.
Leukemia 1999;**13**:335–42.

The study was carried out between 1987 and 1992 by the Pediatric Oncology Group (POG-8704).

Objectives

This study was designed to test the hypothesis that high dose asparaginase consolidation therapy improves survival in paediatric patients with T cell acute lymphoblastic leukaemia and advanced stage lymphoblastic lymphoma.

Details of the study

Eligibility included patients up to 21 years of age. Those with T cell lymphoma were allowed to have received previous mediastinal radiotherapy and up to 7 days of prednisolone as emergency therapy. Standard immunophenotyping was not mandatory but central pathological review was done in all cases. Patients with Murphy stage III and IV disease were eligible.

In the main trial, children with leukaemia and lymphoma were included. For this review, only those with T cell NHL will be considered.

The randomisation site and method are not defined but involved call back to an automated telephone registration system once the patient was in complete remission. No details of the anticipated difference between study arms or number required are given.

The study involved multiagent induction chemotherapy, which included three doses of asparaginase, followed by a consolidation and an CNS directed therapy component. During maintenance therapy, patients were randomised to receive 20 weekly doses of 25 000 units/m^2 of L-asparaginase intramuscularly, beginning on day 99 (Table 9.3).

Measured endpoints were duration of complete clinical remission, (CCR) time from randomisation to relapse, second cancers and death. One-sided analysis of CCR was performed.

Outcome

In the overall study, including ALL, 552 patients were enrolled. Twenty-seven did not meet the eligibility requirement, mainly because central pathology review failed to confirm the diagnosis, 22 did not achieve a documented complete remission, as required for post CR randomisation, and an additional 19 patients were lost due to failure to call the automated telephone registration system to be randomised. Ultimately, 484 patients, 317 ALL and 167 T-NHL, were randomised. For the T-NHL group, 180 of 195 had achieved a complete remission (two were non-evaluable). Of the 167 randomised, 83 received standard treatment and 85 high dose asparaginase.

The 4 year CCR for the standard treatment arm was 64% ± 6%, versus 78% ± 5% for high dose asparaginase (p = < 0·048). Overall, there was no outcome difference between stage III and stage IV NHL.

Table 9.3 Treatment regimen

Induction:	Vincristine 1.5 mg/m² IVP weekly × 5 begin day 1
	Prednisone 40 mg/m²/day PO ÷ tid × 28 days
	Cyclophosphamide 1000 mg/m² IV on day 1
	Doxorubicin 50 mg/m² IV on day 1
	Cytarabine 100 mg/m²/day IVCI for 5 days begin day 22
	Cyclophosphamide 600 mg/m² IV on day 22
	L-asparaginase 10 000 U/m² IM on days 27, 29 and 31
Consolidation:	Teniposide 300 mg/m² IV twice weekly × 4 doses begin day 43
	Cytarabine 150 mg/m² IVP twice weekly × 4 doses after teniposide
	Vincristine 1·5 mg/m² IVP twice weekly × 4 begin day 71
	Prednisone 40 mg/m² PO ÷ tid × 28 days begin day 71
	Doxorubicin 40 mg/m² IV on day 71
CNS prophylaxis:	Intrathecal triple drugs twice weekly × 7 begin day 1, then q 9 weeks throughout maintenance. Cranial RT 2400 cGy begin day 71 for T-ALL patients with WBC > 50K only
Maintenance:	9 week cycle repeated 10 times:
	Cytarabine 150 mg/m²/day IVCI × 3 days begin day 1
	Cyclophosphamide 75 mg/m² IVP q 12 h × 6 doses begin day 1
	Vincristine 2 mg/m² IV on day 22
	Doxorubicin 30 mg/m² IV on day 22
	Prednisone 120 mg/m² PO ÷ tid × 5 days begin day 22
	6-MP 225 mg/m²/day PO ÷ tid × 5 days begin day 22
	Teniposide 300 mg/m² IV q 3 days × 2 doses begin day 43
	Cytarabine 150 mg/m²/dose IVP × 2 doses following teniposide
Randomisation:	L-asparaginase 25 000 U/m² IM weekly × 20 doses begin day 99

IVP, intravenous push; IVCI, intravenous continuous infusion.

In the standard treatment arm, 31 patients relapsed, 8 in the mediastinum alone, 4 in the CNS alone. In the asparaginase arm, 17 relapsed, 3 in the mediastinum alone and 2 with CNS disease. There was one second cancer in the standard arm, compared to 7 in the high dose asparaginase arm. There were 2 deaths, one from bronchiolitis obliterans and one accidental injury.

Details of infection are given only for the whole study group. There was no difference in myelosuppression or sepsis between groups. There were increased incidences of thrombocytopenia (6·2% *v* 2·6%) liver function abnormalities (2·6% *v* 0·9%) hyperbilirubinemia (1·2% *v* 0·05%) and pancreatitis (0·8% *v* 0·1%) in the high dose asparaginase arm. There were no grade 3 or 4 bleeding or thrombotic episodes. Allergic reactions were higher in the asparaginase arm (24% *v* 10%).

Conclusion

It was concluded that despite the surprisingly high level of second malignancy, there was an overall benefit to asparaginase.

Comment

The difference is only marginally significant for NHL. When the ALL data are added, the differences are more marked, with 4 year CCR of 71% ± 3%, versus 58% ± 3%. The authors concluded that in the overall population one could be 95% confident that there was a benefit equal to or greater than 6·8% at 4 years with regard to complete clinical remission. It should be noted that the outcome in T-ALL was poor, with only 30% of patients event free at 7 years, and around 50% of those with NHL survived. Moreover, from the survival curve the differences decreased with follow up time.

Study 12

Murphy SB, Hustu H.
A randomised trial ofcombined modality therapy of childhood non-Hodgkin's lymphoma.
Cancer 1980;**45**:630–7.

This study was carried out between 1975 and 1978 at St Jude Children's Research Hospital.

Objectives

The aim of the study was, first to determine the contribution of involved field radiotherapy in patients with stage III–IV disease and, secondly, to determine the efficacy of "prophylactic" treatment to the central nervous system using cranial irradiation and intrathecal methotrexate in stage II–IV disease.

Details of the study

Eligible patients were all those presenting at St Jude during this period with previously untreated NHL of any histological subtype.

The randomisation method involved a card envelope technique and was carried out at St Jude. Patients were stratified for poor risk features, such as stage IV, mediastinal mass and widespread abdominal disease. No anticipated difference in outcome or numbers required to draw conclusions are detailed.

Induction therapy for stage I–II disease was vincristine, prednisolone, cyclophosphamide and involved field radiotherapy 30–35 Gy. Stage III–IV received the same three drugs plus doxorubicin and were randomised to receive, or not receive, involved field radiotherapy. Involved field was defined as the area involved by the bulky primary tumour. In the case of abdominal disease, the whole abdomen was treated to 20–25 Gy, with the primary site boosted to 30–35 Gy. With thoracic or mediastinal primaries, where the pleura was involved, the affected hemithorax received 12–15 Gy with a boost of 30–35 Gy to the primary area.

If a complete response to induction therapy was documented, children with stage I or completely resected stage II gastrointestinal primaries began two drug oral maintenance chemotherapy and received no CNS prophylaxis. All other children (stage II–IV) who achieved a complete response were randomly selected to receive, or not, the standard regimen of 24 Gy cranial irradiation and five doses of intrathecal methotrexate. Maintenance therapy was then given (Table 9.4).

Primary outcome measures were disease free survival and overall survival.

Outcome

Sixty-nine patients aged 2–19 years were entered, of whom 56 were male. Histological subtype comprised 24 lymphoblastic, 27 undifferentiated, 11 histiocytic and 7 other (Rappaport classification). Twenty-five had abdominal tumours, 18 mediastinal, 12 head and neck, 7 peripheral and 7 other. Twenty-one had stage I and II disease, 48 were stage III and IV.

Forty-six of 48 stage II–IV patients were eligible for the radiotherapy randomisation. One had multifocal disease with no obvious primary and in one follow up was too short at time of

Table 9.4 Treatment outline

Phase I   Induction (6–9 weeks)

For stages I–II:

  Vincristine 1·5 mg/m^2 IV weekly × 6 doses on days 0, 7, 14, 21, 28 and 35

  Cyclophosphamide 1200 mg/m^2 IV on days 0, 21 and 42

  Prednisone 40 mg/m^2 PO × 28 days

  Involved field radiotherapy (3000–3500 rad)

For stages II–IV:

  Same drugs, as above, plus

  Doxorubicin 45 mg/m^2 IV on days 0, 21 and 42

  Randomisation for radiotherapy, as above, versus none

Phase II   CNS prophylaxis (2–3 weeks)

For stage I and stage II with completely resected gastrointestinal primary tumours:

  No prophylaxis

For (other) stages II, III, IV:

  Randomise for cranial irradiation (2400 rad) plus intrathecal methotrexate (12 mg/m^2) × 5 doses, versus no prophylaxis

Phase III   Maintenance (for a total duration of 2 years following diagnosis)

For stages I–IV:

  6-Mercaptopurine 75 mg/m^2 PO daily

  Methotrexate mg/m^2 PO weekly

---

publication. Twenty-one received chemotherapy alone, 25 the addition of radiotherapy.

There was no difference in the observed complete response rate, 17/21 versus 21/25 respectively. Thirty-four patients were randomised for CNS directed therapy: 18 received additional therapy, of whom 4 relapsed (one isolated CNS). Sixteen received no additional therapy: 5 relapsed (4 with isolated CNS disease). Although not statistically significant, it was concluded that there were more CNS relapses in those not given additional CNS directed therapy.

Overall survival was 58% in the group receiving radiotherapy versus 51% in those without, and disease free survival was 42% versus 33% respectively.

Toxicity

The main toxicities were gastrointestinal and/or mucositis, which were observed only in the patients receiving radiotherapy. There was one death due to interstitial pneumonitis, which occurred early in the study before the routine use of septrin prophylaxis.

Conclusion

It was concluded that radiotherapy had no significant benefit on remission rate or overall outcome in patients with stage III and IV disease.

Comment

It should be noted that the study included a range of histological subtypes and the overall high CNS relapse rate could have obscured events at other sites.

10
Hodgkin's disease

Commentary – Tim Eden

In a malignancy like Hodgkin's disease, which has carried with it such a high overall survival rate since the introduction of aggressive systemic as well as localised disease control, the onus has been on physicians to cure patients with least long term toxicity. This is especially so for children where increasing reports of infertility, especially in boys, cardiorespiratory dysfunction and therapeutically induced second malignancies have marred the successful control of the primary disease. The big questions for childhood Hodgkin's disease in the modern era have been:

1   Can cure be obtained without resort to mixed modality therapy, especially in low stage disease?
2   Can a successful chemotherapy regimen(s) be developed which minimises long term toxicity?
3   How much therapy is really needed for advanced disease?

Although the questions to be addressed have been recognised worldwide, what is really surprising is that for such a relatively rare disease comprising only 5–6% of all childhood tumours (corresponding to perhaps 65–75 new cases of all stages per annum in the UK for those in the childhood age range) there has been little attempt to establish international consensus let alone run randomised controlled trials. There has in addition been little adult and paediatric

collaboration. As a consequence, the number of well organised, properly constituted randomised controlled trials for childhood Hodgkin's disease carried out in the past two to three decades has been very small and furthermore the number of patients recruited into each trial is frequently too few to achieve meaningful results. Such recruitment is especially important in a disease with such a long time course where the real benefit of any individual therapy may not emerge for 10–15 years or even longer.

Those trials that have been conducted have also frequently included stratification of patients and assumptions made about long term prognosis on the basis of anecdotal rather than strong evidence, for example, the absence of a mediastinal mass or limited extent of disease in the abdomen, focusing on the number of nodules in the spleen, may constitute more favourable prognostic groups. Once you start to subclassify, the numbers entered into any particular randomisation dwindle dramatically. Finding the actual evidence historically to support such stratification is often extremely difficult.

Study 1 and 2 exemplify some of these problems. Hutchinson *et al* (Study 1) report the CCG-521 study where they compared 12 cycles of alternating mustine, vincristine, procarbazine and prednisolone (MOPP,) (the original successful protocol) and doxorubicin, bleomycin, vinblastine and dacarbazine (ABVD,) (introduced to reduce the long term toxicity of MOPP) versus six courses of ABVD followed by regional irradiation (20 Gy). It is very difficult to find any evidence equating numbers of cycles of therapy required to achieve a favourable outcome and also what dose of irradiation is equivalent to, for example, six cycles of chemotherapy. In essence, when choosing particular chemotherapy regimens you are selecting between different constellations of long term toxicity, for example, with the alkylator based therapy, long term infertility especially in boys and second tumours, whilst with ABVD, potential cardiorespiratory sequelae and some degree of risk of secondary leukaemia. This study, despite a planned recruitment of 50 patients per year for 4 years, ended up with only 125 patients entered. Clearly recruitment to protocols with such different therapeutic approaches is often difficult. Numbers are further reduced by exclusions. They failed to demonstrate any significant difference in terms of event free or overall survival although there was a trend to benefit from combined modality therapy, but what the authors don't report, indeed may not be in a position to assess, are the long term sequelae. What is also not clear from their publication is also whether patients can be salvaged if they relapse having not previously received radiotherapy. It should be mandatory in all future publications of randomised controlled trials in Hodgkin's disease to report explicitly on late sequelae and also for collaborative groups to re-report longer term follow up of studies. Hodgkin's disease is a truly 'long' disease!

Study 2 attempts also in advanced Hodgkin's disease to compare the addition of low dose total-nodal irradiation to therapy containing alternating MOPP and ABVD cycles. Weiner *et al* included a rather broader group of patients in their definition of advanced stage Hodgkin's disease, including patients with stage 2B, and they also did not make the distinction made by the CCG with regard to abdominal stage 3A disease. They used just eight cycles of chemotherapy and similar overall radiation dosages. However, their fraction dosage was lower. Their recruitment was higher, but again they really did not find a significant difference in outcome in terms of event free survival although there was a trend for better survival for those not irradiated. For both these studies you could conclude that irradiation was not required and it may just increase toxicity long term, but the numbers are really too small to draw absolute conclusions. Given the somewhat different selection of patients it is difficult to be sure whether you could put these two trials into a systematic review and come up with any firm conclusions.

Cramer and Andrieu (Study 3) reported on a study conducted between 1972 and 1980 in two categories. They looked at low stage disease treated with three courses of MOPP chemotherapy and then randomised between mantle radiotherapy or involved field radiotherapy. There were only 5 and 10 patients respectively in the randomisation. Again because of some stratification problems, the results are uninterpretable. In the second half of their report they looked at patients with stage 2, 3A and 2B. They compared three courses of MOPP with three courses of CVPP (CCNU, vincristine, procarbazine, prednisone) followed by laparotomy and supradiaphragmatic radiotherapy. In this study only 16 patients were randomised. There was a favourable response to chemotherapy but with the small numbers no conclusions could be drawn. This further confirms the need for proper large and if necessary multicentre international trials to answer important questions.

The fourth study, also from France, reported by Oberlin *et al*, compared ABVD to MOPP plus ABVD plus reduced dose radiotherapy. They limited the number of cycles of therapy and dose of radiation to 20 Gy for good responders and 40 Gy for poor responders. They showed comparability of MOPP plus ABVD to ABVD alone and also demonstrated that there appeared to be no advantage of higher dose irradiation.

Study 5 reported by Sackmann-Muriel *et al* came from a joint adult and paediatric trial but only the paediatric patients were included in the report. They were looking only at favourable patients in their randomised study and included stage IA and B, IIA and B and stage IIIA. They used a fairly complex prognostic index, including age, symptoms, stage and number of involved regions, to classify their patients into favourable, intermediate or unfavourable groupings. The evidence on which they based such stratification is not reported. Their favourable group was randomised between three or six courses of CCVP, their intermediate group between three courses prior to involved field radiation or to AOPE (doxorubicin, vincristine, etoposide, prednisolone) with three courses prior and three courses after involved field radiotherapy. They did make a useful contribution in that they showed that three courses of CVPP chemotherapy was adequate for patients defined as having favourable features. Those were essentially patients who were under the age of 15 with no B symptoms, and stage I disease with less than three nodal regions involved. No patient with bulky mediastinal involvement could be included in that category and slightly older patients could only be if they were symptom free, of either stage I or II, again with limited nodal involvement. Once you start to subcategorise patients in this way you need a lot patients to prove for sure what you are delivering is safe efficacious therapy.

Study 6, reported by Sullivan *et al*, was a worthwhile study in that it particularly reported on a longer follow up, but it was limited to stage III patients and unfortunately involved poor recruitment. They attempted to compare MOPP plus bleomycin versus an alkylating regimen that contained doxorubicin (Adriamycin) (A-COPP). Poor recruitment and a very high number of exclusions detracted from their power to answer the questions that they had raised. The study did report comparison of toxicity, demonstrating excess cardiac complications in the A-COPP arm compared with one malignancy with MOPP and one secondary osteosarcoma with A-COPP. Although the regimens were comparable in terms of 10 year event free and overall survival, no firm conclusions about benefit could be reached.

Finally, Gehan *et al* (Study 7) reported in 1990 on the question of benefit or not of adjuvant MOPP to involved field or extended field radiotherapy in stage I or II disease. They clearly had a problem with randomisation and a high exclusion rate. Five out of 6 second tumours were in the involved field plus MOPP arm. Their conclusion was that involved field irradiation plus combination chemotherapy gave superior disease control but did not influence overall survival and, of course, was associated with the predictable increase in second malignancy.

It is always dangerous to be retrospectively clever, but if some of the collaborative groups throughout the world had worked harder and earlier together to address the questions they were trying to answer they might truly have recruited adequate numbers of patients to have answered all of these questions clearly. We are still left not knowing whether favourable localised disease is best treated with limited chemotherapy or low dose involved field irradiation. Only the truly long term reports of the relative toxicities of the two modalities will help us to answer that question. Whereas for more advanced or unfavourable disease, we again do not know the optimal chemotherapy with least toxicity and how much therapy is really required. Even with more sophisticated statistical analysis and systematic reviews applied to this paucity of randomised trials, non-comparable stratification of patients and poor randomisation rates may not enable us even now to conclude what is the optimal therapy for Hodgkin's disease in childhood.

Studies

Study 1

Hutchinson RJ, Fryer CJH, Davis PC, Nachman J, Krailo MD, O'Brien RT, Collins RD, Whalen T, Reardon D, Trigg ME, Gilchrist GS.
MOPP or radiation in addition to ABVD in the treatment of pathologically staged advanced Hodgkin's disease in children: results of the Children's Cancer Group phase III trial.
J Clin Oncol 1998;**16**:897–906.

The study was carried out between 1986 and 1990 by the Children's Cancer Group (CCG-521).

Objectives

This trial was designed to compare MOPP and ABVD versus ABVD combined with extended field radiotherapy in children and adolescents with stage III and IV Hodgkin's disease.

Details of the study

Patients were less than 21 years of age with stage III and IV disease that was untreated and pathologically staged. Stage 3A patients with no mediastinal mass and disease limited to splenic, celiac or portal nodes were excluded, as were those with less than five splenic nodules. These patients were regarded as having a favourable outcome.

Randomisation site and method are not stated. Patients were balanced for sex, A or B symptoms, favourable histology and mediastinal involvement. The study was designed to detect a 20% difference in 5 year event free survival,

from 60% to 80%. It was planned to recruit 50 patients per year for a 4 year period.

Patients were randomised at presentation to receive either 12 28 day cycles of chemotherapy, alternating between a cycle of MOPP and one of ABVD (regimen A), or six 28 day cycles of ABVD followed by radiation therapy to regions of initial involvement (regimen B). The radiation therapy dose was 21 Gy given in 175 cGy fractions for a total of 12 fractions to one or more of three general regions, based on extent of the disease at time of diagnosis. Regions comprised bilateral neck, bilateral axillae and mediastinum. The pulmonary hila were irradiated in the presence of mediastinal or hilar involvement. Patients with lung involvement were irradiated to 10·5 Gy. Region 2 was the liver, spleen and upper abdominal nodes (above L2). Region 3 was the lower abdominal nodes, which included pelvic nodes. When more than one region required radiotherapy a 2 week interval between treatments was recommended, although it was permitted to treat two adjacent regions concurrently.

Patients who showed significant residual nodal enlargement after chemotherapy were eligible to receive a higher total dose of radiotherapy to those regions. In this situation, it was recommended that there was pathological verification of active disease prior to administration of an additional 1·4 Gy for a total nodal dose of 35 Gy.

Patients were monitored during chemotherapy using cardiac echo and pulmonary function studies.

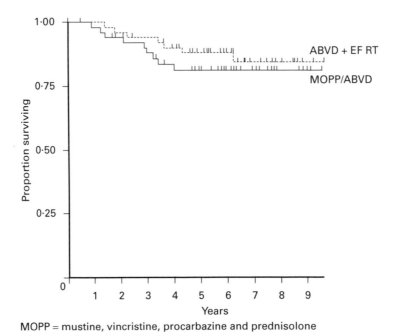

MOPP = mustine, vincristine, procarbazine and prednisolone
ABVD = doxorubicin, bleomycin, vinblastine, dacarbazine
EF RT = extended field radiotherapy

Figure 10.1 Survival by randomised regimens

Major outcome measures were event free survival and overall survival.

Outcome

One hundred and twenty-five patients entered the study, of whom 14 were excluded. In 11 cases this was due to lack of pathological verification, 2 were wrong diagnoses and one patient received prior therapy. There were 71 stage III and 40 stage IV patients. Fifty-seven were randomised to MOPP/ABVD alone and 54 to ABVD plus radiotherapy.

Overall compliance was good, with median dose of the different chemotherapy agents ranging

from 93% to 100%. Eighty-two per cent of radio-therapy was in compliance with the protocol. Six of the eight instances of non-compliance were due to reduced field, and one to reduced dose. One patient was not given radiotherapy, contrary to protocol.

Outcome

Overall survival for the study group was 87% at 4 years, 84% in regimen A and 90% in regimen B. Four year event free survival for regimen A was 77% versus 87% in regimen B (Figures 10.1, 10.2). The relative risk of death was 0·69 for those receiving radiotherapy. It is

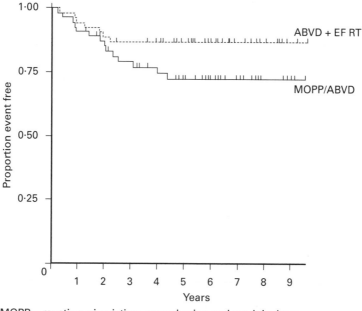

MOPP = mustine, vincristine, procarbazine and prednisolone
ABVD = doxorubicin, bleomycin, vinblastine, dacarbazine
EF RT = extended field radiotherapy

Figure 10.2 Event free survival by randomised regimens

of note that all instances of relapsed disease in regimen A were at sites that would have been included within the radiotherapy field under regimen B. There was no significant difference either for event free or overall survival between the arms (p = 0·45 and p = 0·09 respectively).

Toxicity

There were 190 neutropenic episodes on regimen A, compared to 65 on regimen B. Four patients developed grade 3 or 4 cardiac toxicity and one patient on regimen A had a clinically significant cardiac complication. Eight patients

had grade 3 or 4 pulmonary toxicity, one clinically significant, on regimen A. There was one death due to tuberculosis. No second cancers are described.

Conclusion

It was concluded that the outcome was comparable between both arms, although there did seem to be a somewhat lower event rate in those receiving combined modality therapy. It was suggested that both age and previous medical history should be taken into consideration when determining therapy.

Study 2

Weiner MA, Leventhal B, Brecher ML, Marcus RB, Cantor A, Gieser PW, Ternberg JL, Behm FG, Wharam MD Jr, Chauvenet AR.

Randomized study of intensive MOPP-ABVD with or without low-dose total-nodal radiation therapy in the treatment of stages IIB, IIIA2, IIIB and IV Hodgkin's disease in paediatric patients: a Pediatric Oncology Group study.

J Clin Oncol 1997;**15**:2769–79.

The study was carried out between 1987 and 1992 by the POG group (POG protocol 8725).

Objectives

This study was to determine whether the addition of low dose total nodal irradiation in paediatric patients with advanced stage Hodgkin's disease who have received alternating MOPP–ABVD chemotherapy improves event free and overall survival when compared with patients who received chemotherapy alone.

Details of study

Children and adolescents were eligible (no age specified), presenting with stage IIB, IIIA2, IIIB and IV Hodgkin's disease. Stage IIIA2 was defined as involvement of both upper and lower abdominal nodes. Central pathology review was required for each patient. Staging laparotomy and splenectomy were required only in patients with clinical evidence of stage IA, IIA and IIIA1 disease. Gallium scan was routinely used in this study. If a staging laparotomy was not performed, a minilaparotomy, which consisted of wedge biopsies plus deep-needle biopsy of both lobes of liver, and lymph node sampling were used to confirm the stage of disease. This was performed if the spleen was below the left costal margin or two or more times normal size on imaging or there were gross filling defects detected in the liver or spleen by CT or gallium scan or a greater than 3 cm lymph node was present at the porta hepatis or the splenic hilum on CT scan.

Echocardiography and pulmonary function tests were required during therapy.

Patients were randomised at diagnosis but there are no details of where or what method was used. No details of the difference anticipated or numbers required to demonstrate equivalence are given.

Standard chemotherapy comprised four 1 month cycles of MOPP, alternating with four 1 month cycles of ABVD for a total of 8 months of chemotherapy ± radiotherapy (Figure 10.3). Response was evaluated after three and six cycles of chemotherapy, at the completion of MOPP-ABVD and after radiotherapy in those patients who received this modality. Abnormalities at the end of treatment were to be biopsied and if positive, patients came off study. Radiotherapy was administered at the end of eight cycles of chemotherapy to those patients in complete remission, who were randomised at diagnosis to receive radiotherapy. The radiation field was determined by the pre-treatment evaluation. Patients with clinical evidence of pelvic disease by physical examination, imaging, or laparotomy received total-nodal irradiation.

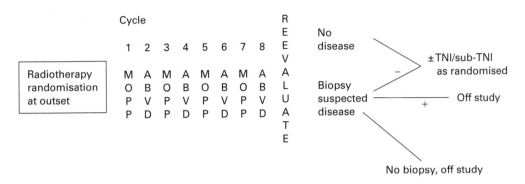

MOPP = mustine, vincristine, procarbazine and prednisolone
ABVD = doxorubicin, bleomycin, vinblastine, dacarbazine

Figure 10.3 Outline of therapy

Patients documented to have no evidence of disease below the aortic bifurcation received sub-total-nodal irradiation (mantle, spleen and para-aortic nodes). All lymphoid tissue, including the spleen, received 21 Gy. Liver, lung parenchyma, pericardium and kidney received doses of up to 10·5 Gy. Three radiation fields were sequentially treated, first the mantle, secondly the para-aortic nodes and spleen and thirdly the pelvis (if necessary). Radiation therapy was given at a dose of 1·5 Gy/day, 5 days per week and the 2 week rest period was provided between each port if haematological recovery was adequate.

Major outcome measures were event free survival and overall survival.

Outcome

One hundred and eighty-three patients were registered, of whom 4 were ineligible; 2 misdiagnoses, one with concurrent brain tumour and one institutional review board problem. The median age of those randomised was 13 years. Eighty-nine were randomised to chemotherapy alone and 90 to radiotherapy. There were 38 stage IIB, 22 stage IIIA2, 52 stage IIIB, 20 stage IVA and 47 stage IVB.

Eight patients failed to complete chemotherapy: there were 2 deaths due to septicaemia, progressive disease in 2, one developed NHL, one was lost to follow up and there were 2 major protocol violations.

At the end of three cycles 54 patients were in complete remission (CR), after six cycles 78 were in complete remission and after eight cycles 132 of 171 patients (77%) attained a clinical CR as determined by physical and radiological examination. Thirty-nine patients had clinical evidence of residual disease. Five of these refused to have a biopsy performed and were removed from the study. Two of these 5 had unequivocal evidence of progressive disease and were censored accordingly. Five patients had a positive biopsy and 29 a negative biopsy. Thus, 161 of 179 patients (90%) were in CR at the completion of chemotherapy.

Eighty-one had been randomised to chemotherapy alone, 80 to receive radiotherapy.

Ten of the 80 randomised to receive irradiation did not, in fact, receive this treatment. Five patients refused, 4 received radiation in non-POG institutions and were excluded and one developed acute myeloid leukaemia prior to radiotherapy. Ultimately, 45 patients received total nodal irradiation, 25 received sub-total TNI, i.e. the pelvic field was omitted.

Toxicity
Overall, chemotherapy was well tolerated. Two patients died of overwhelming sepsis during chemotherapy. Four patients experienced mild asymptomatic cardiac toxicity (ejection fraction < 20% decrease from baseline). Six developed a second malignancy (3 AML, 1 NHL, 1 melanoma).

Outcome
Overall event free survival and survival at 5 years were 79% ± 6% and 92% ± 4% respectively. EFS at 5 years for patients who received chemotherapy plus radiotherapy was 80% ± 8%, compared to 79% ± 9% for chemotherapy alone, with overall survivals of 87% and 96% respectively. Two factors emerged as having prognostic significance, namely, achievement of clinical CR after three cycles (EFS 94%, compared to 78% for those not in clinical CR), and 89% for those under 13 years of age versus 72% for those older than 13 years of age.

Conclusion
It was concluded that there was no difference in outcome whether or not radiotherapy was added.

Study 3

Cramer P, Andrieu J-M.
Hodgkin's disease in childhood and adolescence: results of chemotherapy-radiotherapy in clinical stages IA-IIB.
J Clin Oncol 1985;**3**:1495–1502.

The studies were performed between 1972 and 1980 by the Hopital Saint-Louis and Hopital Laennec, Paris.

Objectives

This is a subgroup analysis of children and adolescents treated on two studies, one comparing mantle involved field irradiation following three courses of MOPP in stage IA to IIA disease, and the second study comparing MOPP and CVPP chemotherapy in stage II, IIIA and IIB disease.

Details of the study

Patients between the ages of 5 and 19 were included in the analysis. They had clinical stage IA–IIB disease. Surgical staging was not performed but lymphangiography was used in all patients.

The randomisation method used is not stated nor where it was done. No planned numbers or differences sought in the study are described.

Study H7701: The patients with stage IA–IIA disease were treated with three courses of MOPP chemotherapy. They were then randomised to either mantle radiotherapy, receiving 35–40 Gy, or involved field, receiving 40 Gy.

Study H7702: The patients with stage II, IIIA and IIB disease were randomised at diagnosis to receive either three courses of MOPP or three courses of CVPP (CCNU, vinblastine, procarbazine and prednisone). At the end of chemotherapy both groups then underwent laparotomy followed by supradiaphragmatic radiotherapy, plus lumboaortic field radiotherapy when there was histologically proven splenic or lumboaortic involvement.

Major endpoints were relapse free survival and overall survival.

Outcome

Study 7701

Five patients received mantle and 10 patients received involved field irradiation. The numerical imbalance was because 8 patients were not stratified by age in the overall study, including adults. In the 5 receiving mantle irradiation there was one abdominal relapse. In the 10 involved field patients, there were 2 abdominal relapses and 1 mediastinal relapse.

Study 7702:

Eight of 8 patients receiving MOPP achieved complete remission and 8 of the 9 receiving CVPP achieved complete remission. There was one abdominal relapse, in a patient who had received CVPP. There were no deaths in complete remission.

Conclusion

The numbers in this study were too small to draw any firm conclusion, although no significant difference was observed between any of the study groups.

Study 4

Oberlin O, Leverger G, Pacquement H, Raquin MA, Chompret A, Habrand JL, Terrier-Lacombe MJ, Bey P, Bertrand Y, Rubie H, Behar C, Zucker JM, Schaison G, Lemerle J.
Low-dose radiation therapy and reduced chemotherapy in childhood Hodgkin's disease: the experience of the French Society of Paediatric Oncology.
J Clin Oncol 1992;**10**:1602–8.

The study was carried out between 1982 and 1988 and was organised by the French Society of Paediatric Oncology.

Objectives

This study was a comparison of ABVD alone to MOPP plus ABVD in favourable Hodgkin's disease with the addition of reduced dose radiotherapy following a good response to chemotherapy.

Details of the study

Eligible patients were aged up to 18 years. There was uniform clinical staging, with CT scan in all and lymphangiography in 95%. Bone marrow biopsy was obtained in children with a clinical stage IIB or more advanced disease. Laparotomy was performed for diagnostic node biopsy in three cases and for staging in one.

The study was designed to include patients with all stages of disease. Those with upper neck IA disease received four cycles of ABVD and those with stage IB, IIB, III or IV disease received three cycles MOPP plus three cycles of ABVD, followed by involved field and lumbosplenic field irradiation. The randomised trial was limited to stage IA and IIA disease, but excluded patients with unilateral nodes localised to the upper neck, who received four cycles of ABVD, and patients with stage IA or IIA who had an ESR >80, who were treated as if they had B symptoms.

The precise randomisation technique is not stated but patients were allocated randomly to treatment arms by telephone.

It was hypothesised that ABVD alone was as effective as MOPP plus ABVD in terms of overall survival and disease free survival in favourable stages. The allowable limit of the true difference between the two arms was 10%. The numbers required are not detailed.

Patients were randomised to receive either four courses of ABVD or alternating two courses of MOPP plus two cycles of ABVD. Response evaluation was performed at the end of chemotherapy. Good remission was defined as complete clinical or radiological disappearance of all tumour (complete remission, CR) or tumour volume reduction of more than 70% (good partial remission, PR). Failure was defined as less than 70% shrinkage or early recurrence before radiotherapy was started.

Good responders received 20 Gy and poor responders 40 Gy. This was given one month after completion of chemotherapy. Involved field irradiation was based on the initial clinical or radiological examination. Bilateral neck irradiation was always performed to avoid asymmetrical growth disturbance. In the supraclavicular field, the external third of the collar bone was excluded to avoid shoulder growth impairment. Lung hila were not irradiated if the patients had only mediastinal disease. For mediastinal disease, radiation was limited to the residual mediastinum after initial chemotherapy.

The major outcome measures were event free and overall survival.

Outcome

One hundred and thirty-six patients with stage IA or IIA disease were registered. Overall, 82% of these achieved a complete remission with chemotherapy and the overall disease free survival at 6 years was 89%.

One hundred and thirty-two patients were randomised, the reason for non-randomisation in the 4 cases is not given. Three patients who were randomised should have been excluded on the basis of elevated ESR or B symptoms.

Sixty-seven were randomised to MOPP plus ABVD and 65 to ABVD alone. There was no significant imbalance between the two groups, although 38% in the hybrid arm had mediastinal involvement, compared to 55% of those receiving ABVD alone. The actuarial risk of relapse at 4 years was 13% for MOPP/ABVD and 10% for ABVD alone.

Toxicity

Treatments were well tolerated. One patient developed acute myeloid leukaemia. Ten per cent of patients developed zoster. No other details of late cardiac or pulmonary toxicity are given.

Conclusion

It was concluded that the treatments are comparable but no recommendation is offered on which should be chosen. The single arm evaluation of reduced dose radiotherapy in good responders suggested this was an appropriate strategy.

Comment

Preliminary data on 174 patients from this trial were also published by Dionet C, Oberlin O, Habrand JL, Vilcoq J, Madelain M, Dutou L, Bey P, Lefur R, Thierry P, LeFloch O, Sarrazin D. Initial chemotherapy and low-dose radiation in limited fields in childhood Hodgkin's disease: results of a joint cooperative study by the French Society of Paediatric Oncology (SFOP) and Hopital Saint-Louis, Paris. *Int J Radiat Onol Biol Phys* 1988;**15**:341–6.

Study 5

Sackmann-Muriel F, Zubizarreta P, Gallo G, Scopinaro M, Alderete D, Alfaro E, Casak S, Chantada G, Felice MS, Quinteros R.
Hodgkin's disease in children: results of a prospective randomized trial in a single institution in Argentina.
Med Ped Oncol 1997;**29**:544–52.

The study was carried out between 1987 and 1994 as part of a national study including adults. The Buenos Aires Group present paediatric data, which was possible because of stratification by centre in the national study.

Objectives

This study compared duration of chemotherapy in favourable disease and two different chemotherapies in an intermediate risk group.

Details of the study

Eligibility had no age limits. Patients were staged clinically, predominantly with CT scanning. A small number had lymphography. Laparotomies were not performed. No central pathology review was performed for this publication.

Randomisation details are not given with regard to method or site. The anticipated numbers of patients required, or the differences sought between study arms, are not detailed.

Patients were grouped on the basis of the Argentine Group for the Treatment of Acute Leukaemias (GATLA) prognostic index for Hodgkin's disease into favourable, intermediate and unfavourable groups. The randomised study applied only to the favourable and intermediate groupings (see Table 10.1 for prognostic

Table 10.1 Score to define the prognostic index

Age(yr)	Symptoms*	Stage	No of involved regions
≤ 15 = 0	A = 0	I = 0	<3 = 0
16–30 = 1	B1 = 1	II = 1	3–4 = 1
31–45 = 2	B2 = 2	III = 2	5–6 = 2
>45 = 3	B3 = 3	IV = 3	>6 = 3

*A, absence; B, presence (number of symptoms).
Staging according to prognostic index:
    Favourable group: score 0–3 (if "bulky" mediastinum, upgrade to intermediate group).
    Intermediate group: score 4–5.
    Unfavourable group: score > 5.

scoring system). Twenty-six patients were in the favourable group. Using conventional staging, there were 21 stage IA and IIA, 3 stage IB or IIB and 2 stage IIIA. There were 64 patients in the intermediate risk group, comprising 32 stage IA, IIA, 12 stage IB, IIB, 18 stage IIIA, IIIB, 2 stage IVA.

The unfavourable group included 24 patients, 19 stage IIIB and 5 stage IVB. These were all given an intensive multiagent chemotherapy regimen, plus involved field radiotherapy.

The favourable group were randomised at presentation between three or six courses of CVPP chemotherapy. This consisted of cyclophosphamide 600 mg/m^2 on days 1 and 8, vincristine 6 mg/m^2 on days 1 and 8, procarbazine 100 mg/m^2 on days 1–14 and prednisolone 40 mg/m^2 on days 1–14.

The intermediate group were randomised between CVPP with three courses prior to involved field radiotherapy or to three courses of AOPE chemotherapy, again three courses prior to and three courses following and after radiotherapy. AOPE comprised doxorubicin 45 mg/m^2 day 1, vincristine 1·5 mg/m^2 day 1, etoposide 150 mg/m^2 days 1 and 3, prednisolone 100 mg/m^2 days 1–5. The radiotherapy dose depended on the initial response to chemotherapy. If there was a greater than 70% reduction in imageable disease a dose of 30 Gy was given. If a less favourable response, 40 Gy was given to the originally involved areas.

The primary outcome measures of the study were the response to chemotherapy and event free and overall survival.

Outcome

The randomised study in the favourable subgroup closed following interim analysis in 1992. This showed no significant differences in either complete response rates (100% and 94% respectively for three or six courses of CVPP) on 80 month event free survival (85% ± 13% for three courses, compared with 87% ± 8% for six courses).

For the intermediate group, response rate was 98% for the CVPP regimen, versus 86% for the AOPE regimen, but the 80 month EFS was 87% ± 5% versus 67% ± 10% respectively (p = <0·04).

Overall, the 80 month EFS for stage IA, IIA was 78% (n = 53), stage IB, IIB 86% (n = 15) and 84% for stage III (n = 39).

Three patients had progressive disease on the AOPE regimen. All achieved a second complete remission with the multiagent regimen used for the unfavourable group.

Toxicity

There was one septic death in the intermediate risk group. No other details of late toxicity are given.

Conclusion

It was concluded that three courses of CVPP is adequate for the good risk group and that the etoposide based regimen is inferior for the intermediate risk group.

Study 6

Sullivan MP, Fuller LM, Berard C, Ternberg J, Cantor AB, Leventhal BG.
Comparative effectiveness of two combined modality regimens in the treatment of surgical stage III Hodgkin's disease in children. An 8-year follow-up study by the Pediatric Oncology Group. *Am J Ped Hematol/Oncol* 1991;**13**:450–8.

The study was carried out by the Pediatric Oncology Group between 1976 and 1982.

Objectives

This study compared two combined modality regimens in children with stage III disease, using either an alkylating regimen, including bleomycin, or an alkylating regimen with an anthracycline.

Details of the study

Eligible patients were under 18 years of age with central pathological review in all cases. Patients were untreated and were both surgically staged and had lymphography.

The randomisation method or location are not detailed. It was anticipated that 69 patients would be required in each of the study arms to give an 80% power to detect a 15% difference in complete response rates. Due to poor recruitment late in the study it was closed prematurely, resulting in an 80% power to detect a 20% difference.

Patients were randomised either to receive sandwich MOPP+B with involved field radiotherapy, which included six courses of MOPP every 28 days either side of involved field radiotherapy (2 before, 4 after), or the alternative,

A-COPP, which again comprised six courses given every 42–56 days (Figure 10.4).

The radiotherapy dose was 35–40 Gy. There was no central review of radiotherapy and few details of the precise fields are given. There was an 8 week rest after radiotherapy prior to continuing chemotherapy.

The primary outcome measure was response rate and event free and overall survival.

Outcome

One hundred and thirty-two patients were entered on the study but 48 were excluded. Thirty seven were from overseas and excluded due to quality of data, 4 had the wrong diagnosis, 4 were lost to follow up, 2 were protocol violations and 1 patient was withdrawn due to toxicity.

Of the 84 patients evaluated, all received over 90% of planned therapy. Forty-five were treated with MOPP, of whom 38 achieved complete remission (84%). Thirty-nine received A-COPP, of whom 36 achieved CR (92%). The precise time at which complete remission was documented is not given.

At 10 years event free survival was 70% for MOPP versus 67% for A-COPP and overall survival 84% and 83% respectively, i.e. no significant difference. No difference was observed for patients with IIIA or IIIB disease or mixed cellularity or nodular sclerosing histology.

Toxicity

Severe infections were documented in 3 patients receiving MOPP, and cardiac complications in 2 patients receiving A-COPP. One

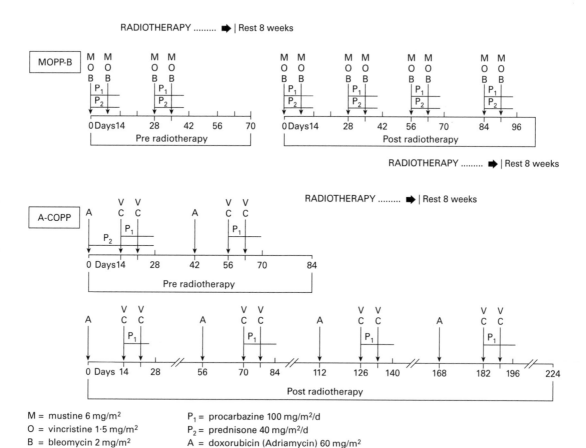

M = mustine 6 mg/m²
O = vincristine 1·5 mg/m²
B = bleomycin 2 mg/m²

P_1 = procarbazine 100 mg/m²/d
P_2 = prednisone 40 mg/m²/d
A = doxorubicin (Adriamycin) 60 mg/m²

Figure 10.4 Chemotherapy regimens MOPP-B v. A-COPP

patient on MOPP developed AML and one patient on A-COPP developed secondary osteosarcoma.

Conclusion

It was concluded that there was no difference between the two regimens with regard to efficacy.

Study 7

Gehan EA, Sullivan MP, Fuller LM, Johnston J, Kennedy P, Fryer C, Gilchrist GS, Hays DM, Hanson W, Heller R, Jenkin RDT, Kung F, Sheehan W, Tefft M, Ternberg J, Wharam M.
The Intergroup Hodgkin's disease in children. A study of stages I and II.
Cancer 1990;**65**:1429–37.

The study was carried out between 1977 and 1981 by the Pediatric Oncology Group, Children's Cancer Group and the Acute Leukemia Group B.

Objectives

This study combined data from two separate studies addressing the issue of the benefit of adjuvant MOPP to either involved field or extended field radiotherapy in children with stage I and II disease.

Details of the study

Eligibility included less than 18 years of age, centrally reviewed pathological diagnosis, pathologically staged I or II disease, and no prior therapy except emergency mediastinal irradiation.

No details of randomisation method or location are given. It was estimated that 47 patients per group were required to provide an 80% power to detect a 22% advantage to the addition of MOPP chemotherapy, with 5% significance level in a one-sided test.

Study outline for first and second line treatment is given in Figure 10.5.

All patients received radiotherapy, which was to be administered within 28 days of pathological diagnosis.

Involved field (IF) radiotherapy included the known involved regions of disease and extended field (EF) included involved regions and continuous uninvolved nodal regions. For stage I and II nodal disease above the diaphragm, the EF volume to be irradiated included the mantle, para-aortic regions to the level of L4, and the splenic pedicle. For stage II

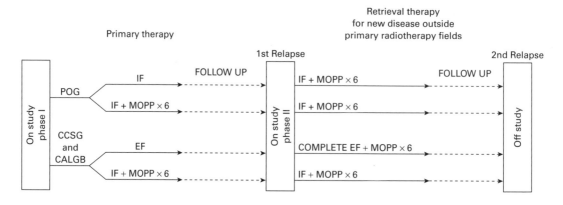

Figure 10.5 Treatment options for initial and recurrent disease. Copyright © 1990 American Cancer Society. Adapted and reprinted from Gehan EA *et al* (full reference above) by permission of Wiley-Liss, Inc., a subsidiary of John Wiley & Sons, Inc.

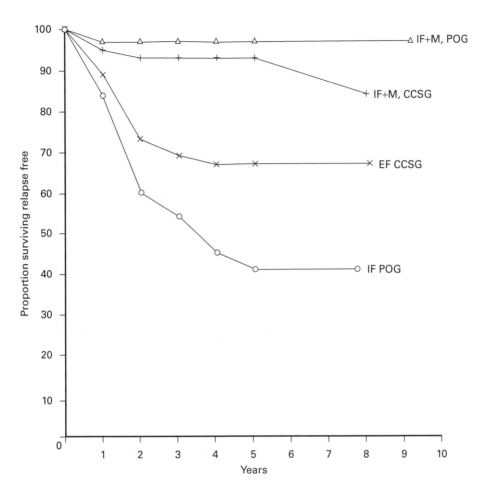

Figure 10.6 Comparisons of relapse free survival by treatment and cooperative group for the randomised, eligible patients. Copyright © 1990 American Cancer Society. Adapted and reprinted from Gehan EA *et al* (full reference p 244) by permission of Wiley-Liss, Inc., a subsidiary of John Wiley & Sons, Inc.

nodal disease in the inguinal and iliac regions without para-aortic involvement, the inverted Y volume was irradiated. Involved regions were given a dose of 35–40 Gy. Residual disease could be given further boost doses at the discretion of the radiotherapist. For EF radiotherapy 35 Gy was recommended as the lower dose limit.

In the combined modality regimen, MOPP chemotherapy followed 4 weeks after IF therapy. Six standard courses were given at 28 day intervals.

Three clinical presentations were excluded from the randomised study, as these were regarded as a favourable subgroup and were treated as elected by the institutional investigators. These comprised stage I unilateral upper neck disease of any histological type other than lymphocyte depleted, stage I unilateral inguinal disease of any histological type and stage I mediastinal disease of the nodular sclerosing type.

The main outcome measures were relapse free survival at 2 years and overall event free survival and overall survival.

Outcome

Three hundred and six patients were registered, of whom 24 were excluded due to lack of data. Two hundred and twenty of 282 were randomised, with 26 excluded after randomisation: 10 wrong staging, 8 refused randomisation, 6 inadequate laparotomy and 2 not Hodgkin's disease. These were excluded from the subsequent analysis. Of the remaining patients in the POG study, 39 patients were randomised to IF radiotherapy alone and 41 to IF plus MOPP. Twenty-one of 39 who received IF alone relapsed, compared to 1 of 41 where MOPP was also given. In the CCSG/CALGB study, 58 patients were randomised to EF radiotherapy, of whom 18 relapsed, and 56 to EF plus MOPP, of whom 5 relapsed.

The 5 year relapse free survival for IF plus MOPP was 97% versus 41% for IF alone ($p = 0.01$) and for EF radiotherapy 67% versus IF plus MOPP 93% ($p = 0.01$). Despite the significant

advantages to the addition of MOPP in both studies, there was no difference in ultimate survival. This was 89% for IF + MOPP, 95% for IF in the POG studies, 90% IF + MOPP and 96% EF in the CCG/ALGB study (Figure 10.6).

Overall, 6 second cancers were reported, 5 had received IF + MOPP, with 3 leukaemias, 1 brain tumour, 1 germ cell tumour and 1 salivary gland carcinoma in a patient receiving extended field radiotherapy alone.

Conclusion

It was concluded that combination chemotherapy with involved field provides a superior relapse free survival but little impact on overall survival. The overall burden of therapy must be taken into account as in most cases further radiation therapy was given following relapse, in addition to further alkylating agent chemotherapy.

Comment

A preliminary report of this study on 223 randomised patients was published by Sullivan MP, Fuller LM, Chen T, Fisher R, Fryer C, Gehan E, Gilchrist GS, Hays D, Hanson W, Heller R, Higgins G, Jenkin D, Kung F, Sheehan W, Tefft M, Ternberg J, Wharam M. Intergroup Hodgkin's disease in children study of stages I and II: a preliminary report. *Cancer Treat Rep* 1982;**66**:937–47.

Study 8

Louw G, Pinkerton CR.
Interventions for early stage Hodgkin's disease in children (Cochrane Review).
The Cochrane Library, Issue 1, 2001.

This is a formal systematic review of randomised data regarding treatment for early stage Hodgkin's disease in children.

Objectives

The objective was to assess the effects of radiotherapy, chemotherapy or combined radiotherapy and chemotherapy on relapse free survival and overall survival rates in children with early stage (I–IIA) Hodgkin's disease.

Details of the study

The search strategy involved search of the Cochrane Library, Medline, 1966–98, Embase, Cinahl, Cancer-CD and reference lists of relevant articles. Three journals were also hand searched.

Selection criteria were randomised controlled trials of involved field radiotherapy, extended field radiotherapy, anthracycline based chemotherapy regimens or alkylating chemotherapy agents in children up to 19 years of age with Hodgkin's disease.

Trial eligibility and quality were assessed and study authors were contacted for additional information.

Outcome

Four trials involving 334 children were included. It was not possible to combine the outcomes as they covered different treatment regimens. The trials were of variable quality. One trial comparing radiotherapy alone showed no discernible difference in relapse free survival (relative risk 0·73, 95% confidence interval 0·49–1·09) or overall survival (relative risk 0·92, 95% confidence interval 0·79–1·07) between involved field and extended field radiotherapy. No discernible difference was found between involved field radiotherapy plus chemotherapy and extended field radiotherapy and chemotherapy (based on one small trial). In another trial, involved field radiotherapy plus chemotherapy appeared to increase relapse free survival compared to either involved field or extended field radiotherapy alone, although a discernible difference was found for overall survival. Extended field radiotherapy alone appeared to increase relapse free survival compared to extended radiotherapy plus chemotherapy (relative risk 0·34, 95% confidence interval 0·14–0·83) but no discernible difference was apparent for overall survival (based on one trial).

Studies included in the review were:

Bayle-Weisgerber C, Lemercier N, Teillet F, Asselain B, Gout M, Schweisguth O. Hodgkin's disease in children, results of therapy in a mixed group of 178 clinical and pathologically staged patients over 13 years. *Cancer* 1984;**54**:215–22.

Cranmer P, Andrieu JM. Hodgkin's disease in childhood and adolescence: results of chemotherapy-radiotherapy in clinical stages IA–IIB. *J Clin Oncol* 1985;**3**:1495–502.

Gehan EA, Sullivan MP, Fuller LM, Johnston J, Kennedy P, Fryer C. The Intergroup Hodgkin's disease in children. A study of stages I and II. *Cancer* 1990;1429–37.

Hutchison G. Radiotherapy of stage I and II Hodgkin's disease. A collaborative study. *Cancer* 1984;**54**:1928–54.

Sullivan M, Fuller L, Chen T, Fisher R, Fryer C *et al.* Intergroup Hodgkin's disease in children. Study of stages I and II: a preliminary report (full report Gehan 1990). *Cancer Treat Rep* 1982;**66**:937–47.

Part II
Leukaemia

AG Shankar

11,12
Acute myeloid leukaemia
Commentary – Judith Chessells

The chances of long term survival for children with acute myeloid leukaemia have improved steadily in the past 20 years. This has been confirmed both by the results of clinical trials, including those reviewed below, and population based registry studies[1,2]. Myeloid leukaemia is a rare disease in childhood and it is difficult to accrue sufficient numbers for randomised trials. Yet the need for such trials is pressing since as survival improves it becomes more important to refine therapy and avoid late effects of treatment. One approach to this problem, adopted by the UK Medical Research Council Working party, is to plan trials for both children and younger adults, another is to develop international studies.

Induction therapy

Can modifications of induction therapy improve remission rates (now in excess of 85–90% in the best studies), improve event free survival and, if possible, minimise late toxicity, especially the cardiotoxicity associated with anthracyclines? The earlier Children's Cancer Group trial reviewed here (Chapter 11, Study 4), CCG-213, which was conducted in 1986-9, compared classic induction therapy for AML comprising three consecutive doses of daunorubicin and a 7 day infusion of cytosine arabinoside (ARA-c) with a 5 drug

regimen (DCTER) containing reduced doses of anthracyclines and including other drugs, even dexamethasone – of questionable efficacy in AML. There was no significant difference in remission rate, which was of the order of 75%, or event free survival, about 32% in both regimens.

For reasons which are not apparent, in the second CCG study, CCG-2891 (Chapter 11, Study 2), the 5 drug DCTER regimen was adopted but patients were randomised to receive the courses at conventional intervals or more intensively to ensure early blast regression. Intensive induction resulted in a higher toxic death rate but less refractory disease and, importantly, a significantly better event free survival than conventional induction.

The MRC AML-10 trial (Chapter 11, Study 3) which included both children and adults, involved slightly higher doses of daunorubicin and more prolonged ARA-C than the CCG protocols and patients were randomised to receive either thioguanine or etoposide, as a third drug. This intensive treatment was designed to produce blast clearance in one course. The overall remission rate was 91%, with no significant difference between protocols in remission rate or event free survival. Induction in the most recent BFM 93 study[3] was also more intensive than the CCG protocols and achieved an 82% remission rate. Despite the authors' conclusions, there was no significant evidence that idarubicin was superior to daunorubicin in induction therapy.

Conclusion

There is no firm evidence that the addition of a third drug during induction of AML adds benefit to the combinations of an anthracycline and intensive ARA-C, but one is often added. The comparison of thioguanine and etoposide (Chapter 11, Study 3) as third induction drugs confounded the myth that etoposide is of special benefit in leukaemia with a monocytic component. Intensive induction therapy, although toxic, improves event free survival (Chapter 11, Study 2). There may be scope for further refinements of induction therapy in AML, for example the use of newer anthracyclines, but in view of the high remission rates now achieved major improvements would seem unlikely and large numbers of patients would be needed to demonstrate a significant benefit.

What next after induction?

The most controversial issue in the management of AML, and the one that lends itself least readily to randomised trials, is the role of allogeneic bone marrow transplant (BMT) in first remission. It is probably true that for many years BMT from a histocompatible sibling donor was regarded as the "gold standard" in treatment of children with AML (Chapter 11, Study 4). Since most children do not have a histocompatible sibling donor, an alternative approach, derived from encouraging single arm unrandomised studies[4],

was the use of high dose therapy and rescue with autologous stem cells. The more conventional approach to treatment, illustrated by several studies reviewed here, is further intensive consolidation therapy. Most protocols for AML do not incorporate continuing (maintenance) therapy and in a randomised comparison in CCG-213 (Chapter 11, Study 4) such maintenance was not beneficial.

Three similar trials in paediatric AML have compared high dose therapy and autologous bone marrow transplantation (ABMT) with conventional post remission consolidation (Chapter 12, Studies 1, 2 and 4) and none found significant evidence of benefit for ABMT. In all three trials, however, the relapse risk was lower and the event free survival superior in patients with a histocompatible sibling donor who were electively treated by BMT.

The fourth trial of ABMT, AML-10 (Chapter 12, Study 3) had a different design, in that after four courses of induction/intensification patients were randomised to receive high dose therapy and ABMT as a fifth consolidation course or to stop treatment. The full results of this trial comprising both children and adults[5] showed that ABMT was associated with a lower relapse rate in all age groups. Survival in children, however, was not improved by ABMT (Chapter 12, Study 3), since children who relapsed after ABMT had a worse survival than those receiving four courses of chemotherapy.

It would seem reasonable to conclude from the available evidence that while there is no established place for high dose therapy and ABMT in paediatric AML there remains scope for additional intensification therapy. Further refinements of chemotherapy under investigation include the use of an additional block of intensification with high dose ARA-C, as in AML-12[6]. The recent BFM Study 83 (Chapter 11, Study 1) involved a randomisation to receive high dose ARA-C and mitoxantrone (HAM) in higher risk patients (defined by clinical and morphological criteria), either after induction or after 6 weeks of lower dose therapy. There was no difference in event free survival between the patients treated with early or late HAM but comparison with historical controls showed an improvement in event free survival.

Recent improvements in event free survival have been achieved in many patients without recourse to BMT in first remission. While a minority of patients have a histocompatible sibling donor, BMT from alternative stem cell sources has become more widely available and safer. However, in general BMT is associated with a higher risk of treatment related death than chemotherapy and an increased risk of late effects of treatment, in particular in respect of growth and fertility. Trials involving BMT are of necessity non-randomised and there are many inherent biases in assessment. One approach is to analyse by intention-to-treat on the basis of comparing outcome for patients with and without a sibling donor. This comparison in the paediatric AML-10 trial showed no significant improvement in EFS for patients with a donor (Chapter 12, Study 3). By contrast, BMT was superior to chemotherapy in recent American trials conducted by the Pediatric Oncology Group (Chapter 12, Study 2) and the Children's Cancer Group (Chapter 12, Study 4), and in the latter compliance with allocated treatment was extremely high.

One recent development in AML, long fashionable in ALL, has been the identification of risk groups – a strategy where BMT might be reserved in first remission to higher risk children as identified by clinical and morphological characteristics[7] or by cytogenetics[8]. It seems justifiable to exempt patients with a good chance of being cured from the risks of BMT, and whether BMT will improve outcome in the worst risk patients remains to be seen.

Conclusion

Results of treatment have improved and for most patients this has been achieved by chemotherapy. There is little evidence to support long term maintenance therapy in management of AML and short term consolidation therapy has proved as effective as high dose therapy and ABMT. The role of BMT is probably evolving and the balance of risk/benefit between BMT and chemotherapy has probably shifted towards chemotherapy in recent years.

References

1 Stiller CA, Eatock EM. Survival from acute non-lymphocytic leukaemia, 1971–88: a population based study. *Arch Dis Childh* 1994;**70**:219–23.

2 Lie SO, Jonmundsson G, Mellander L, Siimes MA, Yssing M, Gustafsson G. A population-based study of 272 children with acute myeloid leukaemia treated on two consecutive protocols with different intensity: best outcome in girls, infants, and children with Down's syndrome: Nordic Society of Paediatric Haematology and Oncology (NOPHO). *Br J Haematol* 1996;**94**:82–8.

3 Creutzig U, Ritter J, Zimmermann M, Hermann J, Gadner H, Sawatzki DB *et al.* Idarubicin improves blast cell clearance during induction therapy in children with AML: results of study AML-BFM 93. AML-BFM Study Group. *Leukemia* 2001;**15**:348–54.

4   Burnett AK, Watkins R, Maharaj D, McKinnon S, Robertson AG, Tansey P *et al.* Transplantation of unpurged autologous bone-marrow in acute myeloid leukaemia in first remission. *Lancet* 1984;**ii**:1068–70.

5   Burnett AK, Goldstone AH, Stevens RF, Hann IM, Gray RG, Rees JKH *et al.* Randomised comparison of addition of autologous bone marrow transplantation to intensive chemotherapy for acute myeloid leukaemia in first remission: results of MRC AML 10 trial. UK Medical Research Council Adult and Children's Working Parties. *Lancet* 1998;**351**:700–8.

6   Webb DK, Harrison G, Stevens RF, Gibson BG, Hann IM, Wheatley K. Relationships between age at diagnosis, clinical features and outcome of therapy in children treated in the Medical Research Council (MRC) trials for Acute Myeloid Leukaemia AML 10 and 12. *Blood* 2001;**98**:1714–20.

7   Creutzig U, Ritter J, Schellong G. Identification of two risk groups in childhood acute myelogenous leukemia after therapy intensification in study AML-BFM-83 as compared with study AML-BFM-78: AML-BFM study Group *Blood* 1990;**75**:1932–40.

8   Grimwade D, Walker H, Oliver F, Wheatley K, Harrison C, Harrison G *et al.* The importance of diagnostic cytogenetics on outcome in AML: analysis of 1,612 patients entered into the MRC AML 10 trial: The Medical Research Council Adult and Children's Leukaemia Working Parties. *Blood* 1998;**92**:2322–33.

11
Induction regimens in acute myeloid leukaemia

Studies

Study 1

Crutzig U, Ritter J, Zimmermann M, Reinhardt D, Hermann J, Berthold F, Henze G, Jürgens H, Kabisch H, Havers W, Reiter A, Kluba U, Niggli F, Gadner H for the Acute Myeloid Leukaemia Berlin–Frankfurt–Munster Study Group.

Improved treatment results in high risk paediatric acute myeloid leukaemia patients after intensification with high-dose cytarabine and mitoxantrone: results of study Acute Myeloid Leukaemia Berlin–Frankfurt–Munster 93.

J Clin Oncol 2001;**19**:2705–13.

AML-BFM 93 was a prospective randomised multicentre study and enrolled patients from January 1993 until June 1998. Two randomisations were incorporated into the study – the first, which was performed at diagnosis and included all eligible patients, ended on 31 December 1997, while patient accrual for the second randomisation (for high risk patients alone) ended 6 months later.

Objectives

The aims of the study were:

- To compare the relative efficacy and toxicity of daunorubicin with Idarubicin in the induction chemotherapy regimen for children with AML.

- To improve the outcome of children with high risk AML with the use of high dose mitoxantrone (HAM) during the post induction phase of therapy.

Details of the study

Previously untreated children and adolescents between the ages of 0 and 17 years with newly diagnosed AML were entered onto the study. All patients who had secondary AML, granulocytic sarcoma, myelodysplastic syndrome or Down's syndrome were excluded from the trial.

Patients were stratified as standard or high risk according to diagnostic morphology of blast cells and blast cell reduction in the bone marrow on day 15. The standard risk (SR) group included FAB M1 or M2 with Auer rods, FAB M3 regardless of bone marrow status on day 15 and FAB $M4E_0$ with $\geq 5\%$ blasts in the marrow on day 15. All other patients were categorised as high risk (HR). Additionally, SR patients who had >5% blasts in the marrow on day 15 were redesignated as HR.

Randomisations were done with permuted blocks. All patients were randomised at diagnosis to an 8 day induction chemotherapy regimen with either ADE (Ara-C 100 mg/m^2 continuous IV infusion on days 1 and 2; daunorubicin 30 mg/m^2

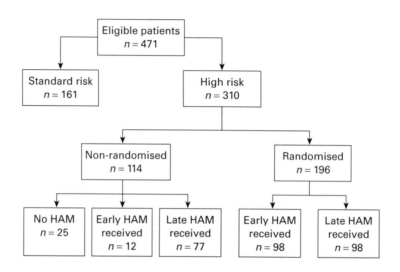

Figure 11.1 Flow of patients entered onto study AML-BFM 93

as 30 minute IV infusion 12 hourly on days 3 to 5 and Etoposide 150 mg/m² as a 2 hour infusion on days 6 to 8) or AIE (Idarubicin 12 mg/m² as 30 minute IV infusion 24 hourly on days 3 to 5 with Ara-C and Etoposide as in the ADE regimen).

High risk patients were randomised to either early HAM (high dose Ara-C 3 g/m² 12 hourly x 3 days and mitoxantrone 10 mg/m² on days 4–5 followed by consolidation therapy) or late HAM (consolidation therapy followed by HAM). Standard risk patients received consolidation therapy without HAM.

Consolidation consisted of 6 weeks of treatment with thioguanine 60 mg/m² PO days 1–43; pred-nisolone 40 mg/m² PO days 1–28; vincristine 1·5 mg/m² IV days 1, 8, 15 and 22; doxorubicin 30 mg/m² IV infusion days 1, 8, 15 and 22; Ara-C 75 mg/m² IV days 3–6, 10–13, 17–20,

24–27, 31–34 and 38–41; cyclophosphamide 500 mg/m² IV days 29 and 43; and intrathecal Ara-C on days 1, 15, 29 and 43.

All patients received an intensification block of high dose Ara-C and etoposide (Ara-C 3 g/m² 12 hourly × 3 days and etoposide 125 mg/m² days 2–5). This was followed by 18 Gy cranial irradiation (in children > 3 years) and maintenance therapy that consisted of daily thioguanine 40 mg/m² PO and Ara-C 40 mg/m² SC × 4 day monthly for a total of 18 months.

Allogeneic bone marrow transplant was recommended for high risk children in CR1 if a matched sibling donor was available.

Outcome measures were 5 year overall survival (OS), event free survival (EFS) and disease free survival (DFS).

Table 11.1 Results of study AML–BFM 93, by HAM group and induction treatment

HAM	Induction	Total no. of patients	<5% blasts on day 15		Complete remission		pEFS ± SE (%)
			No. of patients[a]	%	No. of Patients	%	
Early	Daunorubicin	46	10/21	48	40	87	51·9 ± 7·4
	Idarubicin	52	21/29	72	46	89	51·3 ± 7·0
Late	Daunorubicin	46	14/28	50	37	80	35·6 ± 7·3[b]
	Idarubicin	52	18/28	64	46	89	53·6 ± 7·0

[a] Number of patients with < 5% blasts/total number of patients with data available.

[b] Late HAM after daunorubicin induction versus other groups: p = 0·05, log-rank test.

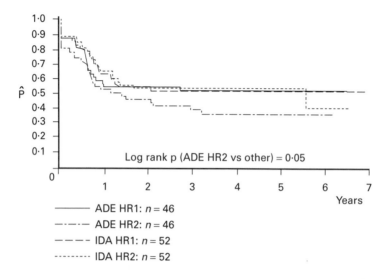

Figure 11.2 Estimated pEFS among high risk patients in study AML-BFM 93. For details of treatments, see text. HR1 = early HAM; HR2 = late HAM

Analysis of all data was performed according to the intention to treat principle.

Outcome

Of the 471 eligible patients enrolled on the AML-BFM 93 trial, 161 patients were categorised as standard risk (SR) and 310 patients as high risk (HR). Figure 11.1 shows the numbers of patients according to treatment and randomisation.

Of the 114 HR patients not randomised, 25 did not receive HAM (18 died of complications, 5 experienced severe toxicity and 2 were assigned to the wrong risk group), 12 were allocated to early HAM and 77 patients to late HAM. Allogeneic bone marrow transplantation was performed in 14 patients, each in the early and late HAM groups.

Complete remission (CR) was achieved in 387 (82%) of 471 patients.

Patients who underwent induction with idarubicin had significantly better blast cell reductions

in the bone marrow on day 15 – 17% patients had > 5% blasts compared to 31% patients on the daunorubicin arm (p = 0·1, χ^2 test). However, 5 year DFS and EFS were similar in both groups of patients. The infection rate was higher in the idarubicin arm (p trend = 0·016), as was the duration of bone marrow aplasia – neutrophil recovery > 0·5 × $10^9/\ell$, which was 2 days longer.

Five year OS, EFS and DFS rates (± SE) were 74% ± 4%, 65% ± 4% and 73% ± 4% respectively in the SR group of patients, while in the HR group it was 52% ± 3%, 44% ± 3%, and 56% ± 3% respectively.

Probability of event free survival (pEFS) was marginally higher among patients treated with daunorubicin and early HAM compared with patients who received daunorubicin and late HAM, whereas results with idarubicin were similar in both the early and late HAM groups of patients (Table 11.1, Figure 11.2).

Conclusion

It was concluded that though idarubicin induction resulted in a significant blast cell reduction in the bone marrow on day 15, this did not translate into improved 5 year event free survival or disease free survival in children with AML. High risk patients who received daunorubicin induction benefited with early HAM intensification. However, idarubicin induction resulted in higher infection rates and a longer duration of neutropenia secondary to bone marrow depression.

Study 2

Woods WG, Kobrinsky N, Buckley JD, Lee JW, Sanders J, Neudorf S, Gold S, Barnard DR, DeSwarte J, Dusenbery K, Kalousek D, Arthur DC, and Lange BJ.

Timed sequential induction therapy improves post remission outcome in acute myeloid leukaemia: a report of the Children's Cancer Study Group.

Blood 1996;**87**:4979–989.

This CCG study (CCG-2891) was a prospective randomised multicentre trial that ran from October 1989 to May 1993.

Objectives

The study aimed to determine whether intensive induction therapy improves long term outcome of children with acute myeloid leukaemia (AML).

Details of the study

Children and adolescents younger than 21 years of age with AML (FAB M0–M7), acute undifferentiated AML or bi-phenotypic leukaemia with myeloid differentiation, myelodysplastic syndrome (MDS) or granulocytic sarcoma were eligible for the study. From April 1992, children with AML M3 were registered on the intergroup APL study (CCG-2911). Patients with known Fanconi's anaemia or Philadelphia positive chronic myeloid leukaemia in chronic phase were excluded from the study. However, for analysis of results, patients with the following conditions were excluded: Down's syndrome ($n = 55$); de novo MDS ($n = 19$); granulocytic sarcoma without bone marrow involvement ($n = 14$); secondary AML ($n = 9$).

Results were analysed on the principle of intention to treat. Accrual goals were set before initiation of the study, with the power to detect 10% difference in DFS at 2 years between the two induction arms of 0·88.

Details of the randomisation method are not specified in the report.

Patients were randomised at diagnosis to one of two induction regimens – standard and intensive – in which identical drugs and doses were used (Figure 11.3). Initial induction chemotherapy consisted of a 5 drug regimen administered over 4 days – dexamethasone, 6-thioguanine, cytosine arabinoside (ARA-C), daunorubicin and etoposide (DCTER). Daunorubicin, etoposide and ARA-c were administered as a continuous infusion for 96 hours. Patients randomised to the intensive arm received a second cycle of DCTER chemotherapy 6 days after completion of cycle 1 irrespective of bone marrow or haematological status. Patients randomised to the standard arm underwent bone marrow evaluation on day 14 and proceeded to cycle 2 (identical to cycle 1) immediately if they had residual leukaemia (> 40% blasts in the bone marrow). However, if leukaemic blast clearance was satisfactory or if the marrow was hypoplastic indicating significant clearance of blasts, cycle 2 was withheld until blood counts recovered or there was clear evidence of disease progression. Patients who showed no response after two cycles were considered protocol failures and were removed from the study. Standard timing induction therapy was closed in May 1993 and GCSF (granulocyte colony stimulating factor) was introduced for all patients thereafter, during the induction phase. The overall time to administer four induction cycles was similar in the two

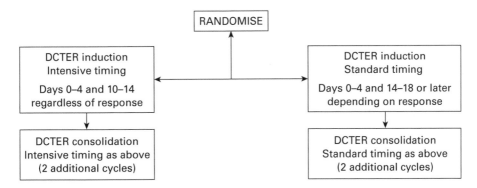

Day 0 through 4: DCTER induction
Dexamethasone 6 mg/m^2/d (0·2 mg/m^2//kg/d) thrice daily
ARA-C 200 mg/m^2/d (6·7 mg/kg/d) continuous infusion
Thioguanine 100 mg/m^2/d (3·3 mg/kg/d) twice daily
Etoposide 100 mg/m^2/d (3·3 mg/kg/d) continuous infusion
Rubidomycin (daunorubicin) 20 mg/m^2/d 20 mg/kg/d (0·67 mg/kg/d) continuous infusion
ARA-C intrathecal (age-based doses)

Post remission therapy

1 Patients randomised to conventional chemotherapy
   (A) Course 1: Days 0 through 2 ARA-C, 3 g/m^2/dose (100 mg/kg) IV over 3 h every 12 h × 4 doses.
        L-asparaginase 6000 IU/m^2 (200 IU/kg) IM, hour 42. Days 7 through 9 ARA-C and L-asparaginase
        repeated exactly as administered days 0 through 2.
   (B) Courses 2 and 3: Two 28–day cycles of 75 mg/m^2 6-thioguanine (2·5 mg/kg) PO daily,
        days 0 through 27; 1·5 mg/m^2 vincristine (0·05 mg/kg) IV, day 0; 75 mg/m^2 ARA-C (2·5 mg/kg)
        IV every day × 4, days 0 through 3; 75 mg/m^2 cyclophosphamide (2·5 mg/kg) IV every day × 4,
        days 0 through 3; 100 mg/m^2 5-azacytidine (3·3 mg/kg) IV every day × 4, days 0 through 3.
   (C) Course 4: 25 mg/m^2/dose ARA-C (0·83 mg/kg) SQ or IV every 6 h × 5 days, days 0 through 4;
        30 mg/m^2 daunorubicin (1 mg/kg) IV day 0; 150 mg/m^2 etoposide (5 mg/kg) IV/dose × 2, days 0 and 3;
        50 mg/m^2/dose 6-thioguanine (1·67 mg/kg) orally every 12 h × 5 days, days 0 through 4;
        2 mg/m^2/dose dexamethasone (0·067 mg/kg) orally every 8 h × 4 days, days 0 through 3.
2 Patients allocated to allogeneic or randomised to autologous BMT. Pre-BMT preparative regimen:
   (A) Busulfan 1 mg/kg/dose, administered orally every 6 h × 16 doses, days − 9 to − 6.
   (B) Cyclophosphamide 50 mg/kg/d IV over 1 h daily × 4 days, days − 5 to − 1.

Doses in parentheses were used for children less than 3 years of age. If a leukaemic response was
documented, all patients received DCTER cycles 3 and 4 in an intensive or standard fashion, based on
initial randomisation, after marrow recovery.

Figure 11.3 Details of therapy for study CCG-2891

arms – 99 days for the intensive arm versus
105 days for the standard arm.

The second randomisation was after four cycles
of induction chemotherapy. Patients who did not

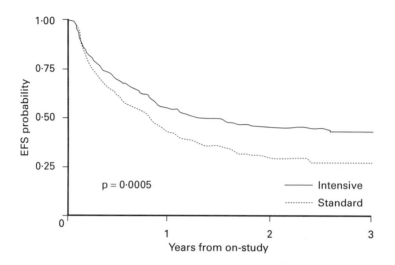

Figure 11.4 EFS from time of study entry for patients with AML, comparing patients randomised to intensive induction timing versus standard induction timing on CCG-2891

have an HLA identical sibling donor were randomised to either autologous BMT (ABMT) or intensive post remission chemotherapy. ABMT patients received a preparatory regimen of 4 days of oral busulphan and 4 days of intravenous cyclophosphamide (200 mg/kg total dose) and had 4-hydroxycyclophosphamide ex vivo purged marrow infused after 1 day's rest. Patients randomised to post remission chemotherapy received four courses of three different chemotherapy regimens, each lasting for 4–6 weeks, (as shown in Figure 11.3). All patients who had HLA identical family donors were allocated to allogeneic BMT with an identical preparatory regimen to ABMT (see Chapter 12, Study 4).

CNS prophylaxis consisted of four doses of intrathecal cytosine asabinoside (IT ARA-C) administered at the start of each DCTER cycle.

Patients with CNS leukaemia had six additional doses of IT Ara-C twice a week.

Main outcome measures were disease free survival (DFS), event free survival (EFS) and overall survival (OS).

Outcome

A total of 589 eligible patients were randomised to either the standard induction arm ($n = 294$) or to the intensive induction arm ($n = 295$). Compliance to induction randomisation was greater than 98%. Thirty-one patients withdrew prior to completion of induction therapy. Of the remaining 558 evaluable patients, 407 successfully completed 4 courses of intensive chemotherapy and were eligible for allocation to allogeneic BMT or randomisation to autologous bone marrow transplantation or intensive

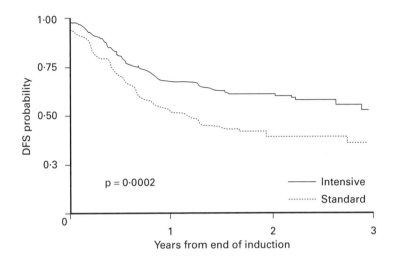

Figure 11.5 DFS from the end of induction for patients with AML enrolled on CCG-2891 and achieving remission, comparing intensively timed induction with standard timed induction therapy

chemotherapy. Seventy-nine patients refused post remission randomisation while data were not available in 2 patients. One hundred and five patients were allocated to allogeneic BMT, 107 were randomised to autologous BMT and 114 patients to intensive chemotherapy. There were no differences between the two groups of patients based on white blood cell counts at diagnosis, FAB subtypes, on the presence of various cytogenetic abnormalities or in the rate of deaths during the first 10 days of the study.

Four hundred and twenty-six patients achieved complete remission after two courses of DCTER therapy. For standard induction ($n = 294$), 195 (70%) patients achieved CR, 71 (26%) failed therapy and 11 (4%) patients died due to chemotherapy toxicity; 17 patients withdrew from the study. For intensive induction ($n = 295$), 212 (75%) patients achieved CR, 38 (14%) had refractory disease while 31 (11%) patients died

due to toxicity; 14 patients withdrew after randomisation. Figure 11.4 shows the 3 year EFS was 42% ± 7% for patients in the intensive arm compared to 27% ± 7% for the standard arm patients ($p = 0.0005$) while the 3 year OS for the intensive and standard arm patients was 51% ± 7% and 39% ± 7% respectively ($p = 0.07$). Comparing the two induction arms, the failure rate was significantly higher in the standard arm ($p = 0.0003$).

Post remission outcome was as follows. The 3 year DFS (median follow up 28 months) from the end of induction for the intensive arm ($n = 212$) patients was 55% ± 8% versus 37% ± 8% (Figure 11.5) for the standard arm ($n = 195$) patients ($p = 0.0002$), and actuarial survival at 3 years was 52% ± 6% compared to 42% ± 6% and at 5 years 49% ± 6% versus. 38% ± 6% ($p = 0.04$) for the intensive and standard arm patients respectively.

In standard induction patients who received a second cycle of chemotherapy within 18 days of cycle 1 (i.e. those with significant residual leukaemia), 3 year EFS was non-significantly better (30% v 26%; p = 0·51).

Toxicity

Patients receiving intensive induction had a significantly higher degree of myelosuppression than those who received standard induction therapy (43% v 24%; p < 0·00001). Intensive arm patients also had increased pulmonary, renal and hepatic toxicity. Death from chemotherapy toxicity was significantly higher in the intensive arm (p = 0·002).

Conclusion

It was concluded that intensively timed induction therapy markedly improved disease free survival, event free survival and overall survival in children with AML, despite significantly higher toxic deaths.

Study 3

Hann IM, Stevens RF, Goldstone AH, Rees JKH, Wheatley K, Gray RG, Burnett AK on behalf of the Adult and Childhood Leukaemia Working Party of the Medical Research Council.

Randomised comparison of DAT versus ADE as induction chemotherapy in children and younger adults with acute myeloid leukaemia. Results of the Medical Research Council's 10th AML Trial (MRC AML 10).

Blood 1997;**89**:2311–18.

The MRC AML-10 trial, which ran from May 1988 to April 1995, was a prospective multicentre randomised study, which involved 41 centres in the United Kingdom, Republic of Ireland and New Zealand.

Objectives

The study compared the relative efficacy and toxicity of thioguanine with etoposide in the induction chemotherapy regimen in children with acute myeloid leukaemia (AML).

Details of the study

All patients below 56 years of age were eligible to be enrolled on the study. In addition to patients who had de novo AML, those with secondary AML or with myelodysplastic syndrome (refractory anaemia with excess of blasts) were also eligible for entry.

There were two randomisations and the details of chemotherapy treatment and randomisations are shown in Figure 11.6. The first randomisation was between two induction regimens – daunorubicin, ARA-C and thioguanine (DAT) and daunorubicin, ARA-C and etoposide (ADE). The second was between autologous BMT and no

further treatment. Children with an identical HLA sibling donor were allocated to allogeneic BMT. In addition, triple intrathecal therapy with methotrexate, cytarabine and hydrocortisone was given as part of each course. Children aged over 2 years who had CNS disease at presentation and not receiving BMT had craniospinal radiotherapy after completion of chemotherapy.

Patients receiving BMT had a preparatory regimen of cyclophosphamide (120 mg/kg total dose over 2 days) and fractionated total body irradiation. For children aged under 2 years, the conditioning treatment was with busulphan (16 mg/kg total dose over 4 days) and cyclophosphamide (200 mg/kg total dose over 4 days).

Outcome measures were complete remission (CR) rate and overall survival (OS).

Outcome

The analysis in this report deals with the outcome in children alone (≤14 years of age) and all analyses were by allocated treatment. Of 286 eligible patients below the age of 15 years, 143 each were randomised to DAT and ADE induction regimens respectively (Table 11.2). There were no significant differences in the distribution of patients by age, gender, secondary AML, diagnostic WBC count, FAB subtype, clonal cytogenetic abnormalities or performance status between the two treatment groups. Seven per cent of children had CNS disease at presentation. Compliance with allocated treatment was 98% in both arms.

Complete remission (CR) was achieved by 91% of patients. There was no significant difference in the CR rate between the DAT arm (89%) and the ADE arm (93%) nor was there any difference in the number of courses required to achieve CR.

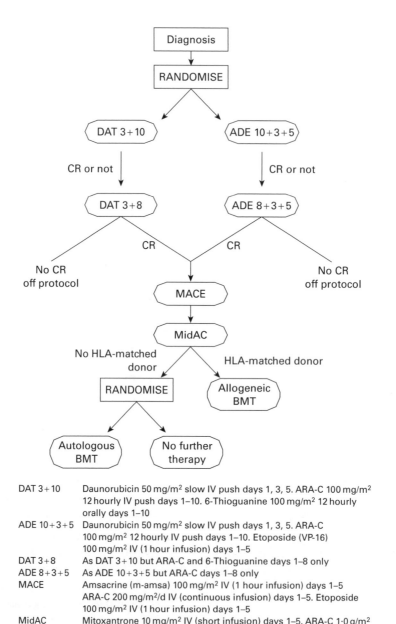

DAT 3 + 10   Daunorubicin 50 mg/m² slow IV push days 1, 3, 5. ARA-C 100 mg/m²
              12 hourly IV push days 1–10. 6-Thioguanine 100 mg/m² 12 hourly
              orally days 1–10
ADE 10 + 3 + 5 Daunorubicin 50 mg/m² slow IV push days 1, 3, 5. ARA-C
              100 mg/m² 12 hourly IV push days 1–10. Etoposide (VP-16)
              100 mg/m² IV (1 hour infusion) days 1–5
DAT 3 + 8   As DAT 3 + 10 but ARA-C and 6-Thioguanine days 1–8 only
ADE 8 + 3 + 5 As ADE 10 + 3 + 5 but ARA-C days 1–8 only
MACE   Amsacrine (m-amsa) 100 mg/m² IV (1 hour infusion) days 1–5
              ARA-C 200 mg/m²/d IV (continuous infusion) days 1–5. Etoposide
              100 mg/m² IV (1 hour infusion) days 1–5
MidAC   Mitoxantrone 10 mg/m² IV (short infusion) days 1–5. ARA-C 1·0 g/m²
              12-hourly IV (2 hour infusion) days 1–3
NB: All doses were reduced by 25% for children less than 1 year old

Figure 11.6 Protocol flow chart for study AML-10

Table 11.2 Presentation features of patients in MRC AML-10

Parameter	Value	No. of patients		% of patients[a]
		DAT	ADE	
Age	0–1	27	25	3
	2–14	116	118	13
	15–24	131	128	14
	> 25	655	661	70
Sex	Male	475	471	51
	Female	454	457	49
Type of AML	De novo	863	859	93
	Secondary	66	69	7
White blood cell count:				
$(\times 10^9/\ell)$	0–9	417	412	45
	10–99	366	385	40
	100–199	84	72	8
	200+	31	38	4
	Unknown	31	21	3
FAB type	M0	16	12	2
	M1	136	172	17
	M2	254	253	27
	M3	143	130	15
	M4	184	184	20
	M5	79	81	9
	M6	28	24	3
	M7	24	18	2
	RAEB-t	13	17	2
	Bilineage	2	0	<1
	All	2	6	<1
	Unknown	48	31	4
Cytogenetic group	Favourable	156	165	17
	Intermediate	466	488	51
	Adverse	53	56	6
	Unknown	232	241	25

[a]Percentages may not add to 100 because of rounding.

Five per cent of the patients had resistant disease with no significant difference between the DAT (6%) and ADE (3%) arms (Table 11.3).

Overall survival (Table 11.4) from entry for patients in the two groups was also similar – DAT (60%) versus ADE (53%). Analysis of survival by FAB subtype showed no differences between thioguanine and etoposide in any subset.

Toxicity

The overall induction death rate was 5% with no statistical difference between the DAT (6%) and

ADE (3%) arms. Haematological toxicity (recovery of neutrophils and platelets) was higher after DAT compared to ADE. In contrast, non-haematological toxicity was more pronounced after ADE (nausea, mucositis, alopecia etc.).

Conclusion

It was concluded that the standard DAT induction regimen was no less effective than the etoposide containing regimen (ADE) in the treatment of children with AML. The regimens were equivalent with regard to toxicity and efficacy and could be used interchangeably.

Table 11.3 Remission outcome in MRC AML-10 by DAT versus ADE (% of patients)

	CR			Induction death			Resistant disease			Survival at 5yr(%)	
	DAT	ADE	Total	DAT	ADE	Total	DAT	ADE	Total	DAT	ADE
All patients	81	83	82	8	9	9	11	9	10	60	53
Age:											
0–14	89	93	91	6	3	5	6	3	5	47	46
15–24	83	88	85	9	5	7	8	7	7	52	46
25–34	81	90	85	9	5	7	10	5	7	33	33
35–44	81	77	79	7	11	9	12	13	12	26	34
45+	75	76	76	11	13	12	14	11	13	41	41

Percentages may not add to 100 because of rounding.

Study 4

Wells RJ, Woods WG, Buckley JD, Odam LF, Benjamin D, Bernstein I, Betcher D, Feig S, Kim T, Ruymann F, Smithson W, Srivatsava A, Tannous R, Buckley CM, Whitt JK, Wolff L, Lampkin BC.

Treatment of newly diagnosed children and adolescents with acute myeloid leukaemia: a Children's Cancer Group study.

J Clin Oncol 1994;**12**:2367–77.

This Children's Cancer Group Study (CCG-213) was a randomised prospective multicentre study that ran from January 1986 to February 1989.

Objectives

The study addressed the following questions:

1   Whether the addition of other chemotherapeutic agents to the standard regimen of cytosine arabinoside (ARA-C) and daunorubicin improved remission rate and clinical outcome in children with acute myeloid leukaemia (AML).
2   Whether allogeneic bone marrow transplantation (Allo BMT) in first complete remission improves disease free survival (DFS) and overall survival (OS) when compared with post remission consolidation chemotherapy.
3   Whether there is a place for "maintenance chemotherapy" in the treatment of childhood AML.

This review focuses on the use of additional drugs in the treatment of childhood AML. The analysis of the results of consolidation therapy (BMT *v* chemotherapy) and maintenance therapy are not within the remit of this review.

Details of the study

All patients below 22 years of age with a diagnosis of AML were eligible to be enrolled on the study. Infants less than 2 years of age with acute monoblastic leukaemia were excluded as they were treated on a different chemotherapy regimen.

No details of the randomisation methodology are given in the report.

Figure 11.7 shows the treatment schema of CCG-213. All patients were randomised at diagnosis to one of two induction regimens. For regimen 1, the first cycle consisted of 7 days of continuous infusion of (ARA-C) and bolus doses of daunorubicin (DNR) on the first 3 days of therapy. The second cycle was shortened to 5 days of ARA-C and 2 days of DNR if reassessment bone marrow showed < 5% blasts after the first cycle otherwise the second and or the third cycles were identical to cycle 1. Regimen 2 consisted of ARA-C, DNR, etoposide (VP-16), dexamethasone (DEX) and thioguanine (TG). Depending on the response to therapy, two or three cycles were given. Patients initially randomised to regimen 1 (7+3) crossed over to receive the 5 drug regimen either after two cycles if in remission (blasts in marrow <5%) or after three cycles irrespective of the marrow status and vice versa.

CNS prophylaxis consisted of intrathecal ARA-C administered on the first day of each induction cycle and throughout the consolidation phase (except during high dose ARA-C therapy) for those not transplanted. Patients who had CNS disease at diagnosis received weekly IT ARA-C during induction and monthly during consolidation.

Post induction, patients who had a HLA–matched donors were assigned to BMT

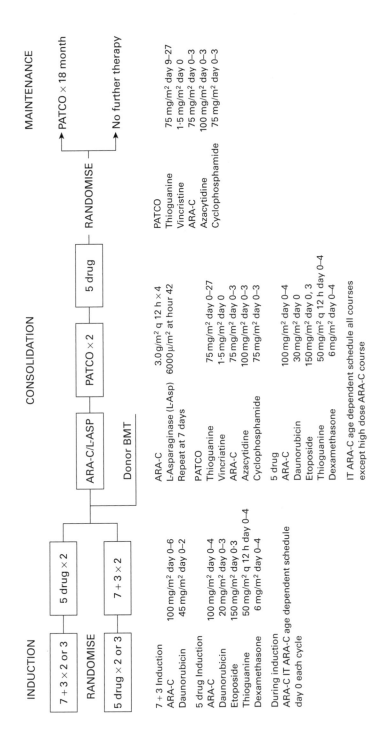

Figure 11.7 Scheme of treatment for study CCG-213. ARA-C, cytosine arabinoside; L-Asp, asparaginase; IT, intrathecal

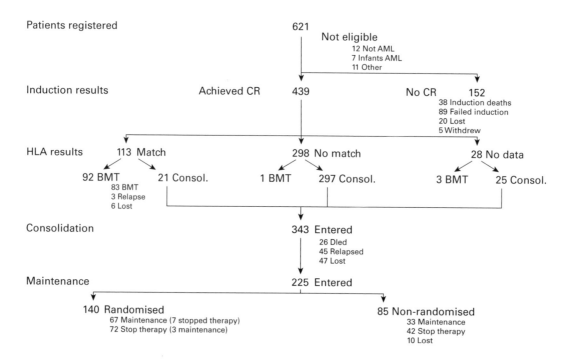

Figure 11.8 CCG-213: patients entering the phases of therapy (induction, BMT, consolidation and maintenance) with explanation for failure to progress to the next phase

after one course of induction if in CR (two or three cycles) or after two courses (five cycles) if marrow had < 16% blasts. BMT conditioning regimen consisted of fractionated total body irradiation and cyclophosphamide. Patients not assigned to BMT received post induction consolidation as shown in Figure 11.7. Following consolidation, patients were randomised either to receive maintenance therapy or stop treatment.

Outcome measures were overall survival (OS) and event free survival (EFS).

Outcome

Figure 11.8 shows the number of eligible patients enrolled and who progressed or failed to progress through the various phases of therapy on the CCG-213 study. Of the 591 patients who were eligible for induction randomisation, 6 were non-randomly allocated to an induction arm and were excluded from analysis of induction outcome.

Both regimens achieved similar rates of remission success: regimen 1 (7 + 3; *n* = 290) 79%

(95% CI 74–84) verses regimen 2 (5 drug; n = 295) 76% (95% CI 71–81), with no significant statistical difference.

After course 1 (two or three cycles of regimens 1 or 2) more patients who received regimen 1 (7 + 3) achieved CR (76%; 95% CI 71–81) compared to 67% (95% CI 60%–72%) for regimen 2 (5 drug) patients (p < 0·02). Early response correlated to improved survival outcome irrespective of treatment regimen as 84% (95% CI 80–88) of patients who had < 16% blasts on day 14 marrow achieved CR. There was no difference in OS or EFS in patients who achieved CR after the first course of induction compared with patients who achieved CR after two courses of therapy

Five year OS for regimens 1 and 2 was 41% (95% CI 35–47) and 37%(95% CI 31–43) (p = 0·16) and 5 year EFS was 32% (95% CI 26–38) and 31% (95% CI 26–36) respectively.

The projected 5 year OS from diagnosis was 39% (95% CI 35–43) and the 5 year EFS was 31% (95% CI 27–35) while the 5 year OS and EFS from the end of induction for all patients irrespective of the post induction therapy were 47% (95% CI 42–52) and 40% (95% CI 35–45) respectively.

Toxicity

Regimen 1 (7+3) patients had a higher degree of bone marrow aplasia and there were more deaths in this arm (25/290 v 13/295; p = 0·06).

Conclusion

It was concluded that the addition of other chemotherapeutic agents to the standard induction regimen of ARA-C and daunorubicin did not improve remission rate, OS or EFS in children and adolescents with AML and early response to induction irrespective of the induction regimen, correlated improved complete remission rates and improved survival.

12

Role of autologous BMT in children with acute myeloid leukaemia in first remission

Studies

Study 1

Amadori S, Testi AM, Aricò M, Comelli A, Giuliano M, Madan E, Masera G, Randelli R, Zanesco L, and Mandelli F, for the Associazione Italiana Ematologia ed Oncologia Pediatrica Cooperative Group.

Prospective comparative study of bone marrow transplantation and post remission chemotherapy for childhood acute myelogenous leukaemia. *J Clin Oncol* 1993;**11**:1046–54.

This was a prospective randomised multicentre trial of the AIEOP Cooperative Group conducted between March 1987 and March 1990.

Objectives

The study aimed to define the role of allogeneic (Allo BMT) and autologous bone marrow transplantation (ABMT) in first remission in children with acute myeloid leukaemia.

Details of the study

Children below 15 years of age with previously untreated AML were eligible for the study. Children with Down's syndrome, secondary AML or AML developing on a background of myelodysplasia were excluded.

Induction therapy consisted of 7 days of continuous infusion of cytosine arabinoside (ARA-C) (200 mg/m^2/d; days 1–7) and 3 days of rapid infusion of daunorubicin (45 mg/m^2/d; days 1–3). If bone marrow showed residual leukaemia on day 21, a second course of daunorubicin (45 mg/m^2/d × 2 days) and ARA-C (200 mg/m^2/d × 5 days) was administered immediately, otherwise it was delayed until recovery of peripheral blood counts. Patients who did not achieve complete remission (CR) after the second course were removed from the study. Consolidation of remission was with the DAT regimen (daunorubicin 60 mg/m^2 day 1; ARA-C 60 mg/m^2 8 hourly

274

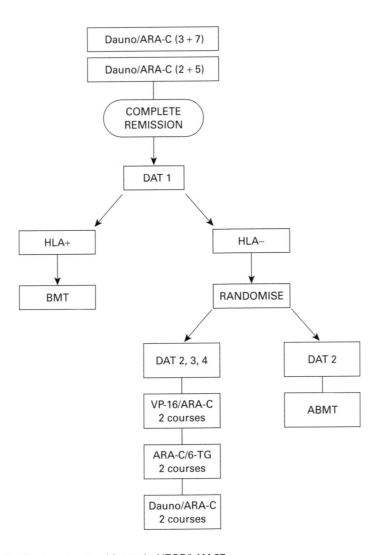

Figure 12.1 Treatment protocol for study AIEOP/LAM 87

SC days 1–5, and thioguanine 70 mg/m²/d 8 hourly PO days 1–5) followed by allogeneic BMT in those who had a matched sibling donor. Children without a matched sibling donor were randomised to either ABMT or six courses of post remission chemotherapy (SPC). CNS prophylaxis consisted of intrathecal chemotherapy (ARA-C and prednisone). The treatment schema shown is in Figure 12.1.

Preparative conditioning for ABMT consisted of carmustine 800 mg/m² over 3 hours from day –5 (BCNU) and followed 24 hours later by 3 day courses each of amsacrine 150 mg/m²/d etoposide

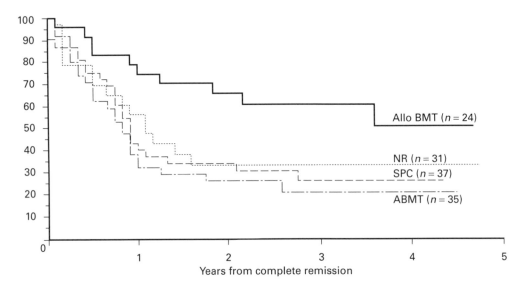

Figure 12.2 Probability of DFS by intended post remission therapy

150 mg/m²/d and ARA-C 300 mg/m²/d as a continuous infusion (BAVC). Cryopreserved unmanipulated marrow was infused 48 hours after completion of ARA-C infusion.

Analysis was performed on the basis of intention to treat.

Outcome

Of the 173 children registered in the trial, only 161 were considered assessable (12 children were excluded due to inadequate documentation or ineligibility). A total of 127 patients (79%) achieved CR. Twenty-four patients were allocated to allogeneic BMT. Of the remaining 103 patients, 72 were randomised to either ABMT (n = 35) or SPC (n = 37). Thirty-one patients were withdrawn from randomisation (NR) because of physician/patient preference in 25, early relapse

in 3, severe induction toxicity in 2, and death in CR in 1.

Sixteen patients switched treatment after randomisation because of parental wishes (n = 15) or late identification of a matched sibling donor in the SPC group. Twenty-three of the 35 (65%) patients randomised to ABMT received the intended treatment and, in contrast, 4 patients in the intensive chemotherapy arm switched treatment.

Risk of leukaemia relapse

There were 9 relapses in the Allo BMT group (n = 24), 25 in the ABMT group (n = 35) and 22 in the chemotherapy group (n = 37). The leukaemia relapse at 5 years was lower in the Allo BMT group compared with either the ABMT or post remission chemotherapy group (45% vs 78% v 70%; p = 0·03).

5 year DFS

Analysis by intention to treat:

Allo BMT group: 51% (SE 13%)
ABMT group: 21% (SE 8%)
SPC group: 27% (SE 8%)
Non-randomised (NR) patients: 34% (SE 10%)
See Figure 12.2.

Analysis by actual treatment received:

Allo BMT group: 56% (SE 13%)
ABMT group: 28% (SE 10%)

SPC group: 17% (SE 8%)
Allo BMT was significantly better than either ABMT or post remission chemotherapy (p < 0·05).

No toxicity data were reported in the study.

Conclusion

It was concluded that autologous bone marrow transplantation was not superior to post remission chemotherapy in preventing leukaemia relapse or extending DFS in children with AML in first remission.

Study 2

Ravindranath Y, Yeagher AM, Chang MN, Steuber CP, Krischer J, Graham-Pole J, Carroll A, Inoue S, Camitta B, Weinstein HJ.
Autologous bone marrow transplantation versus intensive consolidation chemotherapy for acute myeloid leukaemia.
New Engl J Med 1996;**334**:1428–34.

This was a prospective randomised trial carried out by the Pediatric Oncology Group. The study ran between June 1988 and March 1993.

Objectives

The aim of the study was to assess and compare the efficacy of autologous bone marrow transplantation (ABMT) with intensive consolidation chemotherapy in children with acute myeloid leukaemia in first remission.

Details of the study

Eligible patients were under 21 years of age with previously untreated AML (FAB M0 – M7) or isolated granulocytic sarcoma.

All patients received two courses of induction treatment. Course 1 consisted of daunorubicin 45 mg/m^2 on days 1, 2 and 3; cytosine arabinoside (ARA-C) 100 mg/m^2/d by continuous infusion on days 1–7 and thioguanine 100 mg/m^2/d orally on days 1–7. Intrathecal ARA-C was administered on days 1 and 8 of the first course of induction therapy. Additional intrathecal ARA-C was given on days 12 and 19 to patients who had central nervous leukaemia at the time of diagnosis. Course 2 commenced on day 15 if the bone marrow showed residual leukaemia, otherwise it was begun when the ANC was $\geq$ 1 $\times$ 10^9/ℓ and the platelet count was $\geq$ 100 $\times$10^9/ℓ.

The second course consisted of ARA-C 3 g/m^2 as a 3 hour infusion given 12 hourly for six doses.

Patients who attained disease remission M1 (< 5% blasts in the bone marrow) or M2a marrow (5–15% blasts) were eligible for randomisation to intensive chemotherapy or autologous bone marrow transplantation (ABMT) or were allocated to allogeneic (ALLo BMT) where there was an identical HLA sibling donor. All patients then received one course of etoposide 250 mg/m^2 on days 1, 2 and 3 and azacytidine 300 mg/m^2 on days 4 and 5 with intrathecal ARA-C on days 1 and 7. This was followed by either intensive chemotherapy or ABMT in the randomised group, or Allo BMT.

Patients randomised to intensive chemotherapy received six courses of additional chemotherapy at 3-weekly intervals or on recovery of blood counts. Local radiotherapy was given to those with CNS disease or extracranial mass lesions:

Course 1: Daunorubicin 45 mg/m^2 on day 1
ARA-C 3 gm/m^2 12 hourly on days 1, 2 and 3 (six doses)
Course 2: Daunorubicin 45 mg/m^2 on Days 1 and 2 ARA-C 100 mg/m^2/d as a continuous infusion on days 1–5 Thioguanine 100 mg/m^2/d orally on days 1–5
Course 3: Etoposide 250 mg/m^2 on days 1, 2 and 3 Azacytidine 300 mg/m^2 on days 4 and 5
Course 4: ARA-C 3 gm/m^2 12 hourly on days 1, 2 and 3 (six doses)
Course 5: Same as course 2
Course 6: Same as course 3

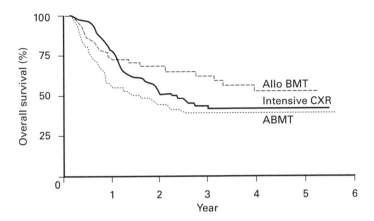

Figure 12.3 Overall survival from time of randomisation or assignment to allogeneic bone marrow transplantation. Adapted with permission, 2002 from Ravindranath Y *et al*, *N Engl J Med* (full reference on p 278). Copyright © 1996 Massachusetts Medical Society.

Patients randomised to ABMT received a regimen consisting of 4 days of oral busulphan ($4\,mg/m^2/d$) and 4 days of intravenous cyclophosphamide (200 mg/kg total dose) and had 4 hydroxy-cyclophosphamide purged cryopreserved marrow infused after 1 day's rest. The chemotherapy preparatory regimen for Allog BMT was identical to ABMT.

Patients who did not achieve remission after the second course of chemotherapy were withdrawn from the trial. It was predicted that 150 randomised patients were necessary to achieve a power of 80% at the 0·05 significance level to detect a difference of 20% in EFS 2 years after randomisation between patients who underwent ABMT and chemotherapy.

The main outcome measures were overall survival (OS) and event free survival (EFS). Calculations of EFS and OS for the entire group started from the date of registration; for the randomised groups it was calculated from the date of randomisation. Analysis was on the basis of intention to treat.

Outcome

Of 666 patients registered, 17 were excluded: wrong diagnosis in (10) protocol violations in (3) withdrawal prior to completion of induction therapy in (4). Only 649 were this considered evaluable for analysis. Of the 552 patients who attained remission (507 M1; 47 M2a marrow), only 232 (68%) patients were randomised to either intensive chemotherapy (117) or ABMT (115). A total of 209 patients were not eligible for randomisation [underwent Allo BMT, 89; non-protocol ABMT, 18; secondary AML, 5; insufficient funds, 64; no beds in transplant unit, 14; death before randomisation, 6; drug toxicity, 5; relapse before transplant, 5; not specified, 3] and a further 111 patients, including 21 with Down's syndrome, declined randomisation.

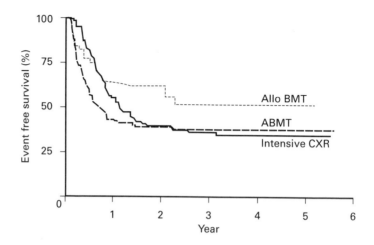

Figure 12.4 Event free survival from the time of randomisation or assignment to allogeneic bone marrow transplantation. Adapted with permission, 2002 from Ravindranath Y *et al*, *N Engl J Med* (full reference on p 278). Copyright © 1996 Massachusetts Medicala Society.

Only 71 of the 115 (62%) patients randomised to ABMT received the intended treatment (withdrawal, 23; relapse before ABMT, 21) and in contrast, only 4 patients in the intensive chemotherapy arm did not receive intended treatment (all 4 underwent ABMT).

The 3 year EFS and OS for the entire group was 34% ± 2·5% and 42% ± 2·6% respectively. However, 3 year OS in the intensive chemotherapy group was 44% ± 6% and in the ABMT group it was 40% ± 6·1% (p = 0·10) (Figure 12.3) and the 3 year EFS was 36% ± 5·8% and 38% ± 6·4% respectively (p = 0·20) The relative risk of failure was 0·81 (95% CI 0·58–1·12) for the chemotherapy group as compared to ABMT

group. The 3 year EFS for Allo BMT patients was 52% ± 8% which was better than both the chemotherapy (p = 0·06) and ABMT groups (p = 0·01) (Figure 12.4).

Toxicity

Procedural deaths were higher in the ABMT group (11/71, 15%) than after chemotherapy (3/113, 2·7%) (p = 0·005).

Conclusion

It was concluded that ABMT was not superior to intensive chemotherapy in the treatment of children with AML in first remission.

Study 3

Stevens RF, Hann IM, Wheatley K, Gray RG on behalf of the MRC Childhood Leukaemia Working Party.

Marked improvements in outcome with chemotherapy alone in paediatric acute myeloid leukaemia: results of the United Kingdom Medical Research Council's 10th AML Trial.

Br J Haematol 1998;**101**:130–40

This was a study by the United Kingdom Medical Research Council Childhood Leukaemia Working Party.

The AML-10 trial ran from May 1988 and March 1995 involving 41 centres in the United Kingdom, Republic of Ireland and New Zealand. It was a randomised trial with a 7 year follow up.

Objectives

- To compare the efficacy of thioguanine with etoposide during remission induction therapy in children with acute myeloid leukaemia.
- To compare high dose therapy followed by autologous bone marrow transplantation with no further treatment in children with acute myeloid leukaemia in first remission after four courses of chemotherapy.

Details of the study

All children below 15 years of age were eligible to be enrolled on the study. In addition to patients who had de novo acute myeloid leukaemia, those with secondary AML or with MDS (refractory anaemia with excess of blasts) were also eligible.

There were two randomisations and the details of chemotherapy treatment and randomisations are shown in Figure 12.5. The first randomisation was between two different induction regimens while the second was between autologous bone marrow transplantation (ABMT) and no further treatment. Children with an identical HLA sibling donor were allocated to allogeneic (Allo) BMT. In addition, triple intrathecal therapy with methotrexate, cytosine arabinoside (ARA-C) and hydrocortisone was given as part of each course.

Children aged over 2 years who had CNS disease at presentation and were not receiving BMT had craniospinal radiotherapy after completion of chemotherapy.

Patients receiving BMT were treated with cyclophosphamide (120 mg/kg total dose over 2 days) and fractionated total body irradiation. For children aged under 2 years, the conditioning treatment was with busulphan (16 mg/kg total dose over 4 days) and cyclophosphamide (200 mg/kg total dose over 4 days).

Outcome measures were disease free survival (DFS) and overall survival (OS).

Outcome

Of 359 eligible patients 341 were considered evaluable for overall outcome and 315 achieved complete remission (CR). A total of 127 were not available for randomisation (30 failed to achieve CR after two courses of chemotherapy; 19 relapsed or died before randomisation; and 78 had a matched sibling donor) and 100 eligible for randomisation were not randomised (5 physician choice, 8 parental choice, 87 electively received ABMT – physician choice 45, parental choice 42).

Only 100 (50%) eligible children in CR were randomised between ABMT and no further

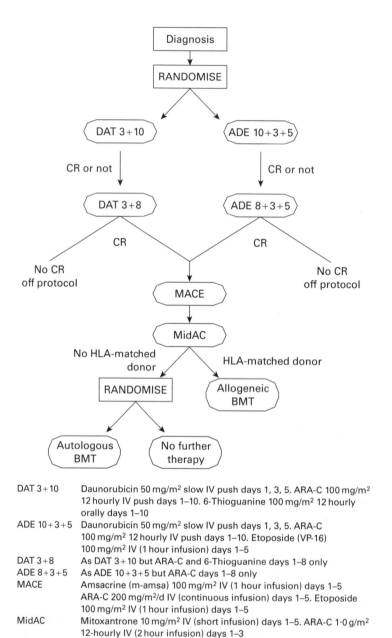

DAT 3+10   Daunorubicin 50 mg/m² slow IV push days 1, 3, 5. ARA-C 100 mg/m²
              12 hourly IV push days 1–10. 6-Thioguanine 100 mg/m² 12 hourly
              orally days 1–10
ADE 10+3+5   Daunorubicin 50 mg/m² slow IV push days 1, 3, 5. ARA-C
              100 mg/m² 12 hourly IV push days 1–10. Etoposide (VP-16)
              100 mg/m² IV (1 hour infusion) days 1–5
DAT 3+8   As DAT 3+10 but ARA-C and 6-Thioguanine days 1–8 only
ADE 8+3+5   As ADE 10+3+5 but ARA-C days 1–8 only
MACE   Amsacrine (m-amsa) 100 mg/m² IV (1 hour infusion) days 1–5
              ARA-C 200 mg/m²/d IV (continuous infusion) days 1–5. Etoposide
              100 mg/m² IV (1 hour infusion) days 1–5
MidAC   Mitoxantrone 10 mg/m² IV (short infusion) days 1–5. ARA-C 1·0 g/m²
              12-hourly IV (2 hour infusion) days 1–3
NB: All doses were reduced by 25% for children less than 1 year old

Figure 12.5 Protocol flow chart for study AML-10. Reprinted from Stevens RF *et al*, *Br J Haematol* (full reference p 281) with permission from Blackwell Science Ltd.

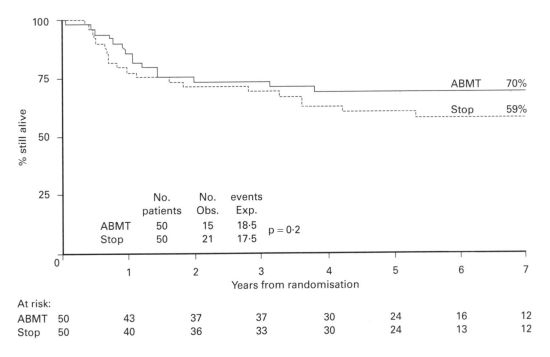

Figure 12.6 Survival by autograft versus stop randomisation. Under number of events, Obs. is the observed number of deaths in each arm and Exp. is the expected number from log-rank analysis. Reprinted from Stevens RF *et al*, *Br J Haematol* (full reference p 281) with permission from Blackwell Science Ltd.

treatment. Of the 50 children randomised to ABMT, only 44 received it – non-compliance was due to infection, death, early relapse, persistent eosinophilia and poor cardiac function (2). Compliance was 100% in the stop arm.

DFS at 7 years in the ABMT group was 68% versus 46% in the stop arm (p = 0·02) while relapse free survival (RFS) at 7 years in the ABMT group was 69% versus 48% in the stop arm (p = 0·03).

OS at 7 years in the ABMT group was 70% versus. 59% in the stop arm (p = 0·2) (Figure 12.6)

Though the DFS and the RFS were lower in patients who were randomised to ABMT, (OS) did not differ between the ABMT and no further treatment groups, and this seems to be related to inferior survival from relapse after ABMT.

Toxicity
The transplant related procedural mortality in the ABMT group was 2%.

Conclusion
It was concluded that ABMT did not improve survival in children with AML in first remission.

Study 4

Woods WG, Neudorf S, Gold S, Sanders J, Buckley JD, Barnard DR, Dusenberry K, DeSwarte J, Arthur DC, Lange BJ, Kobrinsky NL. A comparison of allogeneic bone marrow transplantation, autologous bone marrow transplantation, and aggressive chemotherapy in children with acute myeloid leukaemia in remission: a report from the Children's Cancer Group *Blood* 2001;**97**:56–62.

This was a prospective randomised multicentre trial conducted by the Children's Cancer Group (CCG-2891). It ran from October 1989 to April 1995.

Objectives

The objectives of the study were to compare the efficacy and toxicity of allogeneic bone marrow transplantation, autologous bone marrow transplantation and aggressive post remission chemotherapy in children with acute myeloid leukaemia in first remission.

Details of the study

Children and adolescents younger than 21 years of age with a diagnosis of acute myeloid leukaemia (M0-M7), acute undifferentiated or biphenotypic leukaemia with myeloid differentiation were eligible for the study. Informed consent was obtained from families of patients in all cases. Patients with Fanconi anaemia or Philadelphia postitive chronic myeloid leukaemia were excluded as were children with Down's syndrome. Those who developed secondary AML or had granulocytic sarcoma without bone marrow infiltration or who had be novo myelodisplastic syndrome were also excluded from analysis.

No details of how randomisation was done are given in the report.

The first randomisation was at diagnosis and patients were randomised to two induction regimens – standard and intensive – in which identical drugs and doses were used. Patients randomised to the intensive arm received the second cycle of chemotherapy 6 days after completion of cycle 1 irrespective of bone marrow or haematological status. Initial induction chemotherapy consisted of a 5 drug regimen administered over 4 days – dexamethasone, 6-thioguanine, cytosine arabinoside (ARA-C), daunorubicin and etoposide. Daunorubicin, etoposide and ARA-C were administered as a continuous infusion for 96 hours. Chemotherapy drug doses are not indicated. Standard timing induction therapy was closed in May 1993 and granulocyte colony stimulating factor was introduced for all patients during the induction phase (see Chapter 11, Study 2).

The second randomisation was after four cycles of chemotherapy. Patients randomised to ABMT received a regimen of 4 days of oral busulphan (16 mg/kg total dose) and 4 days of intravenous cyclophosphamide (200 mg/kg total dose) and had 4-hydroxycyclophosphamide ex vivo purged marrow infused after 1 day's rest. Patients randomised to post remission chemotherapy received four courses of three different chemotherapy regimens each lasting for 4–6 weeks. Details of post remission chemotherapy are not available. All patients who had HLA-identical family donors were allocated to Allo BMT with an identical regimen to ABMT.

Main outcome measures were disease free survival (DFS) and overall survival (OS) comparing the three post remission regimens at 4–9 years of follow up.

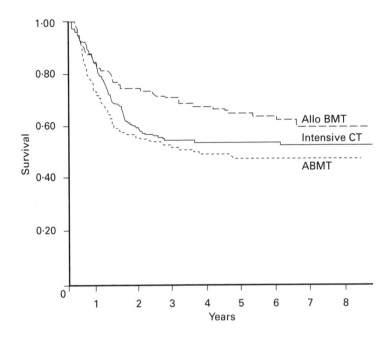

Figure 12.7 Actuarial survival from AML remission, comparing the three post remission regimens from CCG-2891

Table 12.1 Outcome at 8 years actuarial comparing the three post remission regimens from CCG-2891

	Allogeneic BMT	p value (allo v auto)	Autologous BMT	p value (allo v chemo)	Chemotherapy	p value (chemo v auto)
All patients (n = 537)	181		177		179	
Survival	60 ± 90%	0·002	48 ± 8%	0·21	53 ± 8%	0·05
Disease free survival	55 ± 9%	0·001	42 ± 8%	0·31	47 ± 8%	0·01
Patients receiving intensive timing induction (n = 36)	113		115		108	
Survival	70 ± 9%	0·006	54 ± 9%	0·67	57 ± 10%	0·02
Disease free survival	66 ± 9%	0·003	48 ± 9%	0·53	53 ± 10%	0·02

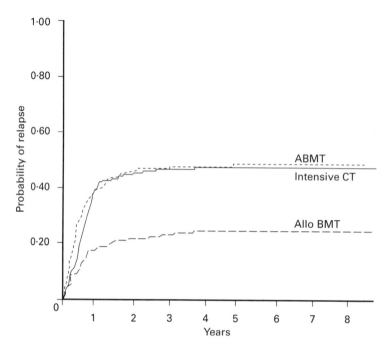

Figure 12.8 Actuarial probability of relapse after AML remission, comparing the three post remission regimens from CCG-2891

Outcome

Of 1114 children registered, 652 patients successfully completed four courses of intensive chemotherapy and were eligible for allocation to allogeneic BMT or randomisation to autologous BMT or intensive chemotherapy. One hundred and fifteen patients refused to participate in the post remission phase of the trial. Analysis was by intention to treat.

A total of 181 patients were allocated to Allo BMT, 177 were randomised to ABMT and 179 patients were randomised to intensive chemotherapy. There was no difference among the three groups of patients based on white blood counts at diagnosis or the various cytogenetic abnormalities. Excluding patients with early relapses and hence not eligible to start actual post remission treatment, compliance rates were between 83% and 97%: 164/181 (94%) Allo BMT; 137/177 (83%) ABMT; 171/179 received post remission chemotherapy.

For the whole group of 537 eligible patients, the 8 year (OS) is 54% ± 4% (SD = 2) and the (DFS) for the same period is 48% ± 4%. Figure 12.7 and Table 12.1 summarise the post remission outcome.

1 Allo BMT: the OS and DFS in this group (*n* = 181) was 60% ± 9% and 55% ± 9%

respectively (p value Allo v Auto 0·002 and 0·001 respectively).

2   ABMT: OS and DFS was 48% ± 8% and 42% ± 8% respectively (p value Auto v Chemo 0·21 and 0·31 respectively).

3   Intensive non-marrow ablative chemotherapy: OS and DFS was 53% ± 8% and 47% ± 8% respectively (p value Chemo v Allo 0·05 and 0·01 respectively).

4   Relapse rates were similar for children randomised to either ABMT or intersive chemotherapy when compared with allogeneic BMT (Figure 12.8).

Toxicity

More gastrointestinal and hepatic toxicity was seen in the Allo BMT group. Average time to neutrophil recovery was 23 days in the Allo BMT arm and 47 days in the ABMT arm. Overall non-leukaemic deaths were 14% in the Allo BMT arm, 5% in the ABMT arm and 4% in the chemotherapy arm. The majority of non-leukaemic deaths in the ABMT arm ($n = 7/9$) and all non-leukaemic deaths ($n = 8$) in the chemotherapy arm were due to infections. There were no apparent differences in toxicity in the post remission arms based on which induction regimen was used.

Conclusion

1   Allogeneic bone marrow transplantation after four courses of intensive chemotherapy reduced the risk for relapse and improved overall and disease free survival in patients with acute myeloid leukaemia.

2   Autologous bone marrow transplantation confers no added advantage over intensive chemotherapy in children with acute myeloid leukaemia.

13–16

Acute lymphoblastic leukaemia

Commentary – Judith Chessells

Acute lymphoblastic leukaemia (ALL), as the commonest type of childhood cancer, is the prototype for clinical trials in paediatric oncology, and the only disease in which there have been significant numbers of large randomised trials. Even these, however, are often insufficiently powered to detect small but important differences in event free survival of the order of 5–10%. Yet this type of improvement is what can be expected in future studies. One way to compensate for this problem is by systematic overviews that involve searching for published and unpublished trials followed by analysis of individual patient data. The childhood ALL collaborative group has already published one such overview about duration and intensity of maintenance chemotherapy in ALL (Chapter 15, Study 8) and another such overview about CNS directed therapy is in preparation (SM Richards, personal communication). A second useful approach is the simultaneous publication of long term follow up results using identical outcome measures and risk groups, as shown in a recent issue of *Leukaemia*[1].

Space does not permit a detailed critique of all the trials which have been reviewed here, and indeed the many others which have been conducted in paediatric ALL. Selected, mostly randomised, trials which illustrate important aspects of management will be briefly discussed.

Induction and intensification therapy

Remission induction can be successfully achieved in over 95% of children with ALL using the simple combination of steroids, vincristine, L-asparaginase and intrathecal methotrexate[2]. The only questions therefore that can be asked about induction therapy are whether the use of additional drugs improves event free survival or whether new drugs or combinations seem effective as initial treatment – so-called "window" studies. The clinical emphasis in ALL moved over 20 years ago to examination of the intensity of therapy during the first few months of treatment and its impact on event free survival. Event free survival is the most important measure of successful treatment in ALL, because although some children may be cured a second time around the results of treatment of relapsed ALL are toxic, stressful and frequently unsuccessful[3].

A strategy which is more established in ALL than AML is the use of "risk adapted" therapy: that is, delivering more intensive therapy to patients at higher risk of treatment failure. Although there are problems in risk group stratification[4], it is clear that some children with ALL have a higher risk of relapse than others. These include infants, older children and those with a high leucocyte count at presentation. Age and presenting white blood cell count formed the basis of a simple and universally applicable basis for stratification developed by the Rome consensus[5], and later refined by the National Cancer Institute (NCI)[6]. The benefit of such a consensus is that it enables international comparisons of outcome[1] without relying on the results of more sophisticated investigations.

It seemed intuitively likely that increasing the intensity of treatment might reduce the chances of relapse in those patients at high risk of relapse on "standard therapy" and this concept lead the Berlin–Frankfurt–Munster (BFM) group to devise more intensive treatment protocols for higher risk patients. This concept had been tried and failed in earlier studies (perhaps because treatment was not sufficiently aggressive) but the BFM group showed that more intensified treatment did benefit these patients, albeit when compared with historical controls[7].

The large American Children's Cancer Group (CCG) have performed prospective randomised trials which showed that intensive therapy cured more high risk children than standard therapy[8] and that additional intensification of treatment in high risk children with a slow response to induction could improve the chance of cure[9]. The results of these trials are confirmed by both randomised and comparative studies performed by other collaborative groups and the reader is referred for details to a recent review of the management of high risk lymphoblastic leukaemia in childhood[10].

Lower risk children, however, also benefit from intensification of therapy. In a small randomised trial the BFM group attempted to omit their winning formula in a subset of lowest risk children with a consequent increase in late marrow relapses[11,12]. At the same time the CCG[13] and the MRC[14] were randomising so-called "average risk" children and all children respectively to receive intensification therapy at 4 weeks, 5 months, both or neither. Results confirm that the addition of blocks of intensified therapy during the first few months improves event free survival in all children with ALL. Analysis of randomised trials of intensive re-induction therapy in seven trials including 3696 patients showed a highly significant reduction in the risk of relapse and a smaller but significant improvement in survival (Chapter 15, Study 8).

Conclusions

Virtually all children with ALL will achieve remission. Twenty-five years ago, some 35–40% of children could be cured after induction therapy, CNS directed treatment and simple continuing (maintenance) therapy with oral mercaptopurine and methotrexate, often with some type of periodic addition of prednisolone and vincristine. The proportion of event free survivals has been doubled by the introduction of some form of intensification therapy for all children and a more aggressive chemotherapeutic approach to those at higher risk of treatment failure.

This blunderbuss therapy has been empirical but successful. There is now the prospect that widespread use of molecular genetics may allow a more sophisticated approach to treatment. Cytogenetic analysis can identify some patients with "standard risk" features who are at high risk of treatment failure[15], for example those with Ph_1 positive leukaemia. Persistent minimal residual disease after the first few months of treatment is highly predictive of subsequent relapse[16–18]. This type of investigation should help in more sophisticated prediction of relapse risk and thus allow more individualised treatment for many children and less toxic treatment for some at least.

CNS directed therapy

Almost 30 years ago randomised trials showed that children with ALL in remission who received no[19,20] or minimal CNS directed treatment with a short course of intrathecal methotrexate injections (Chapter 14, Studies 4 and 9) had a higher CNS relapse rate and ultimately a worse survival than those who received presymptomatic CNS directed therapy. The first widely used form of CNS directed therapy comprised either craniospinal irradiation or cranial irradiation and a short term course of intrathecal methotrexate injections, probably because the former treatment had been used successfully in children with overt CNS relapse. Craniospinal irradiation, being myelosuppressive, was soon abandoned and many protocols relied on cranial irradiation in a dose order of 24 Gy with a course of four to six intrathecal methotrexate injections.

Since then there have been many randomised trials involving various forms of CNS directed

therapy, including those reviewed here, but it is important not to lose sight of the fact that what matters is overall event free survival – not relapse at any particular site. A classic example of the "swings and roundabouts" effect was seen in a seminal trial[21] reported here in long term follow up (Chapter 14, Study 12) performed over 20 years ago by the Cancer and Leukaemia Group B, the forerunner of the Pediatric Oncology Group (POG). All children received intrathecal methotrexate during induction therapy and were then randomised to receive either cranial irradiation or three infusions of modest dose intravenous methotrexate, both treatments being given in association with further short term intrathecal methotrexate. The group who received intravenous methotrexate had a higher CNS relapse rate but a lower rate of other relapses than those having cranial irradiation. The overall event free survival at 37% was poor by today's standards but the contrast in sites of relapse was highly significant. An important difference became apparent long term in the incidence of neuropsychological sequelae, which were more prevalent in patients who had received cranial irradiation[22].

A further example of the interaction of systemic and CNS directed therapy is shown by the early trial from the Cancer and Leukaemia Group B (Chapter 14, Study 9), in which patients randomised to receive dexamethasone during induction and continuing treatment had a lower risk of CNS relapse than those receiving prednisolone.

Concerns about the late effects of treatment prompted alterations in the choice of CNS directed therapy. Children who have received cranial irradiation are at increased risk of growth and endocrine problems[23] and brain tumours[24,25]. The contribution of both cranial irradiation and other forms of CNS directed therapy to neuropsychological sequelae of childhood ALL is more difficult to assess[26].

Comparative, non-randomised studies performed by the CCG (Chapter 13, Study 1) showed that 18 Gy of cranial irradiation was as effective as 24 Gy. Subsequent randomised trials showed that, after an initial course of intrathecal methotrexate injections, regular intrathecal methotrexate throughout therapy was as effective as cranial irradiation in lower risk (Chapter 14, Study 5) and average risk (Chapter 14, Study 11) children, and even in those higher risk children with ALL who showed a satisfactory early response to induction therapy (Chapter 14, Study 14).

Are there any children with ALL who need cranial irradiation? There is no evidence about this issue from randomised trials, although some groups continue to advocate cranial irradiation, often in lower dose, usually for older children with higher WBC counts and possibly T-ALL.

High dose intravenous methotrexate therapy, in doses ranging from 500 mg to 33 g/m[2] has been evaluated in treatment of ALL, both for its CNS protective effects and for prevention of relapse at other sites. It has formed a mainstay of treatment in many countries, notably Scandinavia[27]. It is not clear, however, whether intravenous methotrexate affords additional CNS and bone marrow protection to children who have received both intensified systemic therapy and aggressive intrathecal therapy. Intravenous methotrexate has also been combined with low dose cranial irradiation (12 Gy) (Chapter 14, Study 17) by the BFM group.

Triple intrathecal therapy with methotrexate, hydrocortisone and cytosine arabinoside is as effective as cranial irradiation and intrathecal methotrexate in standard (Chapter 14, Study 1) and higher risk children (Chapter 14, Study 7) and has been extensively used by the POG. However, in a recent report from the POG patients who had received triple intrathecal therapy in association with intermediate dose intravenous methotrexate had an unexpectedly high rate of seizures[28]. There are no published randomised trials comparing efficacy and toxicity of intrathecal methotrexate and triple intrathecal therapy.

Conclusions

Prevention of overt CNS leukaemia can be achieved in most children with ALL by intensive intrathecal methotrexate therapy. Triple intrathecal therapy is also effective but the relative benefits of the two treatments are unclear. Cranial irradiation and short term intrathecal methotrexate therapy are effective but have largely been abandoned because of concerns about the late effects of treatment. It remains uncertain whether there is a small group of high risk patients who may benefit from cranial irradiation. Protocols that include intravenous methotrexate as well as some intrathecal methotrexate are effective but the additional benefit provided by the intravenous methotrexate is uncertain.

Continuing (maintenance) therapy

Long term, relatively low dose, continuing (maintenance) therapy with daily oral mercaptopurine and weekly methotrexate has been part of treatment of ALL for over 30 years. Continuing treatment is unique to ALL and some types of NHL (see Chapter 9) but its precise mode of action is unknown.

It could be argued that, in the era of intensified treatment, there is no role for prolonged maintenance therapy. These considerations lead the Tokyo Children's Cancer Study Group to devise a protocol comprising 6 months of intensive treatment and 6 months of standard oral maintenance[29]. Three hundred and forty-seven children were treated in this way. The relapse rate was high, particularly in lower risk patients, a finding which echoes the outcome of many historic studies when treatment was given for 12–15 months only.

Manipulations of continuing treatment have, in general, not proved effective except for the periodic addition of vincristine and prednisolone (Chapter 16, Study 1). The overview of 1250 children randomised in seven trials showed that the addition of pulses of prednisolone and vincristine significantly reduced relapses, but had a smaller effect on survival (Chapter 15, Study 8). Continuing treatment is immunosuppressive and in an attempt to decrease the risk of serious infections MRC UKALL-V randomised lower risk children to receive mercaptopurine and methotrexate continuously, for 3 weeks in every 4, or pulsed over 5 days every 3 weeks throughout maintenance. In the study 496 children were randomised and the event free survival at 7 years was 48% in patients who received continuous treatment, 46% after semi-continuous treatment and only 35% in the group who received pulsed treatment (Chapter 16, Study 6). By contrast, pulsed therapy was associated with a lower relapse rate than continuous therapy in a trial performed by the Japanese Children's Cancer study group (Chapter 16, Study 5). This trial, however, involved only 115 patients and the methotrexate was given intravenously rather than orally.

Both methotrexate and mercaptopurine are usually given by mouth during the later phases of continuing treatment. The EORTC Trial 58881 included a randomisation to replace oral mercaptopurine with intravenous mercaptopurine for one week per month during continuing treatment. Intravenous mercaptopurine was associated with a higher relapse rate (Chapter 16, Study 7). MRC UKALL-VII (Chapter 16, Study 4) compared oral and intramuscular methotrexate during continuing treatment and found a marginally significant benefit for intramuscular methotrexate on analysis by treatment given. Another British trial[29] showed no difference in outcome between the two routes. Both trials were small, with 80 and 144 patients respectively, hence these results should be interpreted with caution.

A trial from CCG (Chapter 16, Study 3) randomised 164 children to standard continuing treatment with or without additional intravenous methotrexate infusions every 6 weeks. The additional methotrexate was not beneficial. Another approach to more complicated continuing therapy was explored in the St Jude Total XI study[30], which involved a comparison of standard continuing treatment and intensive rotational therapy in standard risk patients. There was no difference in outcome between the two schedules.

It has been suggested that 6-thioguanine, which is more directly activated to thioguanine nucleotides, may be a more effective drug than mercaptopurine[31,32]. The preliminary report from a randomised trial conducted by the COALL study showed that use of thioguanine was not superior to mercaptopurine (Chapter 16, Study 8). The results of other large randomised trials in progress are awaited.

Conclusion

Continuing (maintenance) therapy remains essential in the management of ALL. None of the manipulations reviewed here have proved superior to the combination of mercaptopurine and methotrexate with periodic pulses of steroids and vincristine. This long term outpatient based therapy is more unsupervised than other aspects of treatment. There is evidence that treatment to the level of tolerance reduces the risk of relapse[33,34] and that compliance may be variable[35] in this, as in other forms of oral treatment.

Length of treatment

There have been many trials of duration of therapy in ALL with randomised comparisons varying from 3 with 5 years (Chapter 15, Study 2), to 18 months with 3 years (Chapter 15, Study 1). In general these trials have tended to show that shorter treatment is associated with a marginally higher risk of relapse. Sometimes, as in MRC UKALL-I, which compared 18 months with 3 years, these results have achieved statistical significance. When results of all randomised trials of duration of therapy were included in an overview, data on 3861 patients were available (Chapter 15, Study 8). Longer maintenance therapy decreased the relapse rate in the first year off treatment but had no benefit on overall survival for three reasons. There was an excess of remission deaths in children continuing chemotherapy, an excess of relapses once those children receiving longer therapy stopped treatment and, at the time of analysis, a better response to salvage therapy in children who had received shorter treatment. These results suggest that some relapses at least are deferred rather than prevented by longer treatment. Analysis by age, sex and WBC count did not demonstrate any different effects of treatments within subgroups. There is, however, evidence from several large study groups[36-38] that boys have a higher risk of late relapses than girls. The reason for this difference is unknown, but it has no doubt contributed to the decision in many protocols to give boys 3 rather than 2 years of treatment.

Conclusions

There remains uncertainty about the best length of treatment for lymphoblastic leukaemia, but in general it appears that protocols of shorter than 2 years have been associated with more relapses. There have been few recent trials of duration of therapy, and it is possible that length of total treatment in future studies will be influenced by the intensity of initial treatment and by evaluation of minimal residual disease during therapy.

References

1 Schrappe M, Camitta B, Pui CH, Eden T, Gaynon P, Gustafsson G et al. Long-term results of large prospective trials in childhood acute lymphoblastic leukemia. Leukemia 2000;14:2193–4.

2 Ortega JA, Nesbit ME, Donaldson MH, Hittle RE, Weiner J, Karon M et al. L-asparaginase, vincristine and prednisone for induction of first remission in acute lymphocytic leukemia. Cancer Res 1977;37:535–40.

3 Chessells JM. Relapsed lymphoblastic leukaemia in children: a continuing challenge. Br J Haematol 1998;102:423–38.

4 Chessells JM. Risk analysis in acute lymphoblastic leukaemia: problems and pitfalls. Eur J Cancer 1995;31A:1656–9.

5 Mastrangelo R, Poplack DG, Bleyer WA, Riccardi R, Sather H, D'Angio G. Report and recommendations of the Rome workshop concerning poor-prognosis acute lymphoblastic leukemia in children: biologic bases for staging, stratification, and treatment. Med Pediatr Oncol 1986;14:191–4.

6   Smith M, Arthur D, Camitta B, Carroll AJ, Crist W, Gaynon P *et al.* Uniform approach to risk classification and treatment assignment for children with acute lymphoblastic leukemia. *J Clin Oncol* 1996;**14**:18–24.

7   Riehm H, Gadner H, Henze G, Kornhuber B, Lampert F, Niethammer D *et al.* Results and significance of six randomized trials in four consecutive ALL-BFM studies. *Haematol Blood Transfus* 1990;**33**:439–50.

8   Gaynon PS, Steinherz PG, Bleyer WA, Ablin AR, Albo VC, Finklestein JZ *et al.* Improved therapy for children with acute lymphoblastic leukemia and unfavourable presenting features: a follow-up report on the Children's Cancer Group Study CCG-106. *J Clin Oncol* 1993;**11**:2234–42.

9   Nachman JB, Sather HN, Sensel MG, Trigg ME, Cherlow JM, Lukens JN *et al.* Augmented post-induction therapy for children with high-risk acute lymphoblastic leukemia and a slow response to initial therapy. *N Engl J Med* 1998;**338**:1663–71.

10 Chessells JM. The management of high-risk lymphoblastic leukemia in children. *Br J Haematol* 2000;**108**:204–16.

11 Henze G, Fengler R, Reiter A, Ritter J, Riehm H. Impact of early intensive reinduction therapy on event-free survival in children with low-risk acute lymphoblastic leukemia. *Haematol Blood Transf* 1990;**33**:483–8.

12 Reiter A, Schrappe M, Ludwig W-D, Hiddemann W, Sauter S, Henze G *et al.* Chemotherapy in 998 unselected childhood acute lymphoblastic leukemia patients, results and conclusions of the multicenter trial ALL-BFM 86. *Blood* 1994;**84**:3122–33.

13 Tubergen DG, Gilchrist GS, O'Brien RT, Coccia PF, Sather HN, Waskerwitz MJ *et al.* Improved outcome with delayed intensification for children with acute lymphoblastic leukemia and intermediate presenting features: a Children's Cancer Group Phase III trial. *J Clin Oncol* 1993;**11**:527–37.

14 Chessells JM, Bailey C, Richards SM. Intensification of treatment and survival in all children with lymphoblastic leukaemia: results of UK Medical Research Council trial UKALL X. *Lancet* 1995;**345**:143–8.

15 Harrison CJ. The genetics of childhood acute lymphoblastic leukaemia. *Baillieres Best Pract Res Clin Haematol* 2000;**13**:427–39.

16 Coustan-Smith E, Behm FG, Sanchez J, Torrey Sandland J, Pui C-H, Campana D. Immunological detection of minimal residual disease in children with acute lymphoblastic leukaemia. *Lancet* 1998;**351**:550–4.

17 Cave H, Van Der Werff ten Bosch J, Suciu S, Guildal C, Waterkeyn C, Otten J *et al.* Clinical significance of minimal residual disease in childhood acute lymphoblastic leukaemia. *N Engl J Med* 1998;**339**:591–8.

18 van-Dongen JJ, Seriu T, Panzer GE, Biondi A, Pongers WM, Corral L *et al.* Prognostic value of minimal residual disease in acute lymphoblastic leukaemia in childhood. *Lancet* 1998;**352**:1731–8.

19 Medical Research Council. Treatment of acute lymphoblastic leukaemia: effect of "prophylactic" therapy against central nervous system leukaemia. *Br Med J* 1973;**2**:381–4.

20 Hustu HO, Aur RJA, Verzosa MS. Prevention of central nervous system leukemia by irradiation. *Cancer* 1973;**32**:585–597.

21 Freeman AI, Weinberg V, Brecher ML, Jones B, Glicksman AS, Sinks LF *et al.* Comparison of intermediate-dose methotrexate with cranial irradiation for the post-induction treatment of acute lymphocytic leukemia in children. *N Engl J Med* 1983;**308**:477–84.

22 Hill JM, Kornblith AB, Jones D, Freeman A, Holland JF, Glicksman AS *et al.* A comparativie study of the long term psychosocial functioning of childhood acute lymphoblastic leukaemia survivors treated by intrathecal methotrexate with or without cranial radiation. *Cancer* 1998;**82**:208–18.

23 Leiper AD. Management of growth failure in the treatment of malignant disease. *Pediatr Hematol Oncol* 1990;**7**:365–71.

24 Neglia JP, Meadows AT, Robison LL, Kim TH, Newton WA, Ruymann FB *et al.* Second neoplasms after acute lymphoblastic leukaemia in childhood. *N Engl J Med* 1991;**325**:1330–6.

25 Loning L, Zimmermann M, Reiter A, Kaatsch P, Henze G, Riehm H et al. Secondary neoplasms subsequent to

Berlin–Frankfurt–Munster therapy of acute lymphoblastic leukemia in childhood: significantly lower risk without cranial radiotherapy. *Blood* 2000;**95**:2770–5.

26 Cousens P, Waters B, Said J, Stevens M. Cognitive effects of cranial irradiation in leukaemia: a survey and meta-analysis. *J Clin Psychol Psychiatry* 1988;**29**:839–52.

27 Gustafsson G, Schmiegelow K, Forestier E, Clausen N, Glomstein A, Jonmundsson G *et al.* Improving outcome through two decades in childhood ALL in the Nordic countries: the impact of high-dose methotrexate in the reduction of CNS irradiation. Nordic Society of Pediatric Haematology and Oncology (NOPHO). *Leukemia* 2000;**14**:2267–75.

28 Mahoney-DH Jr, Shuster JJ, Nitschke R, Lauer SJ, Steuber CP, Winick N *et al.* Acute neurotoxicity in children with B-precursor acute lymphoid leukemia: an association with intermediate-dose intravenous methotrexate and intrathecal triple therapy – a Pediatric Oncology Group study. *J Clin Oncol* 1998;**16**:1712–22.

29 Chessells JM, Leiper AD, Tiedemann K, Hardisty RM, Richards S. Oral methotrexate is as effective as intramuscular in continuing (maintenance) therapy of acute lymphoblastic leukaemia. *Arch Dis Childh* 1987;**62**:172–6.

30 Rivera GK, Raimondi SC, Hancock ML, Behm FG, Pui C-H, Abromowitch M *et al.* Improved outcome in childhood acute lymphoblastic leukaemia with reinforced early treatment and rotational combination chemotherapy. *Lancet* 1991;**337**:61–6.

31 Adamson PC, Poplack DG, Balis FM. The cytotoxicity of thioguanine *v* mercaptopurine in acute lymphoblastic leukemia. *Leuk Res* 1994;**18**:805–10.

32 Evans WE, Relling MV. Mercaptopurine *v* thioguanine for the treatment of acute lymphoblastic leukemia. *Leuk Res* 1994;**18**:811–14.

33 Pearson ADJ, Amineddine HA, Yule M, Mills S, Long DR, Craft AW *et al.* The influence of serum methotrexate concentrations and drug dosage on outcome in childhood acute lymphoblastic leukaemia. *Br J Cancer* 1991;**64**:169–73.

34 Dolan G, Lilleyman JS, Richards SM. Prognostic importance of myelosuppression during maintenance treatment of lymphoblastic leukaemia. *Arch Dis Childh* 1989;**64**:1231–4.

35 Davies HA, Lennard L, Lilleyman JS. Variable mercaptopurine metabolism in children with leukaemia: a problem of non-compliance? *Br Med J* 1993;**306**:1239–40.

36 Chessells JM, Richards SM, Bailey CC, Lilleyman JS, Eden OB. Gender and treatment outcome in childhood lymphoblastic leukaemia: report from the MRC UKALL Trials. *Br J Haematol* 1995;**89**:364–72.

37 Shuster JJ, Wacker P, Pullen J, Humbert J, Land VJ, Mahoney-DH Jr, *et al.* Prognostic significance of sex in childhood B-precursor acute lymphoblastic leukemia: a Pediatric Oncology Group Study. *J Clin Oncol* 1998;**16**:2854–63.

38 Pui CH, Boyett JM, Relling MV, Harrison PL, Rivera GK, Behm FG *et al.* Sex differences in prognosis for children with acute lymphoblastic leukemia. *J Clin Oncol* 1999;**17**:818–24.

13

Radiotherapy as CNS directed treatment in acute lymphoblastic leukaemia

Studies

Study 1

Nesbit MEJ, Robinson LL, Littman PS, Sather HN, Ortega J, D'Angio GJ, Denman Hammond G. Presymptomatic central nervous system therapy in previously untreated childhood acute lymphoblastic leukaemia: comparison of 1800 rad and 2400 rad. A report for the Children's Cancer Study Group.
Lancet 1981;i:461–6.

These were prospective randomised multicentre trials that extended from June 1972 to February 1975 (CCG-101 from 1972 and 1974 and CCG-143 from 1974 till 1975). This report focuses only on the patients randomised to either craniospinal radiotherapy (24 or 18 Gy) or to cranial radiotherapy (24 or 18 Gy) plus intrathecal methotrexate.

Objectives

The aim of the study was:

- To evaluate the efficacy of two differing doses of cranial irradiation (RT) with intrathecal methotrexate (IT MTX) in the treatment of childhood acute lymphoblastic leukaemia.
- To compare craniospinal radiotherapy (CS-RT) with cranial radiotherapy (C-RT) plus IT MTX in the prevention of CNS leukaemic relapse.

Details of the study

Previously untreated children and adolescents below the age of 18 years were registered on the trials. Patients who did not achieve remission (< 5% blasts in bone marrow) by day 42 were excluded, as were children who were less than 18 months of age, who were electively allocated intrathecal methotrexate alone.

All patients received identical induction and maintenance treatment consisting of vincristine, L-asparaginase, prednisolone, 6-mercaptopurine and oral (PO) methotrexate. The first trial (CCG-101) used an irradiation dose of 24 Gy, while in the subsequent trial (CCG-143), it was 18 Gy.

CNS prophylaxis in CCG-101 had four arms: craniospinal RT 24 Gy + 12 Gy to gonads; craniospinal RT 24 Gy; cranial RT 24 Gy + IT MTX; and IT MTX alone. In trial CCG-143, there were two arms: craniospinal RT 18 Gy and cranial RT 18 Gy + IT MTX.

The number of children randomised in the four treatment groups was follows:

1   Craniospinal RT 24 Gy = 152 (CCG-101).
2   Craniospinal RT 18 Gy = 86 (CCG-143).
3   Cranial RT 24 Gy + IT MTX = 159 (CCG-101).
4   Cranial RT 18 Gy + IT MTX = 81 (CCG-143).

The randomisation methodology is not specified in the report.

All patients were stratified into three prognostic groups:

(A)   Good prognosis: WBC $< 10 \times 10^9/\ell$; age 3–6 years ($n = 155$).
(B)   Intermediate prognosis: any age and WBC count $10–50 \times 10^9/\ell$ or WBC count $<10 \times 10^9/\ell$ and less than 3 years or more than 6 years of age ($n = 252$).
(C)   Poor prognosis: WBC count $> 50 \times 10^9/\ell$ and any age ($n = 71$).

There were no significant differences between the two study populations (CCG-101 and CCG-143) with respect to initial WBC count, age at diagnosis and sex.

Main outcome measures were

1   CNS relapse rate as the first event in each treatment group.
2   Bone marrow relapse rate as the first event in each treatment group.

3   Event free survival (EFS) in each treatment group stratified according to prognosis.

Outcome

Analyses of results were performed on the basis of intention to treat. Of the 757 patients who achieved remission in the two trials and who were randomised for CNS prophylaxis, the results of the 478 patients who had either craniospinal RT or cranial RT plus IT MTX are reported in this paper.

Thirteen patients who were randomised to receive 18 Gy actually received 24 Gy (6 craniospinal irradiation and 7 cranial irradiation + IT MTX) and their analysis was on the basis of actual treatment received.

CNS Relapse

At 2 years after randomisation, the proportion of patients who experienced CNS relapses was as follows: craniospinal RT 18 Gy 0·05; 24 Gy 0·07; cranial RT + IT MTX, 1800 Gy 0·08; 24 Gy 0·06.

The proportion experiencing CNS relapse in the poor prognostic group at 48 months after randomisation was as follows: craniospinal RT, 24 Gy 0·35; 18 Gy 0·41 (p = 0·84), cranial RT + IT MTX, 24 Gy 0·12; 18 Gy 0·32 (p = 0·45).

Patients in the poor prognostic group who were treated with 18 Gy appeared to have a higher incidence of CNS relapse compared to those treated with 24 Gy, although not statistically significant.

Patients treated with cranial RT + IT MTX had a two fold higher incidence of CNS relapse than those who received craniospinal RT with either 18 Gy and 24 Gy (p = 0·14 and p = 0·20 respectively).

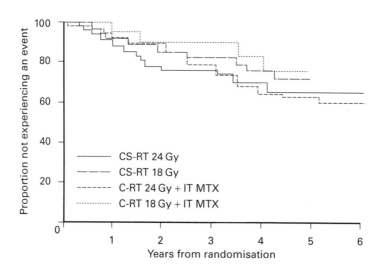

Figure 13.1 Time to first occurrence of relapse in any site or death for patients with good prognosis ALL (see text)

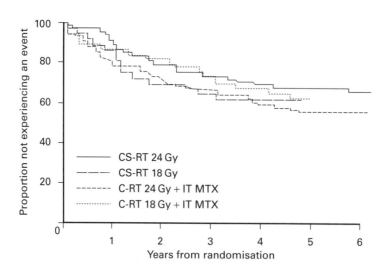

Figure 13.2 Time to first occurrence of relapse in any site or death for patients with intermediate prognosis ALL (see text)

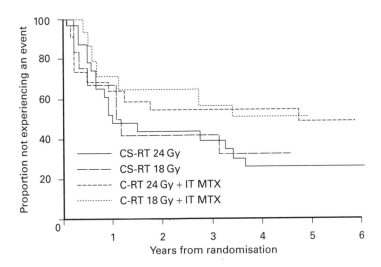

Figure 13.3 Time to first occurrence of relapse in any site or death for patients with poor prognosis ALL (see text)

Bone marrow relapse

Patients who received 18 Gy + IT MTX had fewer marrow relapses or deaths than the group treated with 24 Gy + IT MTX. At 2 and 4 years from randomisation the proportion of patients experiencing marrow relapse or death was as follows:

Marrow relapse: 24 Gy + IT MTX 0·18; 18 Gy + IT MTX 0·12 (2 years).
Marrow relapse: 24 Gy + IT MTX 0·30; 18 Gy + IT MTX 0·21 (4 years).
Death: 24 Gy + IT MTX 0·18; 18 Gy + IT MTX 0·11 (2 years).
Death: 24 Gy + IT MTX 0·29; 18 Gy + IT MTX 0·20 (4 years).

There were no significant differences between the 18 Gy and 24 Gy craniospinal RT groups, neither were there any significant differences between the 24 Gy craniospinal RT and 24 Gy cranial RT + IT MTX groups.

Patients treated with 18 Gy cranial RT + IT MTX appeared to have fewer events than any other combination of therapy.

There were no differences in outcome among the three prognostic groups of patients treated with 18 Gy or 24 Gy for CNS prophylaxis. (Figures 13.1–13.3).

Conclusion

The reduction of the dose of CNS irradiation to 18 Gy did not result in any significant increase in the frequency of CNS relapse, bone marrow relapse or death among any prognostic group of patients.

Study 2

Lilleyman JS, Richards S, Rankin A on behalf of the Medical Research Council's Working Party on Childhood Leukaemia.

Medical Research Council Leukaemia trial, UKALL-VII: a report to the Council by the Working Party on Leukaemia in Childhood. *Arch Dis Childh* 1985;**60**:1050–4.

UKALL-VII was a prospective randomised multicentre trial with enrolment open from April 1979 to March 1980.

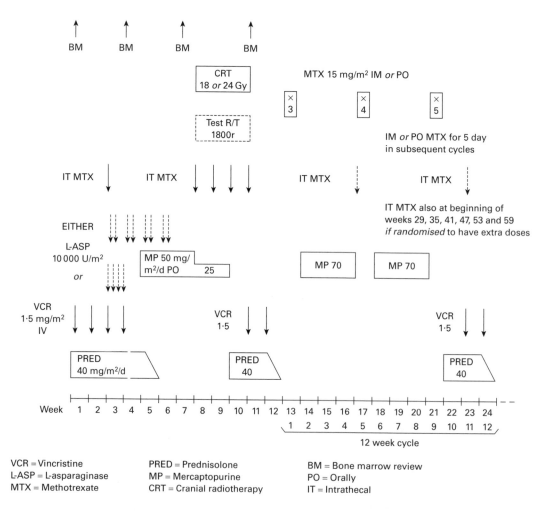

Figure 13.4 UKALL-VII intervention details: treatment time 2 years. Broken lines indicate randomised or allocated variables

Table 13.1 UKALL-VII: randomised variables

Variable		Allocated	Received
Asparaginase	4 doses	40	38
	8 doses	39	41
CNS irradiation	9 fractions	40	41
	12 fractions	39	38
Extra IT MTX	Given	36	34
	Not given	43	43
Methotrexate	IM	40	36
Methotrexate	Oral	39	41
Testicular RT	Given	22	23
	Not given	21	20

IT MTX, intrathecal methotrexate; IM, intramuscular; RT, radiotherapy

Objectives

The study aimed to evaluate the efficacy of a reduction in the dose of cranial irradiation and its impact on the treatment outcome in children with acute lymphoblastic leukaemia. The study also had other objectives, which included evaluation of the need for prophylactic testicular irradiation, the number of doses of asparginase during induction, need for additional intrathecal methotrexate (IT MTX) during maintenance and the use of oral versus intramuscular methotrexate during maintenance.

This review focuses on the CNS prophylaxis treatment alone.

Design of the study

Previously untreated children less than 14 years of age and with the diagnostic white blood cell count $< 20 \times 10^9/\ell$ were enrolled on the trial.

Black children as well as those with T-ALL or B-ALL were excluded from the study.

Remission induction consisted of vincristine, prednisolone and L-asparaginase with intrathecal methotrexate. Drugs, doses, routes of administration and the various randomised treatments are shown in Figure 13.4.

There were two randomisations for pre-symptomatic CNS treatment and both randomisations were independent of each other:

1   Cranial irradiation dose either at 18 Gy in 9 fractions or 24 Gy in 12 fractions.
2   Six additional doses of intrathecal methotrexate at 6-weekly intervals during the first year of maintenance treatment or not.

The methodology of randomisation is not specified in the report.

Outcome measures were:

1   Relapse free survival.
2   Incidence of CNS relapse according to cranial irradiation dose.
3   Incidence of relapse at other sites other than the CNS according to cranial irradiation dose.

Outcome

Of the 87 patients registered in the trial, only 79 were considered eligible for evaluation and subsequent randomisation for CNS prophylaxis (5 were ineligible, 3 failed to remit). Analysis was performed on the basis of intention to treat as well as on the basis of treatment actually received (Table 13.1).

There was no difference in the CNS relapse rate in the children from the two cranial radiotherapy schedules as well as from the differing intrathecal methotrexate schedules when analysed on the basis of intention to treat or by actual treatment received. Six patients had CNS recurrence of disease – 1 patient each in the 18 Gy and extra methotrexate arm as well as 24 Gy and extra methotrexate arm, 2 had 18 Gy and no extra methotrexate, and 2 had 24 Gy and no extra methotrexate. No differences were also evident in the marrow or testicular relapse rates due to the different cranial radiotherapy and intrathecal methotrexate schedules.

Conclusion

A reduction in the cranial irradiation dose from 24 GY to 18 Gy did not increase relapse rates within the CNS. Similarly, additional intrathecal methotrexate during maintenance did not have any significant effect on CNS relapse.

Study 3

Brandalise S, Odone V, Pereira W, Andrea M, Zanichelli M, Aranega V for ALL Brazilian Group, State University of Campinas, São Paulo, Brazil. Treatment results of three consecutive Brazilian co-operative childhood ALL protocols: GBTLI-80, –82 and –85.
Leukaemia 1993;**7**:S142–5.

GBTLI-80 was a prospective randomised multi-centre of the All Brazilian Group study that ran from July 1980 till July 1982.

Objectives

The objectives of the trial were to compare and evaluate the efficacy of 18 Gy cranial irradiation against 24 Gy cranial irradiation in the prevention of CNS relapse of leukaemia in children with good risk ALL.

Details of the study

All children with untreated ALL who were less than 18 years of age and with no previous malignancies were included in the study. All patients with FAB L3 morphology were excluded from the study.

Patients were classified into two prognostic risk groups according to clinical and haematological factors. Good prognosis included patients with WBC count $< 100 \times 10^9/\ell$, with no mediastinal mass or CNS disease. All others were categorised into the poor prognostic group.

Induction therapy consisted of vincristine 1·5 mg/m²/week × 4, daunorubicin 25 mg/m²/week × 4 and prednisone 40 mg/m²/day × 28 days. High risk patients (poor prognosis) also received cyclophosphamide 1200 mg/m² IV on day 1. Good risk patients who achieved remission underwent randomisation between 24 Gy or 18 Gy cranial irradiation for CNS prophylaxis. All high risk patients received 24 Gy cranial irradiation at week 72. Maintenance therapy consisted of daily oral 6-mercaptopurine 50 mg/m² and weekly oral methotrexate 15 mg/m².

Four pulses of cyclophosphamide 150 mg/m²/day × 7 and doxorubicin 35 mg/m² on day 8 were also given during the first year of maintenance therapy. Treatment was continued for 120 weeks for all children.

Details of the randomisation method are not given in the study.

Outcome measures were: CNS relapse rate and event free survival (EFS).

Outcome

Of the 203 patients enrolled on study GBTLI-80, only 185 were eligible for analysis. Exact reasons as to why 18 were excluded from analysis are not stated in the report. It is not clear whether analysis was on the basis of intention to treat.

Of 185 patients analysed, 167 (90%) achieved remission. At the time of analysis (July 1992) 67 patients had relapsed. The incidence of isolated CNS and combined CNS relapse was 6·7%. There was no statistically significant difference in CNS relapse rates between the patients who received 18 Gy and 24 Gy cranial irradiation (p = 0·61).

The 12 year EFS for both the good and high risk groups was 50% (SD 5%).

Conclusion

It was concluded that 18 Gy cranial irradiation was adequate in not only preventing CNS relapse of leukaemia but also had no adverse outcome on EFS in children with good risk ALL.

Study 4

Schrappe M, Reiter A, Zimmermann M, Harbott J, Ludwig W-D, Henze G, Gadner H, Odenwald E, Riehm H.

Long-term results of four consecutive trials in childhood ALL performed by the ALL–BFM study group from 1981 to 1995.

Leukaemia 2000;**14**:2205–22.

ALL-BFM 83 was a multicentre prospective randomised study with treatment stratified according to the BFM (Berlin–Frankfurt–Munster) risk criteria. ALL-BFM 83 began in October 1983 and was closed in September 1986.

Objectives

The study to compared the efficacy of two different doses of presymptomatic cranial irradiation – 12 Gy *v* 18 Gy – in the prevention of CNS relapse of leukaemia in children with high standard risk ALL.

Details of the study

The study was open to all patients less than 18 years of age with previously untreated leukaemia. Children with Down's syndrome who had severe cardiac defects were excluded, as were children who developed ALL as a second malignancy.

Patients were categorised as standard risk (SR: RF < 1·2), medium risk (MR: RF 1·2 < 1·7) or high risk (HR: RF ≥ 1·7) according to the leukaemic cell mass or BFM risk factor at diagnosis. SR patients were further subdivided in ALL-BFM 83 into low-SR (RF 0·8) and high-SR (RF 0·8–1·2) groups.

The duration of induction therapy was 11 weeks. ALL-BFM 83 induction therapy commenced with a 1 week prednisone window with a stepwise increase to full dose of 60 mg/m²/day. The other drugs used during induction therapy (Protocol I) consisted of vincristine (VCR) 1·5 mg/m²/week × 4 prednisone (PDN) 60 mg/m²/day, daunorubicin 30 mg/m²/week × 4 (DNR), L-asparaginase 10 000 U/m²/dose × 8 (ASP), cyclophosphamide (CPM) 1 g/m²/dose × 2, cytosine arabinoside (ARA-C) 75 mg/m²/dose × 16, 6-mercaptopurine (6-MP) 60 mg/m²/day × 28 days and intrathecal methotrexate (IT MTX).

All SR patients of ALL-BFM 83 received 6-MP 25 mg/m²/day and IV MTX 0·5 g/m²/dose × 4 during the consolidation phase.

Re-intensification also consisted of two phases: Phase A – dexamethasone (DEX)/VCR/doxorubicin (DOX)/ASP; Phase B – ARA-C/6-thioguanine (6-TG)/IT MTX (Protocol III, 4 weeks). Low-SR patients were randomised to receive or not the re-intensification block and furthermore did not receive cranial irradiation. High-SR patients were randomised to either 12 Gy or 18 Gy cranial radiotherapy at the end of this block of treatment as part of CNS prophylaxis.

Maintenance phase consisted of daily oral 6-MP and weekly oral MTX for 18 months. Patients in continuous clinical remission were randomised either to stop therapy (18 months) or to continue maintenance treatment for a further 6 months and stop (24 months).

Intrathecal chemotherapy – eight courses of IT MTX – was given to patients in the ALL-BFM 83 study.

The median follow up of patients in continuous complete remission was 11·06 years (8·0 – 16·1 years).

Randomisation details were not specified in the report. Comparisons between the treatment groups were made using the log-rank test.

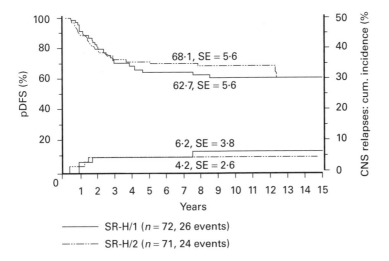

Figure 13.5 Disease free survival and cumulative CNS relapse incident in relation to radiation dose (H/1 = 12Gy, H/2 = 18 Gy). Adapted and reprinted from Schrappe M *et al*, *Leukaemia* with permission from Nature Publishing Group (full reference p 304).

Outcome measures were CNS relapse rate, disease free survival (DFS) and event free survival (EFS).

Outcome

All analyses were based on the principle of intention to treat. The trial registered 653 patients. Of the 397 patients considered as SR (60·8%), 197 (30·2%) were categorised as high SR and 200 as low-SR. Two hundred and eight (31·9%) were categorised as MR and 47 (7·2%) as HR. Of the high SR patients, 143 were randomised to either 18 Gy (*n* = 71) (SR-H/2) or 12 Gy (*n* = 72) (SR-H/l) cranial irradiation for CNS prophylaxis. Reasons for exclusion of the 54 high-SR patients from randomisation are not specified in the report.

Eight year EFS for high-SR patients was 63·8% ± 3·5%. The probability of DFS (pDFS) at 8 years for high-SR patients who received 12 Gy cranial irradiation (SR-H/1) was 62·7% ± 5·6% as compared to 68·1% ± 5·6% for those who received 18 Gy (SR-H/2) (p = 0·68). The cumulative incidence of CNS relapse was also not significant between the two groups of patients (Figure 13.5).

Conclusion

CNS prophylaxis with 12 Gy of cranial irradiation was as effective as 18 Gy in the prevention of CNS relapse of leukaemia and did not have any adverse impact on DFS in high-SR patients.

Study 5

Tsuchida M, Ikuta K, Hanada R, Saito T, Isoyama K, Sugita K, Toyoda Y, Manabe A, Koike K, Kinoshita A, Maeda M, Ishimoto K, Sato T, Okimoto Y, Kaneko T, Kajiwara M, Sotomatsu M, Hayashi Y, Yabe H, Hosoya R, Hoshi Y, Ohira M, Bessho F, Tsunematsu Y, Tsukimoto I, Nakazawa S, for the Tokyo Children's Cancer Study Group.

Long-term follow-up of childhood acute lymphoblastic leukaemia in Tokyo Children's Cancer Study Group 1981–1995
Leukaemia 2000;**14**:2295–306.

Trial L81-10 was a study run by the Tokyo Children's Cancer Group between 1981 and 1984, and was a prospective multicentre randomised trial.

Objectives

The objectives were to compare two differing doses of cranial irradiation (18 Gy *v* 24 Gy) as CNS prophylactic regimens in the treatment of children with standard risk ALL.

Details of the study

Previously untreated children of between 1 and 15 years of age were entered into the study. Children with B-ALL or T-ALL were excluded from the trial. Children were categorised as standard risk (SR) if they were between 1 and 6 years of age with WBC count at diagnosis $< 20 \times 10^9/\ell$. All others were treated as high risk (HR).

Induction therapy consisted of 5 weeks of vincristine $1 \cdot 5$ mg/m^2/week, prednisolone 60 mg/m^2/d and L-asparaginase 6000 U/m$^2 \times 8$ for all patients. This was followed by presymptomatic CNS treatment that consisted of cranial

irradiation plus intrathecal methotrexate 15 mg/m^2 and hydrocortisone 15 mg/m$^2 \times 5$ (IT MH). SR patients were randomised to either 18 Gy or 24 Gy prophylactic cranial irradiation while HR patients received 24 Gy cranial irradiation.

No details of the randomisation methodology are specified in the report.

Maintenance therapy consisted of daily oral 6-Mercaptopurine and weekly oral methotrexate. SR children had mini intensifications every 16 weeks during maintenance with dexamethasone (DEX) 10 mg/m$^2 \times 7$ days and cyclophosphamide (CPM) 150 mg/m$^2 \times 5$ days. In HR patients, the mini intensifications were at 12-weekly intervals during maintenance and they were randomised to either DEX + daunorubicin 30 mg/m^2 (DNR) + CPM, or DEX + DNR alone.

Outcome measures were EFS and probability rate of cumulative isolated CNS relapse and any other CNS relapse.

Outcome

All analyses were performed on the basis of intention to treat. Of the 195 patients enrolled on the study, 86 and 109 patients were classified as SR and HR respectively. Six were excluded from analysis either due to lack of information or incorrect risk classification. Thus 189 were considered evaluable.

Forty-six SR patients received 18 Gy while 40 received 24 Gy cranial irradiation.

The median follow up duration for patients who were free of failure was $15 \cdot 3$ years ($8 \cdot 9$–$17 \cdot 7$ years).

A total of 183 (96·8%) patients achieved complete remission. The overall EFS at 5 years was $56.5 \pm 3.8\%$. The 5-year EFS in the 18 Gy SR group was $81.7 \pm 5.8\%$ compared to $62.3 \pm 8\%$ in the 24 Gy SR group (p = 0.1419). At 15 years, the EFS was $67.2 \pm 7.2\%$ and $53.3 \pm 8.4\%$ respectively. There were three CNS relapses in each arm. No significant differences in EFS were observed in the two HR groups.

Conclusion

In standard risk children with ALL, CNS prophylaxis with 18 Gy cranial irradiation was adequate in preventing CNS relapse of leukaemia with no adverse impact on EFS.

14

Comparisons of methods of CNS directed therapy in acute lymphoblastic leukaemia

Studies

Study 1

Komp DM, Fernandez CH, Falletta JM, Ragab AH, Bennett Humphrey G, Pullen J, Moon T, Shuster J. CNS prophylaxis in acute lymphoblastic leukaemia: comparison of two methods – a Southwest Oncology Group study.
Cancer 1982;**50**:1031–6.

This was part of the AlinC–9 trial (July 1971 – March 1973), which was a prospective randomised multicentre study.

Objectives

The primary aim of the study was to evaluate whether cranial irradiation plus triple intrathecal chemotherapy was superior to triple intrathecal chemotherapy alone as CNS prophylaxis therapy.

Details of the study

All children younger than 15 years of age with leukaemia were enrolled on the trial. This report focuses exclusively on children with acute lymphoblastic leukaemia.

Remission induction therapy consisted of vincristine (VCR) plus prednisone (PDN) or VCR plus PDN along with cyclophosphamide and asparaginase.

Maintenance therapy consisted of 6-mercaptopurine plus regular pulses of PDN. One group of patients also received monthly daunorubicin. Details of the dosing schedules are not specified in the report.

Details of the randomisation methodology are not given. Randomisation of treatment groups was done at the time of initial diagnosis.

Presymptomatic CNS treatment was commenced during maintenance therapy and consisted of intrathecal methotrexate 15 mg/m^2 (max 15 mg), intrathecal hydrocortisone (15 mg/m^2) and intrathecal cytosine arabinoside (30 mg/m^2). During

Table 14.1 CNS relapses versus white blood cell count at diagnosis

WBC count at diagnosis	Treatment	No. patients	No. CNS relapses	p value
<20 ×10^9/ℓ	No RT	67	4	
	RT	53	3	0·87
>20 ×10^9/ℓ	NO RT	35	3	
	RT	39	1	0·35
All patients	No RT	102	7	
	RT	92	4	0·44

RT, radiotherapy; CNS, central nervous system

the first month of maintenance, triple intrathecal therapy was given weekly and thereafter once every 2 months up to a year or till bone marrow or CNS relapse. In addition, one half of the patients were randomised to receive 24 Gy cranial irradiation, which was given at the beginning of maintenance therapy.

Outcome measures were CNS relapse rate, disease free survival (DFS) and overall survival.

Outcome

Of the 194 patients who achieved remission, 102 were randomised to triple intrathecal chemotherapy alone while 92 patients received cranial irradiation plus triple intrathecal chemotherapy. Minimum follow-up for surviving patients was 8 years.

Major violations of CNS prophylaxis protocol occurred in 14 patients.

Eleven patients developed CNS relapses during remission isolated CNS relapse: 6; concurrent with bone marrow or testicular relapse 2; following an earlier testicular relapse 3. Seven of these occurred in non-irradiated patients (n = 102) while four had been radiated (n = 92).

No significant difference was noted in the duration of CNS remission or in the CNS relapse rate between the two groups of patients (p = 0·44) irrespective of the initial WBC count (Table 14.1).

There was no difference in the duration of disease free remission (p = 0·84) or overall survival (p = 0·85) between the two groups of patients. Only 2 of the 6 patients (one patient in each group) who developed isolated CNS relapse remained in haematological remission.

Toxicity
Haematological toxicity was greater in the group that received cranial irradiation (p = 0·05). There were no differences in the occurrence of severe

neurotoxicity or infections between the two
groups of patients.

Conclusion

It was concluded that triple intrathecal
chemotherapy was a satisfactory form of
CNS prophylaxis for children with ALL and
had no adverse impact on CNS relapse rate,
length of haematological remission or overall
survival.

Study 2

Sullivan MP, Chen T, Dyment PG, Hvizdala E, Steuber CP.

Equivalence of intrathecal chemotherapy and radiotherapy as central nervous system prophylaxis in children with acute lymphatic leukaemia: a Pediatric Oncology Study Group.

Blood 1982;**60**:948–58.

South West Oncology Group Study 7420 (AlinC-11) was a prospective multicentre randomised study and ran from September 1974 to October 1976.

Objectives

The study compared the efficacy of intrathecal chemotherapy (IT CT) alone against 24 Gy cranial radiotherapy (CRT) plus intrathecal methotrexate (IT MTX) as CNS prophylaxis regimens.

Details of the study

Previously untreated children and adolescents below 18 years of age were enrolled on the study.

Patients were randomised at diagnosis to one of the four treatment regimens shown in Figure 14.1. Randomisation was according to prognostic groups based on age and WBC count at diagnosis (Table 14.2). Allocation to regimens 1 and 4 (conventional CNS regimen) was weighted 2:1 with the other two regimens. With each regimen, induction was continued for a total of 6 weeks if remission was not achieved in 4 weeks. Maintenance therapy consisted of daily 6-mercaptopurine and weekly methotrexate and was discontinued after 3 years' continuous remission in all regimens.

No details of randomisation method are specified in the study. The Gehan–Wilcoxon test was used to determine the differences among the treatment arms.

Outcome

Of the 408 patients registered in the trial, 11 were excluded from analysis due to ineligibility, wrong diagnosis and other non-specified reasons. Of the remaining 397, 380 patients were considered evaluable (265 were fully and 115 partially evaluable). The numbers of patients fully evaluable in each of the four regimens were as follows: R1 86, R2 55, R3 46, R4 78; while the numbers partially evaluable were R1 42, R2 16, R3 21, R4 36. The reasons for partial evaluability included early death (16), inadequate trial (3), lost for follow-up (34), refused treatment (3), other reasons (59).

The number of CNS relapses, including those combined with marrow relapse in the IT regimens (regimens 1, 2 and 3) was 10/234 (4·3%) compared with 7/105 (6·1%) in the CRT plus IT regimen (Regimen 4).

Figure 14.2 shows the duration of bone marrow remission for each treatment arm. Length of bone marrow remission in the poor prognostic group was better for arm 1 compared to arm 3 (p = 0·04) as well as arm 4 (p = 0·01) (Figure 14.3).

Toxicity

There were no significant differences in the number of patients with severe toxicity in any of the four regimens.

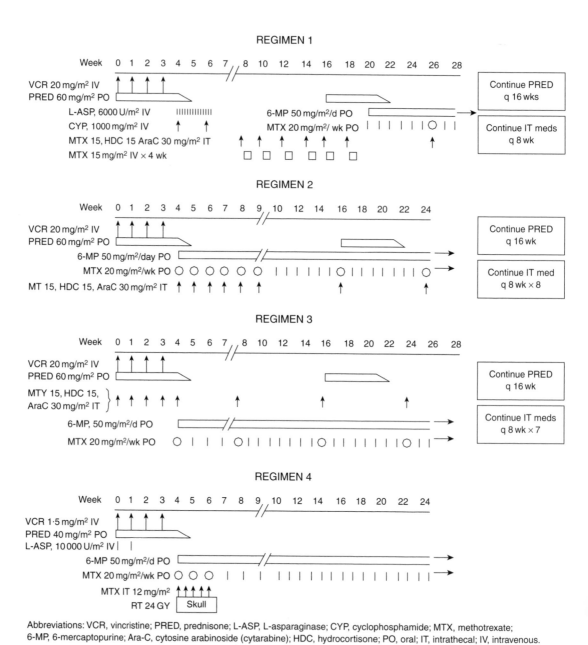

Abbreviations: VCR, vincristine; PRED, prednisone; L-ASP, L-asparaginase; CYP, cyclophosphamide; MTX, methotrexate; 6-MP, 6-mercaptopurine; Ara-C, cytosine arabinoside (cytarabine); HDC, hydrocortisone; PO, oral; IT, intrathecal; IV, intravenous.

Figure 14.1 Treatment regimens 1–4 in SWOG-7420 Acute Leukaemia in Childhood study No. 11

Table 14.2 Staging of acute lymphoblastic leukaemia by age and WBC count at diagnosis

WBC×10⁹/ℓ	Age (yr)				
	1	1–2	3–5	6–10	`10
<10	III	I	I	I	II
10–99	III	II	II	II	III
≥ 100	III	III	II	III	III

Stage I good prognosis.
Stage II average prognosis.
Stage III poor prognosis.

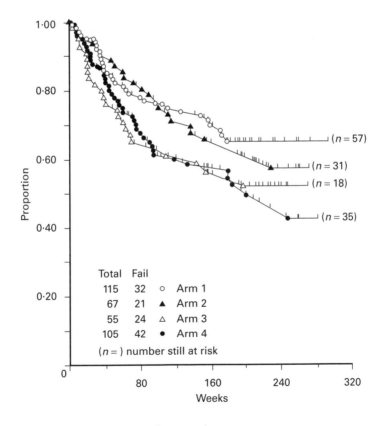

Figure 14.2 Duration of bone marrow remission: all prognostic groups

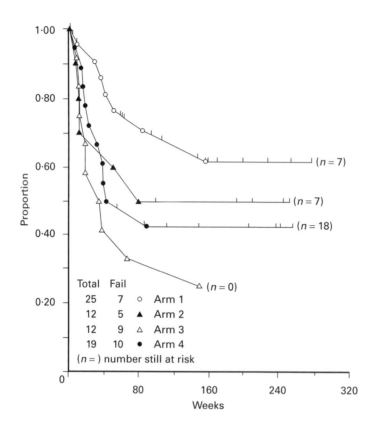

Figure 14.3 Duration of bone marrow remission in poor prognostic group

Conclusion

It was concluded that IT chemotherapy was as effective as cranial radiotherapy plus IT methotrexate in preventing CNS relapse of leukaemia.

Study 3

Bleyer WA, Coccia PF, Sather HN, Level C, Lukens J, Niebrugge DJ, Siegel S, Littman PS, Leikin SS, Miller DR, Chard RL Jr, Denman Hammond G, and the Children's Cancer Study Group.
Reduction in central nervous system leukaemia with a pharmacokinetically derived intrathecal methotrexate dosage regimen.
J Clin Oncol 1983;1:317–25.

The paper was a retrospective analysis of three major Children's Cancer Study Group studies: CCG-141, 141-A and 160 series. Each study had a different method of CNS prophylaxis and this varied from 24 Gy cranial irradiation plus intrathecal methotrexate (IT MTX) during consolidation (CCG-141), 24 Gy cranial irradiation plus IT MTX initiated during induction (CCG 141-A) or 18 Gy cranial irradiation plus IT MTX with or without IT MTX (randomised) during maintenance therapy but with dosage of IT MTX based on CNS volume rather than on body surface area (CCG-160 series). In the CCG-160 series, average risk patients were randomised to maintenance IT MTX (m-IT), low risk patients were randomised to cranial irradiation or m-IT while high risk patients were administered m-IT (Table 14.3).

This review will focus on CCG study 160 (1978 till 1981), which evaluated the influence of maintenance IT MTX on CNS relapse, complete remission duration, haematological remission

Table 14.3 CCSG studies of childhood acute lymphoblastic leukaemia from 1976 to 1981

Study	Years patients entered	No. of patients entered	No. of patients evaluable (%)	Preventive CNS therapies[a]
CCG–141	1976–77	877	818 (93)	Cr + IT
CCG–141A	1977–78	421	387 (92)	Cr + IT
CCG 160 series	1978–81	1943[b]	1797 (93)	
Low risk				
CCG-161		405[b]		IT → Cr / m-IT
Average risk				
CCG-162		1123[b]		Cr + IT → M-IT / No IT
High risk				
CCG-163		415[b]		Cr + IT + m-IT

[a] Arrows denote randomisations. Abbreviations: Cr, cranial irradiation; IT, intrathecal MTX; m-IT, maintenance IT MTX therapy.
[b] As of 29 March 1982.

duration and survival in average risk patients with ALL.

Details of the study

Previously untreated children and adolescents under 18 years of age with ALL were registered on the trial. All children who had CNS leukaemia at diagnosis were kept on the regimen to which they were randomised.

Details of randomisation method are not specified.

Patients were stratified for risk as follows:

Low risk: 3–6 years of age, WBC at diagnosis < 10 ×10^9/ℓ FAB L1 morphology.

Average risk: < 3 or > 6 years of age with WBC count < 50 × 10^9/ℓ or 3–6 years of age and WBC count of 10–50 × 10^9/ℓ or low risk patients with FAB L2 morphology.

High risk: any age or FAB morphology with WBC count > 50 × 10^9/ℓ.

Remission induction therapy consisted of Vincristine (VCR), Prednisone (PDN) and L-asparaginase (ASP). Consolidation therapy differed in the form of CNS treatment. Maintenance therapy (standard maintenance therapy consisted of VCR + PDN + MTX + 6-MP) depended on the randomisation and risk group. Low risk patients were randomised to a reduction in therapy with VCR and PDN deleted. A third of the average risk patients had standard maintenance therapy similar to that in the earlier trials, a third received periodic pulses of VCR, PDN and ASP added to the standard maintenance therapy every 6 months and a third received pulses of cytosine arabinoside, doxorubicin or cyclophosphamide added at monthly

intervals to the standard maintenance therapy. Children who were randomised to receive maintenance IT, were given IT MTX every 12 weeks during maintenance therapy.

Neither drug dosages nor the chemotherapy schedule are specified in the paper.

IT MTX doses were age adjusted: 6 mg, 8 mg, 10 mg and 12 mg for ages <1, 1, 2 and 3 years or greater respectively.

Outcome measures were CNS relapse rate and duration of haematological remission.

Outcome

CCG-160 enrolled 1943 patients, of whom 1123 were categorised as average risk. However, only 1024 patients were randomised to receive maintenance IT MTX or not. The actual number of patients randomised to each arm is not specified. Details regarding the number of patients who were excluded, who failed remission induction therapy, who relapsed prior to commencement of maintenance therapy or who died in remission etc, are not available.

Patients who were randomised to receive maintenance IT MTX had a lower CNS relapse rate but the difference was only marginal (p = 0·06). This was most evident in children over 10 years of age.

The incidence of bone marrow relapses, remission deaths and deaths after relapse were higher in the maintenance IT MTX group.

Conclusion
It was concluded that maintenance intrathecal methotrexate did not significantly reduce CNS relapse rate in children with average risk ALL.

Study 4

Ortega JA, Nesbit ME, Sather HN, Robinson LL, D'Angio GJ, Denman Hammond G.
Long term evaluation of a CNS prophylaxis trial – treatment comparisons and outcome after CNS relapse in childhood ALL: a report from the Children's Cancer Study Group.
J Clin Oncol 1987;**5**:1646–54.

This was a Children's Cancer Study Group (CCG-101) prospective randomised multicentre study that extended from June 1972 to July 1974.

Objectives

The study aimed to determine the effectiveness of four different CNS prophylaxis regimens and also their relationship to bone marrow relapse and survival.

Details of the study

Previously untreated children and adolescents with ALL below the age of 18 years were included in the trial. Children less than 18 months of age were not randomised but allocated to regimen 4 – intrathecal methotrexate (IT MTX) alone. Protocol violations or marrow relapse on treatment were criteria for exclusion from the study.

No details regarding randomisation are specified in the report.

Induction therapy consisted of vincristine, prednisone and L-asparaginase. Those who achieved complete remission were randomised to any one of four CNS prophylaxis regimens:

Regimen 1: 24 Gy craniospinal irradiation plus extended field radiation (12 Gy) to include liver, spleen, kidneys and gonads.
Regimen 2: 24 Gy craniospinal irradiation only.

Regimen 3: 24 Gy cranial irradiation + IT MTX 12 mg/m^2 twice a week ×6 doses.
Regimen 4: IT MTX 12 mg/m^2 twice a week × 6 doses.

Maintenance therapy consisted of daily 6-mercaptopurine (6-MP), weekly oral MTX and monthly pulses of vincristine and prednisone. Lumbar punctures were performed at bone marrow relapse and prior to discontinuation of maintenance therapy. Patients with CNS disease at diagnosis were given IT MTX 12 mg/m^2 twice a week (minimum two doses) until the CSF was clear.

Interim analysis showed that children on regimen 4 had a high incidence of CNS relapse and hence 93 regimen 4 patients, who had not developed CNS disease, were recalled for additional CNS prophylaxis. Those with WBC count $\geq 20 \times 10^9/\ell$ were treated with regimen 2 while all others were treated with Regimen 3. Twelve children chose not to have additional CNS prophylaxis.

Outcome measures were CNS relapse rate, disease free survival (DFS) and overall survival.

Outcome

Analysis of results was on an intention to treat basis. The median follow up was 132 months (maximum of 161 months). Of the 736 patients enrolled on the study, only 675 patients completed induction and achieved remission. Five hundred and ninety were subsequently randomised to one of the four CNS prophylaxis regimens:

Regimen 1: 135
Regimen 2: 152
Regimen 3: 159
Regimen 4: 144
Regimen 4: 34 (Non-random allocation because of age).

Table 14.4 Comparison of relapse/death rates in the CNS prophylaxis groups

Type of event	Regimen 4 (IT MTX)		Regimens 1, 2, and 3 (radiotherapy)		
	Observed events (O_1)	Expected no. $(E_1)^a$	Observed events (O_2)	Expected no. $(E_2)^a$	Adjusted difference[b]
Isolated CNS relapse as initial event	55	19·4	29	64·6	71·2
Isolated marrow relapse as initial event	18	24·4	88	81·6	−12·8
Other initial events	10	16·7	65	58·3	−13·4
Any first relapse or death in remission	83	60·5	182	204.5	45·0
Marrow relapse at any time	54	47·0	133	140·0	14·0
Death	67	57·7	168	177·3	18.6

[a] "Expected" number of events (calculated by life table methods) if both groups actually had the same risk of the event.

[b] Calculated by $(O_1 - E_1) - (O_2 - E_2)$; this adjusts for the discrepancy in the size of the two groups and provides an estimate of the excess number of events between the two groups. A positive value indicates an excess for the IT MTX regimen; a negative value, an excess for the radiotherapy regimens.

For outcome analysis, patients were categorised into two groups. The first group included all patients who had IT MTX alone (regimen 4) and the second group comprised all patients who had cranial irradiation (Regimens 1, 2 and 3).

Isolated CNS relapse as the first event was higher in regimen 4 patients compared to patients who had cranial irradiation (55 v 29, (p<0·0001, Figure 14.4). Isolated bone marrow relapses as the first event were higher in the radiotherapy group (Table 14.4).

Figure 14.5 shows the difference in DFS for the two groups, again indicating a large difference (p<0·001).

The overall survival between the two groups was not significantly different (p = 0·16, Figure 14.6).

Of the 26 patients in regimen 4 who developed one isolated CNS relapse with no subsequent CNS relapses, 14 died and 12 remained alive (11 with no further relapses) (survival rate 46%). This compared to 4 in the irradiation group who

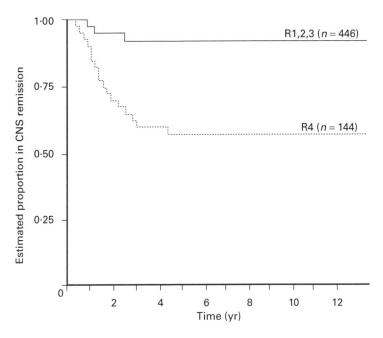

Figure 14.4 Time to isolated CNS relapse (as an initial event) from randomisation

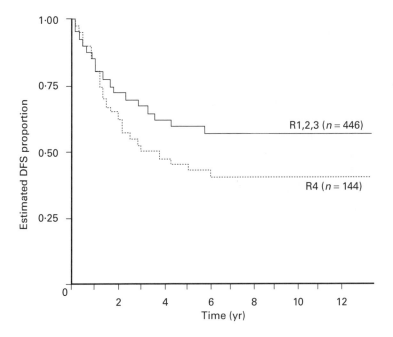

Figure 14.5 Disease free survival from randomisation

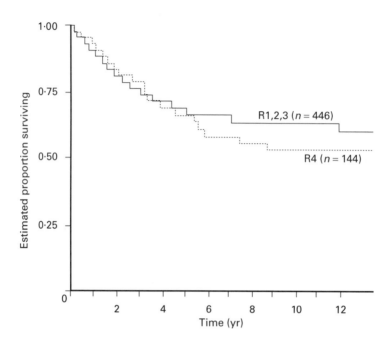

Figure 14.6 Overall survival from randomisation

remained alive (3 with no further relapses of any type) of the 17 who developed one isolated CNS relapse (survival rate 24%).

Conclusion

It was concluded that although short treatment with intrathecal methotrexate alone as CNS prophylaxis was unsatisfactory in preventing CNS relapse of leukaemia, this did not impact significantly on overall survival due to a higher incidence of marrow relapses in the radiotherapy group.

Study 5

Littman P, Coccia P, Bleyer WA, Lukens J, Siegel S, Miller D, Sather H, Denman Hammond G. Central nervous system (CNS) prophylaxis in children with low risk acute lymphoblastic leukaemia (ALL).
Int J Rad Oncol Biol Phys 1987;**13**:1443–9.

Trial CCSG-161 of the Children's Cancer Study Group was a prospective randomised study for children with low risk ALL that ran from April 1978 to May 1983.

Objectives

The study addressed whether maintenance intrathecal methotrexate (IT MTX) can be substituted for cranial irradiation (CR RT) as CNS prophylaxis treatment.

Details of the study

Only previously untreated children aged between 3 and 6 years inclusive, with a total WBC count $<10 \times 10^9/\ell$ at diagnosis and with less than 25% FAB L2 cells (low risk group) in the bone marrow were enrolled on the study.

Median follow up for surviving patients at the time of data analysis was 54 months from randomisation – start of CNS intensification.

Details of the randomisation method used are not reported.

All patients were treated on a standard induction regimen that consisted of vincristine (VCR), L-Asparaginase (ASP) and prednisone (PDN) for a 4 week period. In addition, two doses of IT MTX were given to all patients on day 0 and day 14 of induction therapy. At the end of induction

therapy (day 28), patients who attained remission or M2 marrow (< 25% blasts) were randomised to one of four treatment groups with regard to intensification and maintenance:

Regimen 1: CR RT CNS prophylaxis plus maintenance chemotherapy of oral 6-Mercaptopurine (6-MP) and MTX.

Regimen 2: CR RT CNS prophylaxis plus maintenance chemotherapy of oral 6-MP, MTX with additional pulses of VCR and PDN every 12 weeks.

Regimen 3: IT MTX CNS prophylaxis plus maintenance chemotherapy of oral 6-MP, MTX and IT MTX during maintenance at 12 week intervals.

Regimen 4: IT MTX CNS prophylaxis plus maintenance chemotherapy of oral 6-MP, MTX with additional VCR and PDN and IT MTX during maintenance therapy at 12 week intervals.

Patients randomised to CR RT received 18 Gy in 10 fractions with four doses of IT MTX on days 0, 7, 14 and 21 of the intensification block, and those randomised to IT MTX received four doses of IT MTX (on the same days) and then every 84 days (8 or 12 doses, depending on the duration of maintenance) during maintenance therapy.

Patients who proceeded to maintenance therapy either had M1 or M2 marrow at the end of the intensification block. Those who were in continuous remission for 2 years were randomised either to continue maintenance therapy for an additional year (four additional maintenance cycles) or to stop therapy.

Outcome measures were disease free survival (DFS), CNS relapse (isolated or concurrent) as a

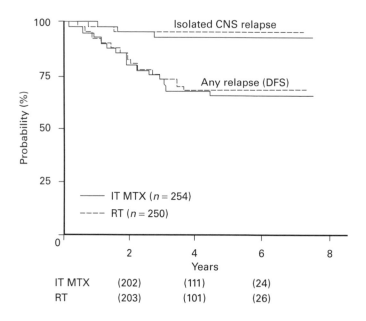

Figure 14.7 Isolated CNS relapse and any relapse (disease free survival) from the time of randomisation. Comparison of CNS prophylaxis groups. Numbers in parentheses indicate the number of patients disease free that have reached various follow up times. Reprinted from Littman P *et al*, *Int J Rad Oncol Biol Phys* (full reference p 321) with permission from Elsevier Science.

first disease recurrence, and bone marrow relapse.

Outcome

Analyses of outcome were on the basis of intention to treat. The exact details regarding the number of patients enrolled on the study, induction failures, protocol violations, toxic deaths during induction therapy, relapse prior to randomisation etc. are not specified in the report.

Of the 504 patients who were randomised to the two different CNS prophylaxis regimens, 250 patients were randomised to CR RT and 254 to IT MTX.

The last CNS relapse occurred at 41 months post CNS randomisation and 76·1% of all disease free patients were beyond that point.

CNS relapse rate (isolated or concurrent) was 6% in the CR RT group compared to 8% in the IT MTX group (p = 0·48) while the isolated CNS relapse rate from randomisation was 5% and 7% respectively (p = 0·44). The eventual cumulative incidence of CNS relapse as a first event was estimated to be 6·1% and 8·4% with CR RT and IT MTX respectively.

Bone marrow relapse rate was 21% and 22% in the CRT RT and IT MTX groups respectively (p = 0·88).

The DFS at 54 months was 67·4% and 66·5% for CR RT and IT MTX groups respectively (p = 0·82) (Figure 14.7).

Conclusion

It was concluded that as both modalities of CNS prophylaxis had similar CNS relapse rates and DFS, intrathecal methotrexate could be substituted for cranial radiotherapy.

Study 6

Ortega JJ, Javier G, Olive T.
Treatment of standard- and high-risk childhood acute lymphoblastic leukaemia with two CNS prophylaxis regimens.
Haematol Blood Transfusion 1987;**30**:483–91.

This was a prospective randomised study – both pilot and a parallel multi-centre (11 hospitals) trial – and is reported to have run from April 1978 to December 1983. Minimum follow up was 25 months with a median of 62 months.

Objectives

The study aimed to compare the efficacy of intrathecal chemotherapy (IT CT) alone versus cranial irradiation (CRT) plus intrathecal methotrexate (IT MTX) in the prevention of CNS relapse of leukaemia in children. The other objectives were to improve outcome in patients with high risk acute lymphoblastic leukaemia and to detect occult testicular disease in boys who were in continuous complete remission at 2 years.

This review focuses on the comparative efficacy of the two forms of CNS prophylactic regimens alone.

Details of the study

All children with ALL (B-ALL excluded) below 15 years of age were enrolled on the study.

Patients were classified as standard risk (SR) and high risk (HR) according to a risk index that was based on clinical and haematological factors.

CNS prophylaxis regimens were as follows:

Regimen A: cranial irradiation (24 Gy/12 fractions) plus six doses of IT MTX.

Regimen B: Six doses of intrathecal MTX and cytosine arabinoside (ARA-C) plus four additional monthly doses during the first year of maintenance.

All children received induction therapy that consisted of vincristine (VCR) 1·5 mg/m^2/week × 4, prednisolone (PDN) 40 mg/m^2/d × 4 weeks and L-asparaginase (ASP) 10 000 U/m^2 × 6 doses for the SR group and the same plus daunorubicin (DNR) 30 mg/m^2/wk × 2 for the HR group.

Pre-symptomatic CNS treatment consisted of CRT plus IT MTX (regimen A) or IT MTX 10 mg/m^2 (max. dose 10 mg) and ARA-C 30 mg/m^2 (max. dose 30 mg) (regimen B) along with 6-Mercaptopurine (6-MP) 40 mg/m^2/d in both regimens.

Maintenance treatment consisted of oral 6-MP 60 mg/m^2/d and IM MTX 15 mg/m^2/wk. HR patients also received 2 week intensification blocks of PDN, VCR (two doses) and DNR (one dose) every 12 weeks for 3 years. Duration of maintenance therapy was 3 years for girls and 5 years for boys.

Testicular biopsies were performed in all boys in CR at 2 years and those who had disease had testicular irradiation and 4 weeks of re-induction with VCR and PDN.

Outcome measures were disease free survival (DFS) and CNS relapse rate.

Outcome

Pilot study (Hospital Infantil Vall d'Hebrón)

The number registered on the study was 87 (SR 65, HR 22). One HR patient was excluded

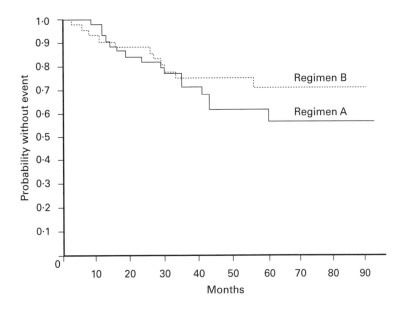

Figure 14.8 Disease free survival with two regimens of CNS prophylaxis

who died in remission due to cranial trauma. There were 86 evaluable patients, comprising 34 SR and 10 HR patients in regimen A (*n* = 44) and 31 SR and 11 HR patients in regimen B (*n* = 42).

Five year disease free survival (DFS) for all patients was 65% (SD 6%). For SR patients the probability of continuous complete remission (CCR) was 67% and for HR patients it was 58%.

Five year DFS in regimen A patients was 56·4% versus. 71·4% in regimen B patients. This was not statistically significant. (Figure 14.8).

Regimen A patients had more relapses (*n* =16) than those in regimen B (*n* =10), but this was not statistically significant. The proportion who relapsed within the CNS was low: regimen A-2 (4·5%) *v* regimen B-1 (2·4%). The bone marrow was the predominant site of relapse.

Toxicity

Two patients treated on regimen A developed encephalopathy while a third developed akinetic seizures. One patient on regimen B developed transient paraparesis after the sixth IT treatment. Psychomotor evaluation showed a lower mean IQ in the irradiated group.

Multicentre trial

Of 256 evaluable patients, 95% attained CR (243). Of these 114 (86 SR; 28 HR) patients had regimen A CNS prophylaxis while 129 (97 SR; 32 HR) were treated on regimen B. There were

108 relapses, of which 19 were CNS relapses. No significant differences according to CNS prophylaxis regimen were found. No further details are given in the report.

Conclusion

It was concluded that CNS prophylaxis with intrathecal chemotherapy (methotrexate and cytosine arabinoside) was effective in preventing CNS relapse of leukaemia.

Study 7

Van Eys J, Berry D, Crist W, Doering E, Fernbach D, Pullen J, Shuster J and Wharam M. A comparison of two regimens for high-risk acute lymphocytic leukaemia in childhood. *Cancer* 1989;**63**:23–29.

This was a Pediatric Oncology Group trial (AlinC-12) and was a prospective randomised study. Enrolment was from 1976 to 1979.

Objectives

The study compared the efficacy of triple drug intrathecal chemotherapy (IT CT) against cranial irradiation plus IT methotrexate (IT MTX) as prophylaxis against CNS relapse of leukaemia in children with high risk acute lymphoblastic leukaemia.

Details of the study

Previously untreated children and adolescents aged below 21 years with high risk ALL according

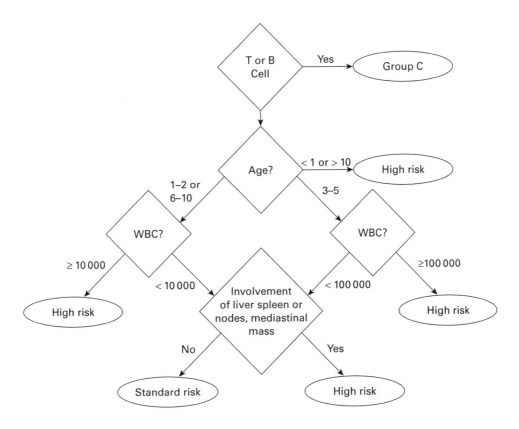

Figure 14.9 Decision tree for risk classification. Copyright © 1989, American Cancer Society. Adapted and reprinted from Van Eys J *et al* (full reference above) by permission of Wiley-Liss, Inc., a subsidiary of John Wiley & Sons, Inc.

to the POG criteria (Figure 14.9) were enrolled on the study. Excluded from the trial were patients with T-ALL, B-ALL (SIg⁺) or with CNS disease at diagnosis.

Details of the randomisation methodology are not given in the report.

All patients were randomised at diagnosis to receive either arm 1 or arm 3. For arm 1 patients, induction therapy consisted of IV vincristine 2 mg/m²/wk (max. dose 2 mg), oral Prednisone 60 mg/m²/d and IV L-asparaginase 10 000 IU/m² weekly × 2. If remission was not achieved after 4 weeks, two additional weeks of vincristine and prednisone were given.

In arm 3, induction was similar to arm 1 except that L-asparaginase 6000 IU/m² daily for 14 days was given during consolidation along with cyclophosphamide 1 g/m² on days 30 and 43.

CNS prophylaxis was as follows. In arm 1 the dose of cranal irradiation (CRT) was age dependent: > 2yr 24 Gy, 1–2 yr 20 Gy and < 1 yr 15 Gy. Five doses of IT MTX were given during CRT. Treatment was given in daily fractions of 180–200 cGy, five fractions per week. CNS prophylaxis in arm 3 consisted of triple IT CT given on the day preceding each 4 day intravenous MTX every 2 weeks for six courses, and also during the entire maintenance phase of treatment at 8 weekly cycles. Doses of intrathecal drugs were methotrexate 15 mg/m² (max. 15 mg), cytosine arabinoside 30 mg/m² (max. 30 mg) and hydrocortisone 15 mg/m² (max 15 mg).

Maintenance therapy consisted of oral 6-mercaptopurine 50 mg/m², weekly oral methotrexate 15 mg/m² with pulses of prednisone and vincristine every fourth month during the maintenance phase. Treatment was stopped at 3 years from date of remission. Figures 14.10a and 14.10b show the scheme of the two regimens.

For an expected 5 year actuarial disease free survival, a sample size of 290 patients was required to detect a relative risk (RR) of below two-thirds or above 1·5 with 80% power (p < 0·05 two-sided by Cox regression).

$$RR = \frac{\text{Instantaneous failure rate of Group 3}}{\text{Instantaneous failure rate of Group 1}}$$

Outcome measures were CNS relapse, bone marrow relapse and other extramedullary relapse (EMD).

Outcome

Two hundred and seven eligible patients were randomised for arm 1 treatment and 223 for arm 3 treatment. Of those, 10 children were ineligible and a further 29 partially evaluable in arm 1 while 7 were ineligible and 38 children were considered partially evaluable in arm 3. Reasons for partial evaluability were early death (arm 1 = 5, arm 3 = 3), toxicity (arm 1 = 2, arm 3 = 7), lost for follow up (arm 1 = 10, arm 3 = 20), inadequate data (arm 1 = 6, arm 3 = 3), refusal of chemotherapy (arm 1 = 3, arm 3 = 4) and other non-specified reasons (arm 1 = 3, arm 3 = 1).

Analysis was based on all eligible patients irrespective of evaluability.

A total of 167 randomised patients treated on arm 1 (n = 197) achieved CR against 175 (n = 216) patients in arm 3. Complete remission rate for arm 1 was 85% versus 81% for arm 3.

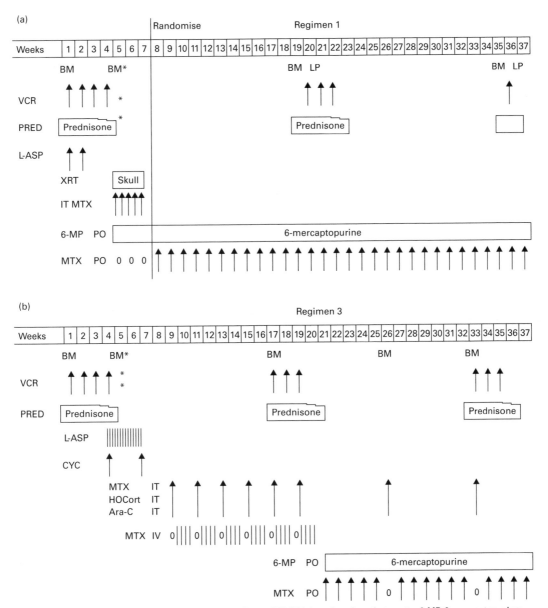

VCR, vincristine; PRED, prednisone; L-ASP, L-asparaginase; IT MTX, intrathecal methotrexate; 6-MP, 6-mercaptopurine; CYC, cyclophosphamide; HOCort, hydro + cortisone; Ara-C, cytosine arabinoside; PO, orally; XRT, radiotherapy

Figure 14.10 Schema for (a) treatment arm 1 and (b) treatment arm 3. (*If not M-1 marrow then V + P is continued for an additional 2 weeks; if still not in remission, the patient is off the study). Copyright © 1989 American Cancer Society (as with Figure 14.9).

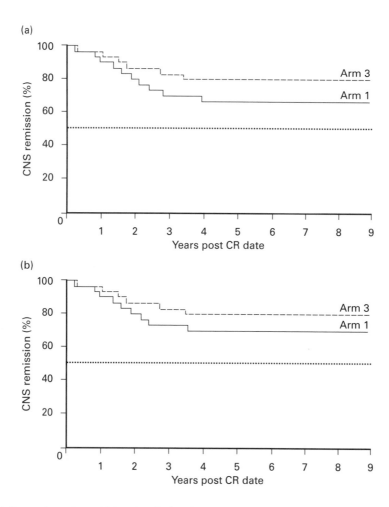

Figure 14.11 (*a*) Comparison of overall duration of central nervous system remission between arm 1 and arm 3. (*b*) Comparison of the incidence of isolated CNS relapse between treatment 1 and arm 3. Copyright © 1989 American Cancer Society (as with Figure 14.9).

There were 37 CNS relapses in arm 1 patients against 26 in arm 3 (RR 0·59; 95% CI 0·36–0·98, p = 0·04). Triple intrathecal chemotherapy was better than cranial irradiation plus intrathecal methotrexate as prophylaxis against CNS relapse of leukaemia (Figure 14.11).

There were 54 relapses at other EMD sites in arm 1 patients versus 39 in arm 3 (RR 0·60; 95% CI 0·39–0·90, p = 0·013). This reflected a higher incidence of testicular relapses in arm 1 (*n* = 12) compared to arm 3 (*n* = 5) (p = 0·01).

There were no significant differences in bone marrow relapses between the two arms (p = 0·13).

During maintenance therapy, toxicities were similar in both arms.

Toxicity

Toxicity during induction was greater in arm 3 (34/216) with one fatality than in arm 1 (6/197). The incidence of life threatening toxicity was also greater in arm 3 patients (12/216 v 1/197).

Conclusion

It was concluded that triple intrathecal chemotherapy provided adequate protection against CNS relapse of leukaemia in children with high risk leukaemia.

Study 8

Zintl F, Malke H, Reimann M, Dörffel W, Domula M, Eggers G, Exadaktylos P, Kotte W, Krause I, Kunert W, Mittler U, Möbius D, Reddemann H, Weinmann G, Weissbach G.

Results of acute lymphoblastic leukaemia therapy in childhood: GDR experiences 1981–1987. *Haematol Blood Transfusion* 1990;**33**:478–82.

The GDR Haematology and Oncology Working Group conducted this prospective multicentre randomised trial using a modified BFM (Berlin-Frankfurt-Munster) protocol. This study (ALL-VII 81) ran from September 1981 till December 1987.

Objectives

The study compared the efficacy of moderate dose intravenous methotrexate (MDMTX) plus intrathecal methotrexate (IT MTX) against cranial irradiation (CRT) plus intrathecal methotrexate (IT MTX) in the prevention of CNS relapse of leukaemia in standard risk patients.

Details of the study

Children with previously untreated ALL (excluding B-ALL) were enrolled on the study. All patients were divided into three risk groups: standard risk (SR), medium risk (MR) and high risk (HR) according to the BFM risk criteria (see Study 17).

Chemotherapy treatment details are not been specified in the report.

SR patients were randomised to either 18 Gy CRT/IT MTX (SR-A) or MDMTX (500 mg/m^2) + IT MTX (SR-B) as CNS prophylaxis. Randomisation was stopped in 1986 due to high CNS failure rate

in the MDMTX group. Seventy patients received an additional 18 Gy CCRT after MDMTX (SR-C). During maintenance therapy, patients were once again randomised (after 78 weeks) either to receive MTX and 6-mercaptopurine (6-MP) for another 6 months or a late intensification protocol.

No details are given of the randomisation method used.

Outcome

Of the 524 children registered on the study, 342 (65%) were classified as SR according to the BFM risk criteria. One hundred and eighty-seven children were randomised to 18 Gy CRT + IT MTX (SR-A) and only 43 to MDMTX (SR-B). The reduced number of patients in SR-B was due to stopping randomisation in 1986 and 70 children had MDMTX and 18 Gy CRT (SR-C).

Of the 524 registered patients, 503 achieved remission (96%). Among the SR group, 330 out of 342 achieved remission (96%).

CNS relapse rate is shown in Figure 14.12. Twenty-three patients in the SR group relapsed within the CNS, of whom 11 had isolated CNS relapse while the remaining 12 also had bone marrow relapse. Only 6 of 187 SR-A patients had CNS relapse (3%).

The 5 year event free interval with regard to CNS prophylaxis regimens in the SR group was SR-A 62%, SR-B 57% and SR-C 72%.

Nine patients in the SR group developed testicular relapse. There were no testicular relapses in the MDMTX group.

No toxic effects were reported.

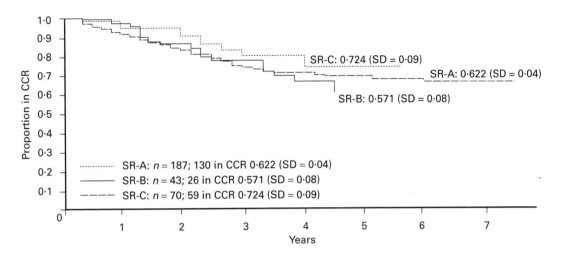

Figure 14.12 Probability of event free interval for standard risk patients with different CNS prophylaxis

Conclusion

It was concluded that moderate dose intra-venous methotrexate was less effective than cranial irradiation in preventing CNS relapse of leukaemia in standard risk patients.

Study 9

Jones B, Freeman AI, Shuster JJ, Jacquillat C, Weil M, Pochedly C, Sinks L, Chevalier L, Maurer HM, Koch K, Falkson G, Patterson R, Seligman B, Sartorius J, Kung F, Haurani F, Stuart M, Burgert EO, Ruymann F, Sawitsky A, Forman E, Pluess H, Truman J, Hakami N, Glidewell O, Glicksman AS, Holland JF.

Lower incidence of meningeal leukaemia when prednisone is replaced by dexamethasone in the treatment of acute lymphocytic leukaemia. *Med Paediatr Oncol* 1991;**19**:269–75.

CALGB trial 7111 was a prospective multicentre randomised trial and enrolled patients from February 1971 to March 1974.

Objectives

The study objectives were:

- To compare the efficacy of dexamethasone against prednisone in improving outcome in children with acute lymphocytic leukaemia (ALL).
- To compare the efficacy of intrathecal Methotrexate (IT MTX) alone versus cranial irradiation (CRT) plus IT MTX in the prevention of CNS relapse of leukaemia in children.
- To assess the efficacy of asparaginase during induction therapy.

Details of the study

All patients with previously untreated ALL up to the age of 20 years were eligible for entry. Lumbar punctures were not routinely performed at diagnosis nor were they were performed at the time of any haematological relapse.

Treatment details were as follows:

Induction: At diagnosis, all patients were randomised to receive vincristine (VCR) 2 mg/m^2/week IV and either prednisone (PDN) 40 mg/m^2/d or dexamethasone (DEX) 6 mg/m^2/d with or without L-asparaginase (ASP) (prior to, simultaneously or subsequent to a 3 week course of VCR and steroids). Patients who did not receive ASP received 4 weeks of VCR and steroids.

Interim maintenance: Prior to July 1971, patients who achieved remission received two courses of methotrexate (MTX) 15 mg/m^2/d IM × 5 days, with 9 days of rest between each course. After another 9 day rest they then received two courses of 6-mercaptopurine (6-MP) – 600 mg/m^2/ IV × 5 days with a similar period of rest between each course. From July 1971, patients were randomised either to the parenteral regimen of 6-MP and MTX or to daily oral (PO) 6-MP 90 mg/m^2 and weekly PO MTX 15 mg/m^2 with a monthly pulse of VCR and 7 day pulse of steroids.

CNS prophylaxis: Patients in remission were randomised to either IT MTX 12 mg/m^2 weekly for 3 weeks alone or with 24 Gy given in 12 fractions of cranial irradiation.

Maintenance phase: Three doses of IT MTX was given every 2 weeks at the beginning of maintenance therapy. Patients who were randomised to parenteral 6-MP and MTX were switched to PO 6-MP and PO MTX after one year of therapy. Additionally, pulses of VCR and steroids were given at 3-monthly intervals. All patients who remained in CR continued antileukaemia treatment for 5 years, at which time they were randomised to continue treatment for a further 2 years or discontinue treatment. The treatment schema is shown in Figure 14.13.

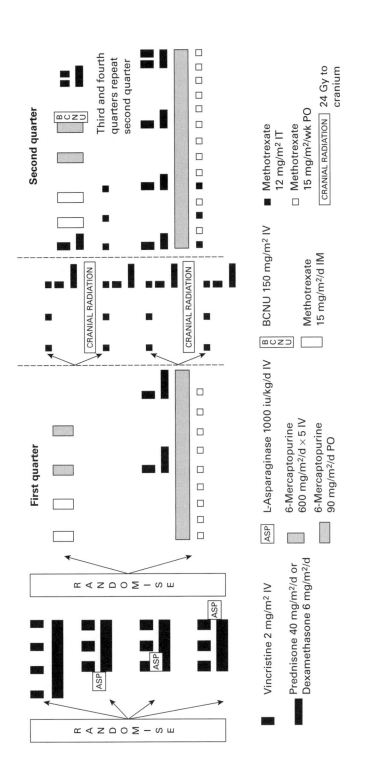

Figure 14.13 Treatment schema. The top arm is arm A (parenteral course) and the lower arm is arm B (daily oral therapy). IV, intravenous; PO, orally; IM, intramuscular; IT, intrathecal

This review focuses on the randomised arms of the CNS prophylaxis regimens alone as well as on the comparative efficacy of dexamethasone against prednisone.

No details of the randomisation method used are given in the study.

Outcome measures were CNS relapse rate and complete remission duration.

Outcome

Of 673 patients enrolled on the trial, 27 were excluded (ineligible 7, protocol violation 8, early loss 2, inadequate records 7 and non-random entry 3). Of the remaining 646, 554 (85·7%) achieved remission.

Sixty-one were excluded from analysis of the CNS prophylaxis therapy (49 relapsed prior to CNS prophylaxis; 12 were disqualified during maintenance due to inadequate data). Thus 493 patients were randomised for CNS therapy: 255 were randomised to IT MTX alone and 238 to CRT plus IT MTX.

Evaluation of CNS relapse revealed the following outcome. With the CNS prophylaxis regimens, CNS relapse occurred in 30 of 238 (12·6%) patients who received CRT plus IT MTX compared to 70 of the 255 (27·5%) patients who received IT MTX alone (p < 0·001). Patients who were treated with CRT plus IT MTX also had a longer duration of complete remission (p = 0·037).

In those given steroids (DEX v PDN), use of DEX also decreased the incidence of CNS relapse – 33 of 231 (14·3%) patients in the DEX arm versus 67 of 262 (27·5%) patients in the PDN arm (p < 0·017). Asparaginase had no effect on the incidence of CNS relapse.

Conclusion

It was concluded that cranial irradiation plus intrathecal methotrexate offered greater protection against CNS relapse of leukaemia compared to intrathecal methotrexate alone. Dexamethasone also offered increased protection against CNS relapse as first site of failure compared to prednisone.

Study 10

Niemeyer CM, Reiter A, Riehm H, Donnelly M, Gelber RD, Sallan SE.

Comparative results of two intensive treatment programs for childhood acute lymphoblastic leukaemia: the Berlin– Frankfurt–Munster (BFM) and Dana-Farber Cancer Institute (DFCI) protocols.

Ann Oncol 1991;**2**:45–9.

This was a comparative study of the ALL-BFM 81 and the DFCI 81–01 treatment protocols for childhood acute lymphoblastic leukaemia (ALL). The BFM 81 trial ran from 1981 to 1983 in 37 centres in West Germany and Austria. The DFCI trial 81–01 was conducted in seven centres within the USA between 1981 and 1985.

Objectives
- The BFM 81 trial compared the efficacy of intermediate dose intravenous methotrexate (IDMTX) against cranial irradiation (CRT) in the prevention of CNS relapse of leukaemia in standard risk patients.
- The studies compared the efficacy of the two CNS prophylaxis regimens.

Details of the study

Only children and adolescents with ALL (excluding B-ALL) below 18 years of age enrolled in both the trials were included in the analysis.

No details of the BFM randomisation method are specified in this report.

Risk criteria used to assign treatment were different in the two protocols. Standard risk (SR) patients in the DFCI group were between 2 and 9 years of age, with WBC < 20 × 10⁹/ℓ, no CNS disease, no mediastinal mass or T cell disease. All others were categorised as high risk (HR). The BFM risk classification was based on the BFM risk factor assessment. To compare outcome, BFM patients were categorised to the same risk groups according to the DFCI criteria. Study populations in the two groups were comparable and there were equal percentages of SR and HR patients in both groups of patients.

The other main differences between the two protocols were:

1 All DFCI patients received CRT for CNS prophylaxis.
2 Standard risk patients in the BFM protocol were randomised between IDMTX and CRT for CNS prophylaxis.
3 The total duration of treatment was 24 months for the DFCI patients whereas BFM children were randomised to either 18 or 24 months of treatment.

Outcome measures were CNS relapse rates in the standard risk BFM patients.

Outcome

A total of 611 patients enrolled in the BFM study and 286 patients (3 excluded as they were over 18 years of age) in the DFCI trial were considered evaluable. In the BFM SR treatment group, 177 were randomised to ID MTX arm and 180 to the CRT arm.

Overall event free survival at 6 years was 69% (± 2%) for BFM and 70% (± 3%) for the DFCI patients. Comparing the IDMTX and CRT arms in the BFM group, isolated CNS relapses in the IDMTX arm ($n = 177$) were higher than in the

CRT arm ($n = 180$): 6·8% ($n = 12$) v 2·2% ($n = 4$). Combined CNS relapses were similarly high in the IDMTX arm compared to the CRT arm: 7·3% ($n = 13$) v 1.7% ($n = 3$).

Comparison of the incidence of CNS relapses between the BFM and DFCI groups showed there was a higher incidence of CNS relapses in the BFM group ($n = 57$, 9·5%) compared to the DFCI ($n = 19$, 6·9%) group (p = 0·004).

No toxicity details are specified in the report.

Conclusion

Intermediate dose methotrexate was not an adequate substitute in preventing CNS relapse of leukaemia compared to cranial irradiation in patients with standard risk ALL.

Study 11

Tubergen DG, Gilchrist GS, O'Brien RT, Coccia PF, Sather HN, Waskerwitz MJ, Denman Hammond G.
Prevention of CNS disease in intermediate risk acute lymphoblastic leukaemia: comparison of cranial irradiation and intrathecal methotrexate and the importance of systemic therapy: a Children's Cancer Group Report.
J Clin Oncol 1993;**11**:520–6.

This was a Children's Cancer Group Study (CCG-105) and was a prospective randomised trial that ran from May 1983 to April 1989. The trial was based on a 2 × 4 factorial design in which the first factor refers to the two types of CNS prophylaxis and the second factor refers to the four systemic regimens.

Objectives

- To compare the efficacy of 18 Gy cranial radiotherapy (CRT) + intrathecal methotrexate (IT MTX) during the first 6 months of treatment versus IT MTX alone throughout the duration of treatment as CNS prophylaxis regimens.
- To compare the efficacy of the standard CCG regimen with the BFM regimen or modified BFM regimens.

In this report we will focus on the comparative merits of the two forms of CNS prophylaxis regimens alone.

Details of the study

Previously untreated children and adolescents with intermediate risk ALL aged between 1 and 21 years were enrolled on the CCG-105 study.

Table 14.5 Eligibility criteria for CCG-105

Age (mth)	WBC count (× $10^9/\ell$)	FAB (% L2 cells)	Percent of study population
12–23	< 50	≤ 10	10
24–119	< 10	> 10[a]	29
24–119	10–49.9	≤ 10	39
120–251	< 50	≤ 10	22

Abbreviation: FAB, French-American-British.

[a] Also eligible were boys in this age and WBC count group who had < 10% FAB L2 cells, but who had platelet counts of < 100 × $10^9/\ell$. Patients were excluded from CCG-105 if they had a lymphomatous presentation.

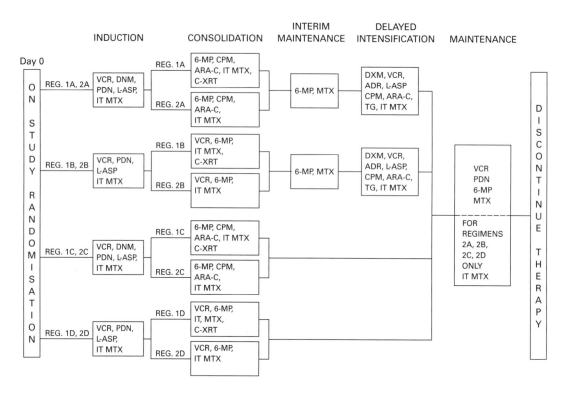

Figure 14.14 Schematic diagrams of the therapy in CCG-105. The 2 x 4 design tests two forms of CNS prophylaxis and four systematic regimens. VCR, vincristine; DNM, daunorubicin; PDN, prednisone; L-ASP, asparaginase; 6-MP, 6-mercaptopurine; CPM, cyclophosphamide; ARA-C, cytosine arabinoside; DXM, dexamethasone; TG, thioguanine

Children with lymphomatous features or with greater than 10% lymphoblasts of FAB L_2 morphology were excluded. (See Table 14.5)

Randomisation to one of four systemic treatment arms and to the two CNS prophylactic regimens was as shown in Figures 14.14 and 14.15. Regimen A was the most intense arm and regimen D the least. CRT 18 Gy in 10 fractions commenced on day 28 (regimens B and D) or Day 35 (regimens A and C). IT MTX was given on days 1, 14, 28, 35, 42 and 49 and every 12 weeks during maintenance for patients randomised to IT MTX. Patients randomised to regimen A or C received additional IT MTX on day 56 of the consolidation block. The duration of maintenance therapy was 3 years for boys and 2 years for girls.

The median follow up was 74 months after completion of induction therapy (range 4 months to 9 years). CNS randomisation was stopped for children between 1 and 9 years in November 1987 as sufficient numbers had been randomised. Analysis was performed on the basis of intention to treat.

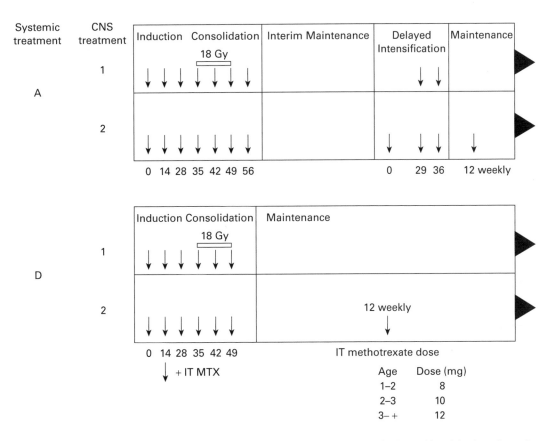

Figure 14.15 Timing and dose of CNS therapy for the most intensive systemic arm (regimen A) and the least intensive systemic arm (regimen D). CNS treatment 1 is cranial radiotherapy; CNS treatment 2 provides IT MTX during all phases of treatment

Outcome measures were relapse free survival (RFS), disease free survival (DFS) and event free survival (EFS).

Outcome

The total number of patients registered on the trial was not specified, however 2·4% were considered ineligible, 1·7% were not randomised for reasons unspecified and 2% were excluded because they had CNS leukaemia at diagnosis and were not randomised for CNS treatment. A total of 1388 patients were randomised to the two CNS regimens: 697 in the CRT arm and 691 in the IT MTX arm.

Seven year survival estimates for all randomised patients were:

CRT arm (*n* = 697): CNS RFS 93%, DFS 69%; EFS 68%.

IT MTX arm (*n* = 691): CNS RFS 91%, DFS 67%, EFS 64%.

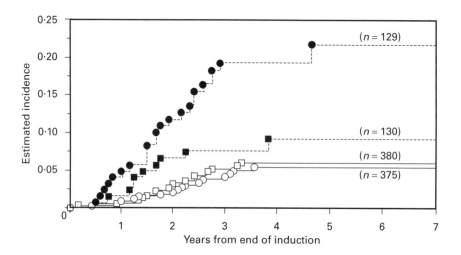

Figure 14.16 Cumulative incidence life-table curves for isolated CNS relapse as an initial event by type of CNS and systemic therapy. ● IT MTX plus standard chemotherapy; ■ cranial radiotherapy plus standard chemotherapy; ○ IT MTX plus intensive chemotherapy; □ cranial radiotherapy plus intensive chemotherapy

Seven year survival by age groups was as follows:

CRT arm (1–9 yr): CNS RFS (n = 515) 94%, DFS (n = 515) 72%, EFS (n = 526) 70%.

IT MTX (1–9 yr): CNS RFS (n = 507) 91%, DFS (n = 507) 71%, EFS (n = 518) 68%.

CRT (10–21 yr): CNS RFS (n = 169) 91%, DFS (n = 169) 61%, EFS (n = 171) 60%.

IT MTX (10–21 yr): CNS RFS (n = 169) 90%, DFS (n = 169) 54%, EFS (n = 173) 53%.

There was no significant difference in outcome for the two CNS regimens when the entire population was considered. In children 10 years or older, however, the CRT treatment group had a better 7 year EFS (60% v 53%; p = 0·04). This difference was due to fewer bone marrow and testicular relapses in the CRT treatment group.

The CNS relapse rate was also directly related to the intensity of the systemic therapy as higher CNS relapse rates were observed in those who received standard systemic therapy in both the CNS regimens, especially so in the IT MTX arm (p < 0·001). (Figure 14.16).

No toxicity was reported.

Conclusion

- IT MTX alone given during the entire duration of therapy affords protection from CNS relapse equivalent to CRT plus IT MTX.
- In children aged over 10 years, CRT reduced the incidence of systemic relapse.
- CNS relapse rate was also dependent on the intensity of systemic therapy.

Study 12

Freeman AI, Boyett JM, Glicksman AS, Brecher ML, Leventhal BG, Sinks LF, Holland JF. Intermediate-dose methotrexate versus cranial irradiation in childhood acute lymphoblastic leukaemia: a ten-year follow-up.
Med Pediat Oncol 1997;**28**:98–107.

This was a prospective randomised multicentre trial (CALGB 7611) which enrolled patients from November 1976 until July 1979.

Objectives

The aim of the study was to evaluate whether intermediate dose methotrexate IV could substitute cranial irradiation (CRT) as CNS prophylaxis therapy.

Details of the study

Previously untreated children and adolescents less than 20 years of age with ALL were enrolled on the study. All patients with hepatic or renal dysfunction, CNS disease at diagnosis or hyper-uricaemia were excluded from entry until these abnormalities normalised. Patients were stratified as standard or high risk according to age and diagnostic white cell count. Standard risk (SR) children were between 2 and 8 years of age and had a diagnostic white cell count of $< 30 \times 10^9/\ell$. All others were categorised as high risk (HR).

A sample size of 300 patients was chosen to provide 95% power ($\alpha = 0.05$) to detect a 15% difference in the relapse rates of the observation and end intensification arms.

Remission induction therapy was identical for all and consisted of IV vincristine 2 mg/m^2/dose/week (VCR) × 4 weeks (max. dose 2 mg) oral prednisone 40 mg/m^2/d × 4 weeks (PDN), IV asparaginase 1000 IU/kg/d × 10 doses (ASP) and intrathecal methotrexate (IT MTX) 12 mg/m^2/dose × 3 doses (max. dose 15 mg). All patients who did not achieve remission within 4 weeks (< 5% blasts) had treatment continued for a further 2 weeks (VCR, PDN and ASP). Patients not in remission at 6 weeks were taken off the trial.

Complete responders were randomised for CNS prophylaxis to either cranial irradiation (CR RT) plus IT MTX or intermediate dose intra-venous methotrexate (IDMTX) plus IT MTX. The dose of IDMTX was 500 mg/m^2/dose at 3-weekly intervals × 3. A third was given as IV bolus and the remaining two-thirds was given as 24-hour intravenous infusion. IT MTX was given concurrently with IDMTX on all three occasions. Folinic acid was given 24 hours after completion of IDMTX (single dose of 12 mg/m^2; max. dose 15 mg).

Cranial irradiation was given as 24 Gy in 12 fractions over a period of 16 days with concurrent administration of 3 doses of IT MTX (12 mg/m^2). All patients also had reinforcement with VCR and PDN at weeks 6, 12, 16, 20 and 24 after commencement of CNS prophylaxis.

Maintenance therapy consisted of oral mercaptopurine (90 mg/m^2/d) plus oral methotrexate (15 mg/m^2/week). Two-weekly doses of vincristine and 2 weeks of oral prednisolone were also given (from week 28) every 12 weeks for the duration of maintenance treatment. At the end of 3 years of maintenance therapy, patients were randomised to stop treatment or receive a late intensification similar to the initial induction plus three doses of IT MTX.

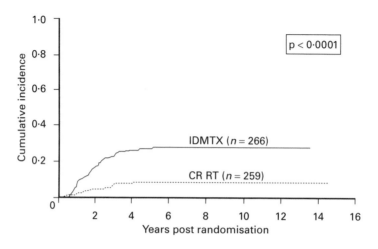

Figure 14.17 Cumulative incidence functions of CNS relapse as a first event for the IDMTX and CR RT arms

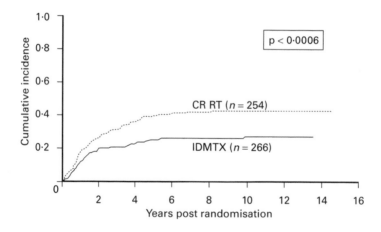

Figure 14.18 Cumulative incidence functions of haematologic relapse as a first event in the IDMTX and CR RT arms

Outcome measures were continuous clinical remission, CNS relapse rates, bone marrow relapse rates and survival. Median follow up of patients at risk for failure was 8 years.

Outcome

Of the 634 patients enrolled on the trial, only 596 were evaluable for response to induction therapy.

Of the 546 patients who achieved remission, only 525 patients were randomised to either CR RT (259) or IDMTX (266). (Eleven patients were never randomised, 6 were lost before CNS prophylaxis, 2 patients refused randomisation and 2 patients had inadequate records.) Patient characteristics in both arms were similar except that twice as many children were under 2 years

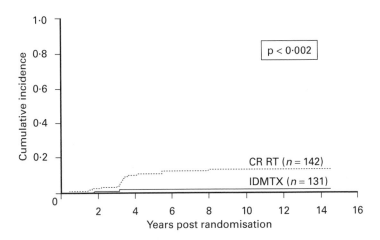

Figure 14.19 Cumulative incidence functions of testicular relapse as a first event in male children with ALL treated with the IDMTX and CR RT arms

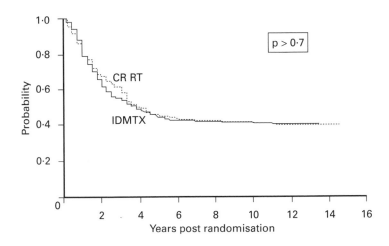

Figure 14.20 Duration of continuous clinical remission in the IDMTX and CR RT arms

old in the IDMTX arm. All analyses were performed on the basis of intention to treat.

Patients in the CR RT arm had a lower incidence of CNS relapse compared to the IDMTX arm (p < 0·0001). The 12 year CNS relapse rate for the IDMTX and CR RT arms were 28% ± 3% and 8% ± 2% respectively (Figure 14.17). There were no differences in CNS relapse rates between the sexes (p > 0·2).

The IDMTX regimen afforded greater protection against marrow relapse compared to CR RT (p < 0·0006). This was most evident in the SR patients. The 12 year incidence rates were 27% ± 3% and 43% ± 3% for the IDMTX and CR RT arms respectively (Figure 14.18).

Boys randomised to IDMTX had a lower incidence of testicular relapse (p = 0·002) (Figure 14.19).

There were no differences in survival after relapse in both treatment arms. The 12 year continuous clinical remission rates for the IDMTX and CR RT arms were 40% ± 5·4% and 40% ± 5·9% respectively (p > 0·7) (Figure 14.20).

Toxicity

No significant toxicity was reported. Two patients developed second malignancy after salvage treatment. Survivors who received CR RT had a lower IQ and also performed poorly on the Wide Range Achievement Test.

Conclusion

It was concluded that IDMTX offered superior protection against testicular relapse and bone marrow relapse but offered less protection against CNS relapses than cranial irradiation.

Study 13

Steinherz PG, Ganyon PS, Breneman JC, Cherlow JM, Grossman NJ, Kersey JH, Johnstone HS, Sather HN, Trigg ME, Uckun FM, Bleyer WA.
Treatment of patients with acute lymphoblastic leukaemia with bulky extramedullary disease and T-cell phenotype or other poor prognostic features. *Cancer* 1998;**82**:600–12.

Trial CCG-123 was a randomised prospective multicentre trial of the Children's Cancer Group that commenced in April 1983 and closed to patient recruitment in April 1989.

Objectives

The primary objective of this randomised trial was to evaluate the effectiveness of three different chemotherapy regimens so as to improve the event free survival in children with high risk acute lymphoblastic leukaemia. The secondary objective was also to evaluate the need for cranial radiotherapy as CNS prophylaxis in the treatment of high risk ALL. This review examines the latter objective alone.

Details of the study

All patients entered into the study were between 1 and 20 years of age and had at least one site of bulky disease (mediastinal mass > 33% of transthoracic diameter, splenomegaly or lymphadenopathy > 3 cm) and either also had T-cell disease and/or WBC > $50 \times 10^9/\ell$ or Hb > 10g/dℓ. All aged less than 1 year of age and those with FAB L3 leukaemia were excluded from the study.

The study was conducted in two periods, each involving randomisation among three regimens: (1) randomisation to regimens A, B or C until

regimen C was dropped from the study (disproportionately high CNS recurrences in patients on regimen C) in October 1985 and a later period of randomisation (December 1985) to regimens A, B and D (regimen B was closed to patient entry before closure of trial in April 1987). Details of randomisation are not specified in the report.

Children with CNS disease at diagnosis were not eligible for Regimen C treatment.

Regimen A: (CCG modified Berlin–Frankfurt–Munster regimen) consisted of five phases of treatment and included: (1) induction; (2) consolidation including 18 Gy cranial irradiation plus intrathecal methotrexate; (3) interim maintenance; (4) re-induction/re-intensification; and (5) the maintenance phase. No irradiation was given to sites of bulky disease.

Regimen B (LSA₂-L₂ with cranial irradiation) consisted of intensive induction with irradiation (15 Gy) to sites of bulky disease and also 18 Gy cranial irradiation plus IT MTX as CNS prophylaxis at the end of induction therapy.

Regimen C (LSA₂-L₂ without cranial irradiation) was similar to regimen B except that no cranial irradiation was given for CNS prophylaxis.

Regimen D (the New York regimen) was a based on a five drug induction therapy combined with 15 Gy irradiation to bulky extra-abdominal sites, and 18 Gy cranial irradiation plus IT MTX was given during the consolidation phase of therapy. IT MTX was given on the first day of each new maintenance cycle during the maintenance phase of treatment (Figures 14.21–14.23).

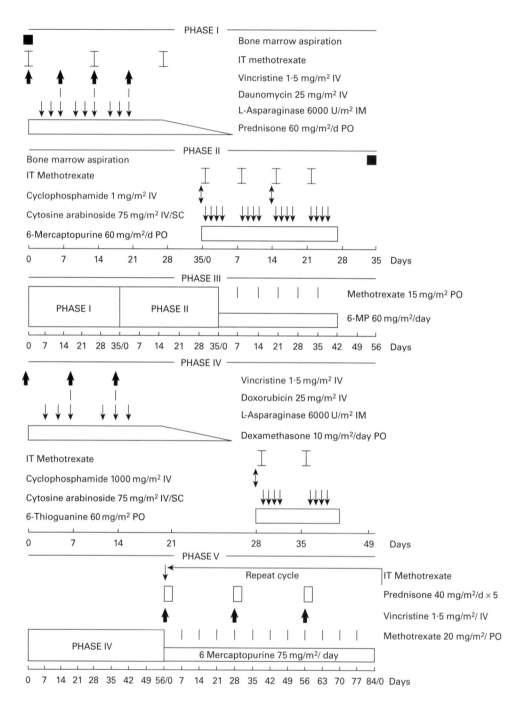

Figure 14.21 Overview of regimen A: CCG modified BFM 76/79. The dose of IT MTX is not given. IV, intravenously; IM, intramuscularly; PO, orally; SC, subcutaneously

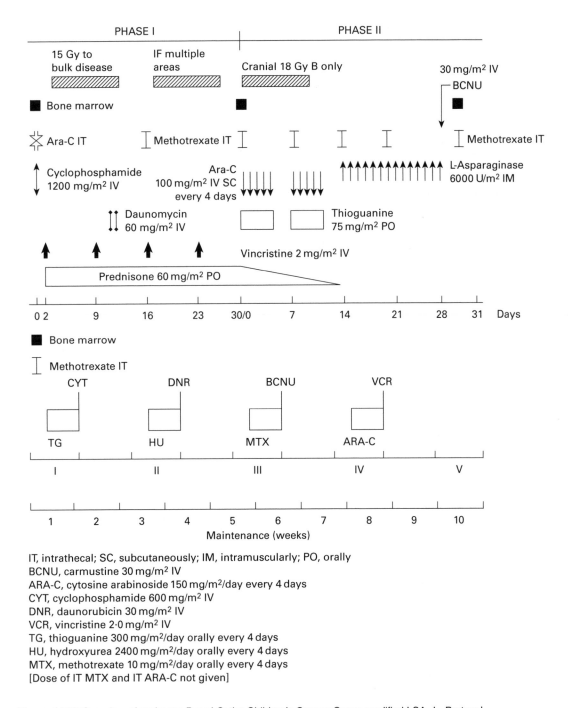

PHASE I | **PHASE II**

15 Gy to bulk disease

IF multiple areas

Cranial 18 Gy B only

30 mg/m² IV
— BCNU

■ Bone marrow

Ara-C IT   Methotrexate IT   Methotrexate IT

Cyclophosphamide 1200 mg/m² IV

Ara-C 100 mg/m² IV SC every 4 days

L-Asparaginase 6000 U/m² IM

Daunomycin 60 mg/m² IV

Thioguanine 75 mg/m² PO

Vincristine 2 mg/m² IV

Prednisone 60 mg/m² PO

0 2   9   16   23   30/0   7   14   21   28   31   Days

■ Bone marrow

Methotrexate IT

CYT   DNR   BCNU   VCR

TG   HU   MTX   ARA-C

I   II   III   IV   V

1   2   3   4   5   6   7   8   9   10

Maintenance (weeks)

IT, intrathecal; SC, subcutaneously; IM, intramuscularly; PO, orally
BCNU, carmustine 30 mg/m² IV
ARA-C, cytosine arabinoside 150 mg/m²/day every 4 days
CYT, cyclophosphamide 600 mg/m² IV
DNR, daunorubicin 30 mg/m² IV
VCR, vincristine 2·0 mg/m² IV
TG, thioguanine 300 mg/m²/day orally every 4 days
HU, hydroxyurea 2400 mg/m²/day orally every 4 days
MTX, methotrexate 10 mg/m²/day orally every 4 days
[Dose of IT MTX and IT ARA-C not given]

Figure 14.22 Overview of regimens B and C: the Children's Cancer Group modified LSA$_2$-L$_2$ Protocol

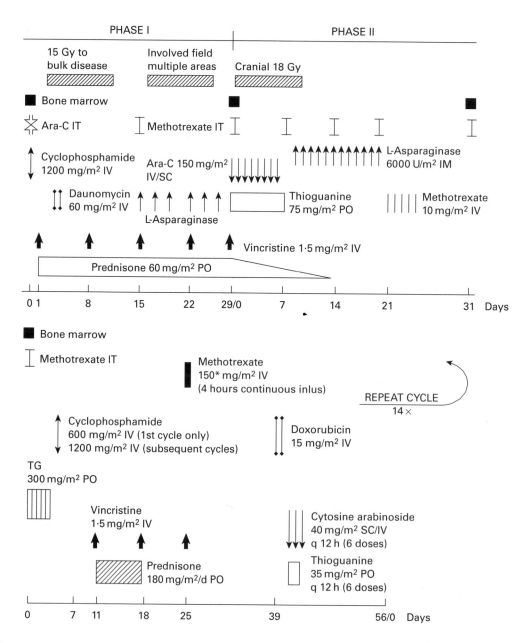

Figure 14.23 Overview of regimen D: the New York protocol. The lower half of the figure depicts the repeating 56 day maintenance cycles. Doxorubicin (Adriamycin) was discontinued after the first 10 maintenance cycles for a maximum total anthracycline dose of 300 mg/m² of doxorubicin and 120 mg/m² of daunomycin. The dose of IT MTX and IT ARA-C is not given

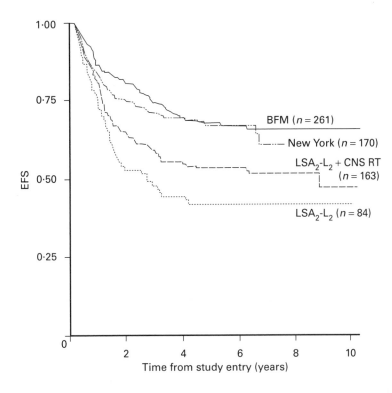

Figure 14.24 Event free survival (EFS) of each treatment regimen. A, Berlin–Frankfurt–Munster; B, LSA$_2$-L$_2$ with cranial RT; C, LSA$_2$-L$_2$ without cranial RT; D, New York. P values: A v B, 0·004; A v C, 0·0001; A v D, 0·97; B v C, 0·34: B v D, 0·01; D v C, 0·001

Outcome measures were event free survival (EFS), overall survival (OS) and relapse free survival (RFS).

All analyses were based on intention to treat. Seven hundred and eight patients were entered into the trial, of whom only 694 were considered eligible for analysis. Of the 694 eligible patients, 678 (16 refused randomisation) were randomised to one of the four chemotherapy regimens. From April 1983 to October 1985, 260 patients were randomised – 88 to regimen A, 89 to regimen B, 83 to regimen C. Final randomisation tally when

the study closed was regimen A 261, B 163, C 84, D 170. The patient characteristics of the four regimen groups were similar. T cell phenotype comprised 65% of the total patients, 20% had WBC count > 200 × 10^9/ℓ and 59% had Hb > 10g/dℓ at diagnosis. There was non-compliance in 5 of 678, who switched to another treatment arm in the study (2 in regimen B2 and 1 each in regimens A, C and D).

Outcome measures were bone marrow relapse rate, event free survival (EFS), CNS relapse free survival (RFS) and overall survival (OS).

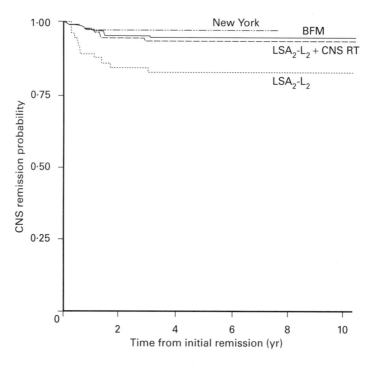

Figure 14.25 Freedom from isolated CNS recurrence on the four therapeutic regimens. CNS control on the three regimens containing 18 Gy cranial irradiation was significantly better than on LSA$_2$-L$_2$ without cranial irradiation. P values: A *v* B, 0·69; A *v* C, 0·0007; A *v* D, 0·3; B *v* C, 0·01; B *v* D, 0·2; and D *v* C, 0·0002

Outcome

EFS at 6 years from diagnosis for the entire cohort was 60% ± 4% and OS was 67 ± 4%. EFS was similar for both the modified BFM (A) and New York regimens (D) (67% ± 6% and 67% ± 7% respectively, and was significantly better than either of the two LSA$_2$-L$_2$ regimens (B 53% ± 8% and C 42% ± 0%).

Comparing regimens B and C only, the difference in EFS was small (p = 0·34, Figure 14.24). The 6 year CNS RFS was 94% for regimen B patients compared to 84% for regimen C patients (p = 0·02, Figure 14.25).

Bone marrow relapse rate for regimen B patients was 32% ± 8% versus 39% ± 12% for regimen C

patients at 6 years from diagnosis. Overall survival for regimen B patients was 59% ± 8% compared to 53% ± 11% for regimen C patients.

Toxicity

Toxicity was similar in all four regimens. No significant difference in toxicity was observed between regimens B and C.

Conclusion

It was concluded that LSA$_2$-L$_2$ chemotherapy with cranial irradiation as CNS prophylaxis resulted in lower CNS relapse rates compared to the same regimen without cranial radiotherapy. However, this did not translate into better overall survival.

Acknowledgements

Figures 14.21–25 are Copyright © 1998 American Cancer Society. Adapted and reprinted from Steinherz PG *et al* (full reference on p 347) by permission of Wiley-Liss, Inc., a subsidiary of John Wiley & Sons, Inc.

Study 14

Nachman J, Sather HN, Cherlow JM, Sensel MG, Gaynon PS, Lukens JN, Wolff L, Trigg ME.
Response of children with high risk acute lymphoblastic leukaemia treated with and without cranial irradiation: A report of the Children's Cancer Study Group.
J Clin Oncol 1998;**16**:920–30.

This Children's Cancer Group Study (CCG-1882) was a prospective randomised multicentre study which ran from May 1989 to June 1995.

Objectives

The study aimed to determine whether cranial irradiation could be omitted for presymptomatic CNS therapy in a select subgroup of children with high risk acute lymphoblastic leukaemia without compromising survival.

Details of the study

Eligible patients were:

1 Aged 1–9 years and WBC $\geq 50 \times 10^9/\ell$ or aged ≥ 10 years.
2 Patients who achieved rapid early response (RER), i.e. < 25% blasts in bone marrow on day 7 and bone marrow remission by day 28.

Patients with lymphomatous features or CNS disease at diagnosis were excluded.

Results were monitored at 6 monthly intervals after patients reached 18 months of follow up and continued for a maximum of 10 analyses. At the fifth interim analysis in July 1993, as the outcome difference favoured regimen A, randomisation was discontinued and the study committee recommended that all patients (except those less than 10 years of age and with a WBC count $< 100 \times 10^9/\ell$) who were

6 months or less on the study be recalled for cranial irradiation as for regimen A.

Details of the methodology of randomisation are not specified.

Randomisation for presymptomatic CNS therapy was at the end of induction therapy.

Treatment consisted of five phases (Figure 14.26): induction (5 weeks), consolidation (5 weeks), interim maintenance (8 weeks), delayed intensification (7 weeks) and maintenance (multiple 12 week courses). Maintenance therapy cycles continued for 2 and 3 calendar years for girls and boys respectively.

Induction therapy consisted of vincristine (VCR) 1·5 mg/m^2 IV, prednisone (PRED) 60 mg/m^2 orally, daunomycin (DNM) 25 mg/m^2 IV and L-asparaginase (ASP) 6000 U/m^2 IM. Intrathecal cytosine arabinoside (IT ARA-C) was administered on day 0 and IT methotrexate (MTX) on days 14 and 28.

Consolidation consisted of cyclophosphamide 1000 mg/m^2 (CPM), 6-mercaptopurine 60 mg/m^2 (6-MP) and ARA-C 75 mg/m^2 IV/SC. All patients also had weekly doses of IT MTX $\times 4$ while regimen A patients also received 18 Gy CRT in 10 fractions.

Presymptomatic CNS therapy consisted of IT MTX given during induction and consolidation, delayed intensification and maintenance with 18 Gy CRT during consolidation (Regimen A), or regimen A IT MTX (without CRT) plus additional doses of IT MTX given during interim maintenance, delayed intensification and the first four cycles of maintenance therapy (Regimen B) (Table 14.6).

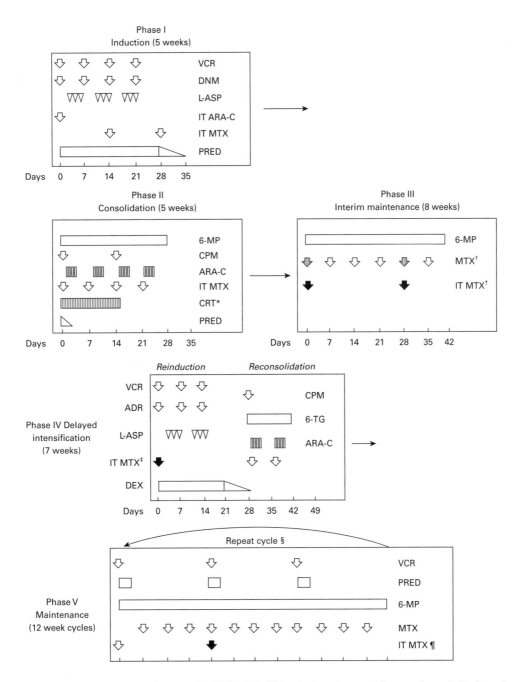

Figure 14.26 Schematic diagram of therapy for CCG 1882. White, both regimens; stripes, regimen A; black, regimen B. *Regimen A only. ‡Regimen B, IT MTX on days 0 and 28. †Regimen B, IT MTX on day 0. §Cycles continued for 2 years (girls) or 3 years (boys). ¶Regimen B, IT MTX on days 0 and 28, courses 1–4

Table 14.6 Presymptomatic treatment for prevention of CNS disease according to regimen

Phase	Regimen A (CRT+)	Regimen B (CRT-)
Induction	IT ARA-C × 1	IT ARA-C × 1
	IT MTX × 2	IT MTX × 2
Consolidation	IT MTX × 4	IT MTX × 4
	CRT 1·8 Gy × 10	
Interim maintenance	None	IT MTX × 2
Delayed intensification		
Re-induction	None	IT MTX × 1
Re-consolidation	IT MTX × 2	IT MTX × 2
Maintenance		
Courses 1–4	IT MTX × 1	IT MTX × 2
Courses 5–end	IT MTX × 1	IT MTX × 1

Interim maintenance therapy consisted of oral 6-MP 60 mg/m^2 (daily) and MTX 15 mg/m^2 (weekly) for regimen A patients, while regimen B patients also had two additional doses of IT MTX.

Delayed intensification therapy consisted of dexamethasone 10 mg/m^2 orally (DEX), VCR 1·5 mg/m^2 IV, doxorubicin 25 mg/m^2 IV (ADR), LASP 6000 U/m^2 IM, CPM 1000 mg/m^2 IV, 6-thioguanine 60 mg/m^2 (6-TG) and ARA-C 75 mg/m^2 IV/SC. Regimen A patients received two doses of IT MTX while regimen B patients had 3 doses of IT MTX (three doses).

Maintenance therapy was with monthly pulses of VCR and PRED with weekly oral MTX and daily 6-MP with IT MTX given on the first day of each 12-weekly cycle (Regimen A).

Patients on regimen B received the same regimen of oral MTX except that IT MTX was substituted for oral MTX on day 28 of courses 1 to 4. Regimen B patients also received IT MTX on day 0 of each cycle.

Intrathecal chemotherapy doses were age adjusted: ARA-C 30 mg, 50 mg, 70 mg, and MTX 8 mg, 10 mg, 12 mg for ages 1, 2 and 3 years or greater respectively.

Outcome measures were CNS relapse rate, and event free survival (EFS).

Outcome

The number of patients entered on the trial was 1021. There were 702 RER patients (day 7 marrow), of whom 5 patients died before day 28 and 1 had M3 marrow on day 28 while 29 had CNS disease at diagnosis and were non-randomly assigned to CRT. This left 667 RER patients eligible for randomisation. Thirty-one

Table 14.7 Trends in occurrence of events during late follow up

Analysis period	No. of events		RHRa	
	Regimen A (CRT+)	Regimen B (CRT−)	≤ 2 yr Follow up	> 2 yr Follow up
January 1994	33	54	1·97	0·86
September 1994	47	57	1·54	0·53
January 1995	62	62	1·41	0·47
September 1995	68	66	1·44	0·41
January 1996[b]	76	72	1·38	0·50

[a] Relative hazard rate (RHR) for regimen B versus regimen A for patients in follow up ≤ 2 years or > 2 years.

[b] Kaplan–Meier estimates at 5 years of follow up were 69·1% and 75·0% for regimens A and B, respectively (P = 0·50, using a two-sided test).

patients were not randomised (no reasons are given), leaving a total number randomised of 636. Three hundred and seventeen were randomised to regimen A and 319 to regimen B.

At the time of the fifth interim analysis in July 1993, the numbers of events were as follows: regimen A 28, regimen B 48, relative hazard rate (RHR) = 1·85 for B compared with A, p = 0·004. Three year EFS was 82·1% ± 4·0% for regimen A and 70·4% ± 4·2% for regimen B.

At the time of the tenth analysis in January 1996, the numbers of events were as follows: regimen A 76, regimen B 72; RHR = 0·5 for B compared with A (where follow up was > 2 years) (Table 14.7).

Five year EFS was 69·1% ± 3·4% and 75·0% ± 2·7% for regimens A and B respectively (p = 0·5) (Figure 14.27).

The most frequent event in either group was bone marrow relapse – 57 (54 isolated) in regimen A and 43 (41 isolated) in regimen B. CNS relapses were more frequent in regimen B, 11 (isolated 10) compared to 8 in regimen A (isolated 5). The temporal sequence of the events differed in both groups of patients. During the first 2 years of follow up the number of bone marrow relapses for patients on both regimens A and B were similar (31 v 33) but between 2 and 6 years of follow up regimen A patients had more bone marrow relapses (26 v 10). Eight of the 10 CNS relapses in regimen B patients occurred within the first 2 years of follow up.

Analysis on intent to treat showed that by 5 years of follow up probability of isolated CNS relapse was 2·3% ± 1·1% and 3·6% ± 1·1% (p = 0·72) for regimens A and B respectively (Figure 14.28).

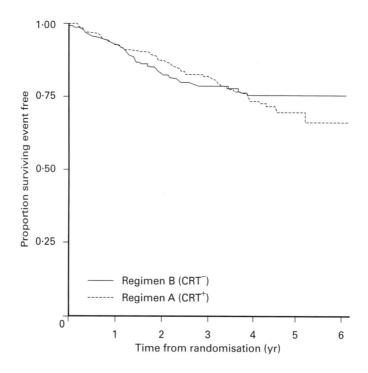

Figure 14.27 Event free survival of children with high risk ALL treated with regimens A and B for presymptomatic treatment of the CNS

By intention to treat analysis, survival after isolated CNS relapse was better in patients on regimen B (p = 0·009). All 10 patients who had an isolated CNS relapse on regimen B were alive compared to only 2 out of 5 patients on regimen A.

Toxicity

There were 18 seizures during post induction therapy – 7 in regimen A and II in regimen B. Two patients treated on each regimen developed leukoencephalopathy. There were 23 deaths in remission – 9 in regimen A and 14 in regimen B.

Conclusion

It was concluded that (1) Presymptomatic CNS therapy with intensified IT MTX is a satisfactory form of CNS prophylaxis in children with high risk acute lymphoblastic leukaemia if they have a rapid early response to induction chemotherapy. (2) Intensified IT MTX afforded protection against late bone marrow relapse.

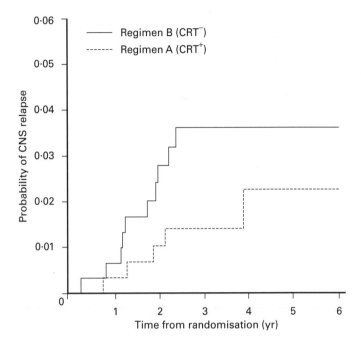

Figure 14.28 Probability of isolated CNS relapse in children with high risk ALL treated with regimens A and B for presymptomatic treatment of the CNS

Study 15

Vilmer E, Suciu S, Ferster A, Bertrand Y, Cave H, Thyss A, Benoit Y, Dastugue N, Fournier M, Souillet G, Manel AM, Robert A, Nelken B, Millot F, Lutz P, Rialland X, Mechinaud F, Boutard P, Behar C, Chantraine JM, Plouvier E, Laureys G, Brock P, Uyttebroeck A, Margueritte G, Plantaz D, Norton L, Francotte N, Gyselinck J, Waterkeyn C, Solbu G, Philippe N, Otten J.

Long term results of three randomised trials (58831, 58832, 58881) in childhood acute lymphoblastic leukaemia: a CLCG–EORTC report. *Leukaemia* 2000; **14**:2257–66.

Trial 58832 was a prospective randomised trial carried out from 1983 to 1989.

Objectives

The aim of the trial was to determine whether omission of cranial irradiation in children with medium or high risk acute lymphoblastic leukaemia treated with high dose intravenous methotrexate plus intrathecal methotrexate adversely influenced CNS relapse rate or treatment outcome.

Details of the study

Only medium and high risk patients below 18 years of age were eligible to be registered on this study. Patients with CNS disease at diagnosis were not eligible for the trial. Risk factor (RF) calculation was according to the BFM (Berlin–Frankfurt–Munster) criteria based on three initial factors: circulating peripheral blasts, size of liver and spleen. $RF = 0.2 \times \log_{10}(\text{blasts/mm}^3 + 1), + 0.06 \times \text{cm hepatomegaly} + 0.04 \times \text{splenomegaly}$. Standard risk patients had a RF score < 1·2, in medium risk patients it was between 1·2 and 1·69, and high risk patients had a score ≥ 1·7.

No details of randomisation method are given in the study.

Treatment commenced with a pre-phase of 7 days of prednisone/prednisolone and one dose of intrathecal methotrexate (IT MTX), followed by induction therapy that consisted of vincristine (VCR) 1·5 mg/m²/week × 4, daunorubicin 30 mg/m²/week × 4 weeks, daily prednisolone 60 mg/m²/d × 4 weeks and daily IV L-asparaginase (ASP) 5000 U/m²/d × 21 days. Four weeks of consolidation followed and included 6-mercaptopurine (6-MP) 60 mg/m²/d × 28 days, cytosine arabinoside (ARA-C) 75 mg/m²/d for 4 days of each week and cyclophosphamide (CPM) 1 g/m² on days 1 and 29. All patients also received five doses of IT MTX during the first 8 weeks of induction/consolidation treatment. Interim maintenance consisted of an 8 week course of oral (PO) 6-MP 25 mg/m²/d, high dose IV MTX 2·5 g/m²/dose × 4 plus IT MTX × 4. Re-induction therapy consisted of dexamethasone 10 mg/m²/d × 21 days, VCR 1·5 mg/m²/week and doxorubicin 30 mg/m²/week × 4, ASP 10 000 U/m² ×4 doses, two cycles of ARA-C 75 mg/m²/dose, CPM 1 gm/m², 2 weeks of daily PO thioguanine (6-TG) 60 mg/m²/d and IT MTX × 1. After completion of re-induction all patients were randomised to receive 24 Gy prophylactic cranial irradiation or not. Children between the ages of 1 and 2 years received 20 Gy. Maintenance therapy consisted of daily PO 6-MP 50 mg/m² and weekly PO MTX 20 mg/m². The total duration of treatment for all patients was 2 years.

Outcome

All analyses were performed on the basis of intention to treat. Only patients who remained failure free were censored on the date of last contact.

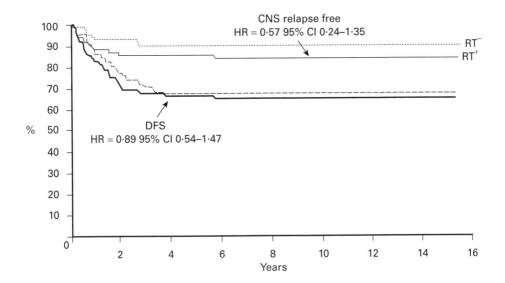

Figure 14.29 Comparison of disease free survival and CNS relapse free interval in medium and high risk patients randomly assigned to receive or not receive cranial radiotherapy (RT). Adapted and reprinted from Vilmer E *et al*, *Leukaemia* with permission from Nature Publishing Group (full reference p 360).

A total of 267 meduim and high risk patients were registered on the study. Details regarding the number of patients who achieved remission by the end of induction–consolidation, number of patients who had CNS disease at diagnosis, number of induction failures or of toxic deaths etc. are not available. Of the 183 patients who underwent randomisation for cranial irradiation, 90 patients were treated with high dose (HD) MTX and prophylactic cranial irradiation while 93 received HDMTX alone.

Outcome measures were CNS relapse rate and disease free survival DFS.

The CNS relapse rates in patients randomised to cranial irradiation plus HDMTX were 15% ± 4% compared to 9% ± 3·2% in patients without

cranial irradiation. The hazard ratio (no radio-therapy *v* radiotherapy) was 0·57, 95% CI 0·24–1·35. The isolated CNS relapse rates for patients treated with HDMTX alone was 7% ± 2·8% compared to 7% ± 2·9% for those who had cranial irradiation plus HDMTX.

Six year DFS was 66% ± 5% and 68% ± 4·8% for patients with and without cranial irradiation respectively (Figure 14.29).

Conclusion
It was concluded that the omission of cranial irradiation in medium or high risk children did not increase the risk of CNS relapse and had no significant impact on DFS.

Study 16

Koizumi S, Fujimoto T.

Improvement in treatment of childhood acute lymphoblastic leukaemia: a 10-year study by the Children's Cancer and Leukaemia Study Group. *Int J Hematol* 1994;**59**:99–112.

Protocol 874 of the Children's Cancer and Leukaemia Study Group was a prospective randomised trial carried out between 1987 and 1990.

Objectives

The aim of this trial was to determine whether the omission of presymptomatic cranial irradiation in children with either low risk or intermediate risk acute lymphodlastic leukaemia, adversely influenced CNS relapse rate or treatment outcome.

Previously untreated children with ALL were registered in the trial. Children with low or intermediate risk ALL were randomised to either cranial irradiation (CRT) with intrathecal chemotherapy (IT CT) or high dose IV methotrexate (HD MTX) plus IT CT. All eligible patients were randomised by a block random method that balanced assignment within and across institutions. All children with high risk ALL received cranial irradiation. Risk factor calculation was based on age and WBC count at diagnosis (Table 14.8).

Remission induction therapy consisted of IV vincristine (VCR) 2·0 mg/m^2/week, oral prednisone (PDN) 60 mg/m^2/d and L-asparaginase 2000 Us/m^2/dose IV. The duration of the remission induction phase is not unavailable from the report.

For CNS prophylaxis patients who attained complete remission were randomly assigned to 18 Gy CRT plus IT CT (regimen A) or HDMTX (2–4·5 g/m^2) plus IT CT (regimen B). IT CT comprised of methotrexate 12 mg/m^2 and hydrocortisone 50 mg/m^2. The total number of doses of IT CT is not specified in both risk groups of patients.

Maintenance chemotherapy consisted of intermittent cyclic administration of IV intermediate dose methotrexate 225 mg/m^2 and alternating biweekly oral 6-mercaptopurine (6-MP) 175 mg/m^2 ×5 days. All patients also received VCR/PDN pulses including late intensification with high-dose MTX. Patients with intermediate risk ALL also received Doxorubicin, VCR and L-asparaginase during maintenance.

Outcome

Of the 370 eligible patients enrolled in the trial, 80 were considered to have low risk ALL and 109, intermediate risk. Ninety-seven patients (42 low risk and 55 intermediate risk) were randomised to receive CRT plus IT CT while the remaining 92 patients (38 low risk and 54 intermediate risk) received HDMTX plus IT CT.

Outcome measures were CNS relapse rate and event free survival (EFS).

The CNS relapse rates were lower in patients randomised to CRT (3/97, 3%) compared to patients who did not receive CRT (9/92, 9·7%).

Five year EFS rate was 75·6% ± 5·7% and 70·5% ± 6·1% for low and intermediate risk patients who received CRT compared to 69·2% ± 5·5% and 67·5% ± 5·9% for the same risk groups of patients respectively who did not receive CRT. This was not statistically significant.

Table 14.8 Stage of acute lymphoblastic leukaemia according to age and WBC count at diagnosis

WBC count (×10⁹/l)	Age (yr)				
	<1	1–< 4	4–< 6	6–< 10	≥ 10
≤ 50	IV (II)	I	I	II	III
50–≤ 10	IV (II)	I	II	III	III
10–≤ 50	IV (III)	II	II	III	III
> 50	IV (III)	III	III	III	III

I, low risk group; II, intermediate risk group; III, high risk group; IV, infant group; I + II standard risk group. Parentheses indicate the staging system for the 811 protocol.

Conclusion

It was concluded that the omission of cranial irradiation in low or intermediate risk children with ALL had no significant impact on EFS despite a slightly higher rate of CNS relapse.

Study 17

Schrappe M, Reiter A, Henze G, Niemeyer Ch, Bode U, Kühl J, Gadner H, Havers W, Plüss H, Kornhuber B, Zintl F, Ritter J, Urban Ch, Niethammer D, Riehm H, for the ALL- BFM study group.

Prevention of CNS recurrence in childhood ALL: results with reduced radiotherapy combined with CNS-directed chemotherapy in four consecutive ALL-BFM trials.

Klin Padiatr 1998;**210**:192–9.

ALL-BFM trials 81, 83, 86 and 90 were prospective randomised multicentre trials that were conducted between 1981 and 1995 in Austria, Switzerland and Germany. Data was collected and updated on a regular basis in Hannover and Vienna.

Objectives

The study aims were:

- To determine whether cranial irradiation could be omitted for pre-symptomatic CNS therapy in standard risk children with acute lymphoblastic leukaemia (ALL) without adversely affecting the CNS relapse rate (ALL-BFM 81 study).
- To evaluate the efficacy of a reduction in the dose of cranial irradiation and its impact on the treatment outcome in children with high standard risk ALL (ALL-BFM 83 study).

This review focuses on the BFM 81 and 83 trials alone.

Details of the study

Children and adolescents up to the age of 18 were enrolled in the four ALL-BFM trials. Patients were stratified into risk groups according to the BFM risk factor (BFM-RF), which was based on the diagnostic peripheral blood blast count and hepato-splenic enlargement. Those patients with Philadelphia chromosome positive ALL were categorised as high risk. In study ALL BFM 81, patients were categorised into three risk groups according to the BFM risk factor (RF): standard risk (RF < 1·2), medium risk (RF 1·2–< 1·7) and high risk (RF ≥ 1·7). In BFM ALL 83 study, standard risk group patients were further subdivided into low standard risk (RF < 0·8) and high standard risk (RF 0·8–< 1·2). Medium and high risk groups were as defined in the earlier BFM ALL 81 study.

Chemotherapy details regarding induction, consolidation, intensification and maintenance blocks have not been specified in this report.

CNS prophylaxis treatment for ALL-BFM 81 was as follows. Standard risk patients (BFM-RF score 0·8–1·2) were randomised to 18 Gy cranial irradiation plus oral methotrexate (0·02 g/m^2 ×8) and intrathecal methotrexate (IT MTX) × 6 (SR-A), or to ID MTX (0·5 g/m^2 × 4) and IT MTX × 6 alone (SR-B).

In ALL-BFM 83, in patients with high standard risk ALL (BFM-RF 0·8 < 1·2) were randomised to 18 Gy cranial irradiation plus ID MTX (0·5 g/m^2) × 4 and IT MTX × 8 or 12 Gy cranial irradiation plus ID MTX (0·5 g/m^2) × 4 and IT MTX × 8.

The outcome measure was CNS relapse rate.

In the ALL-BFM 81 trial (BFM–RF 0·8–< 1·2) 142 patients were randomised to cranial irradiation plus oral MTX and IT MTX while 137 received ID MTX and IT MTX alone.

In the ALL-BFM 83 trial, of the 143 high standard risk patients (BFM-RF 0·8–<1·2), 72 patients

Table 14.9 Relapse according to the BFM (81 and 83) CNS prophylaxis regimens

	BFM 81		BFM 83	
	SR-A (pts with RF 0·8–<1·2 only)	SR-B (pts with RF 0·8–<1·2 only)	SR-H/1 RF 0·8–<1.2	SR-H/2 RF 0·8–<1·2
Treatment				
CRT (GY)	18	–	12	18
MTX (g/m²)	8 × 0·02 PO	4 × 0·5 IV	4 × 0·5 IV	4 × 0·5 IV
IT MTX (no. of inj.)	6	6	8	8
Patients randomised	80	74	72	71
Patients (%)				
All relapses	28·8	37·8	34·7	28·2
Isolated CNS	1·3	10·8	2·8	2·8
Combined CNS/BM	1·3	10·8	2·8	1·4

Table 14.10 Trial ALL–BFM 81: randomised comparison fo preventive cranial irradiation versus intermediate dose methotrexate in standard risk ALL patients (BFM-RF <1·2)

	SR-A	SR-B
Treatment		
CRT (Gy)	18 y	–
MTX (g/m²)	8 × 0·02 (PO)	4 × 0·5 (IV)
IT MTX (no. of inj.)	6	6
Patients randomised	142	137
Relapses (%)		
All relapses	21·8	30·6
Isolated CNS	0·7	6·6
Combined CNS/BM	1·4	7·3

Standard risk (SR) = BFM-RF 0·8–1·2.
CRT, cranial radiotherapy; BM, bone marrow; PO, orally; IV, intravenous.

were randomised to 12 Gy cranial irradiation (SR-H/1) and 71 patients to 18 Gy cranial irradiation (SR-H/2).

Outcome

BFM-81 trial

The incidence of CNS relapses was higher in SR-B group patients (Tables 14.9 and 14.10). Again, though the incidence of CNS relapse was small in low standard risk ALL patients (BFM-RF < 0·8) treated with ID MTX without cranial irradiation (SR-B 1·6% isolated and 3·2% combined CNS relapses), nevertheless, the incidence of all relapses was lower in the irradiated group (SR-A) of low standard risk ALL patients compared to the unirradiated group (all relapses 12·9% v 22·2% in SR-B).

BFM-83 trial

Both cranial irradiation regimens were equally effective in the prevention of CNS relapses. There was a slightly increased rate of systemic relapses in the group who received 12 Gy cranial irradiation but the difference was not statistically significant (Table 14.10).

Comparing the results of the patients in the BFM 83 study (SR-H/1 and SR-H/2) with the matching subset of patients in the BFM 81 study (SR-A), the addition of ID MTX and two additional doses of IT MTX did not improve overall outcome or reduce the incidence of CNS relapse.

Conclusion

BFM-ALL 81 trial

It was concluded that intermediate dose intravenous methotrexate plus intrathecal methotrexate without cranial irradiation in high standard risk (BFM-RF 0·8–1·2) ALL patients was unsafe as it resulted in a significantly increased rate of CNS relapse. However, in low standard risk patients (BFM-RF < 0·8), cranial irradiation could be omitted without any increased incidence of CNS relapse.

BFM-ALL 83 trial

The dose of CNS irradiation can be reduced to 12 Gy in high standard risk ALL patients (BFM-RF 0·8–<1·2) without an increased frequency of CNS relapses when combined with intermediate dose methotrexate and intrathecal methotrexate.

15

Duration of continuing (maintenance) therapy in acute lymphoblastic leukaemia

Studies

Study 1

The Medical Research Council's Working Party on Leukaemia in Childhood.
Duration of chemotherapy in childhood acute lymphoblastic leukaemia.
Med Paed Oncol 1982;**10**:511–20.

This report analyses the results of the first three multicentre UKALL (I, II and III) randomised trials and describes the differences in remission duration and survival in the three trials. Details regarding the exact period when each trial was conducted are not mentioned.

Objectives

The primary objective of this analysis was to determine the minimal effective length of maintenance therapy for children with acute lymphoblastic leukaemia.

Details of the study

Criteria for enrolment onto the three UKALL trials were not specified. In UKALL-III patients were categorised into standard risk (age 1–13 years, WBC $< 20 \times 10^9/\ell$) or high risk (> 14 years or WBC $> 20 \times 10^9/\ell$) according to age and WBC count at diagnosis.

Chemotherapy protocol details for any of the three trials are not given in the report (detailed reports *Br Med J* 1977;**2**:495 and *Br Med J* 1978;**2**:787). The only substantial difference between these trials during the first 12 weeks of therapy was in the dosage and timing of asparaginase, which was given for 4 weeks daily from weeks 7 until 11 at 6000 U/m^2 IV in UKALL-I, and at 10 000 U/m^2 for four doses over 8 days during weeks 1, 4 or 5 in the subsequent trials. However, in all three of the trials, patients who completed the shorter period of treatment (84 weeks in UKALL-I, 108 weeks in UKALL-II and III) and were still in first remission were then randomised either to stop or continue treatment up to a total of 156 weeks.

Analyses of allocated duration of therapy were restricted to patients who were in first remission

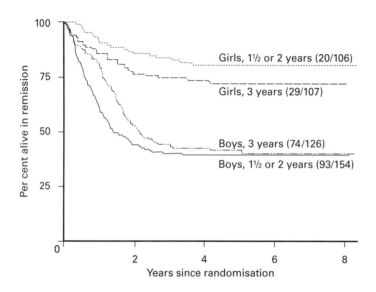

Figure 15.1 Disease free survival according to sex and allocation to stop or continue treatment, from the time of randomisation to stop or continue

and on chemotherapy at 80 weeks (UKALL-I) or 104 weeks (UKALL-II and III). These cut off points (4 weeks before the randomisation) were chosen because randomisations were performed in advance and a few patients stopped treatment early.

Outcome measures were disease free survival (DFS), testicular relapse rate and non-testicular relapse rate.

Methodology of randomisation is not detailed in the report for any of the three trials.

Outcome

The numbers of patients enrolled in each of the three trials is not specified nor are details of actual numbers of patients in each trial who were randomised to stop or continue treatment specified.

For boys, the relapse rate increased with stopping treatment (p < 0·001) whereas in girls it was non-significantly lower when treatment was discontinued. The 5 year DFS after randomisation to stop or continue treatment was 76% for girls compared with 40% in boys (Figure 15.1). This difference appeared only after stopping treatment. The DFS rate 2 years after the start of treatment for patients in remission at 12 weeks was 64% for boys versus 70% for girls (UKALL-I patients censored at 84 weeks).

Testicular relapse was initially significantly higher in those allocated to stop treatment (p < 0·001) but a similar incidence occurred among those who stopped treatment after 3 years (Figure 15.2). Eventual cumulative incidence was slightly higher in the longer treatment group.

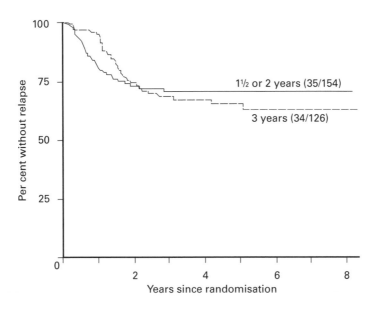

Figure 15.2 Testicular relapse as a first event, according to allocation to stop or continue treatment

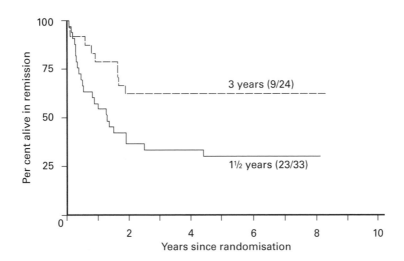

Figure 15.3 Disease free survival for UKALL-I males, ignoring testicular recurrence, according to allocation to stop or continue maintenance

Non-testicular relapse was higher in boys in UKALL-I who were randomised to stop treatment at 84 weeks compared to those who continued treatment (p = 0·02) (Figure 15.3). DFS 5 years after randomisation was 31% and 63% respectively. No significant differences in non-testicular

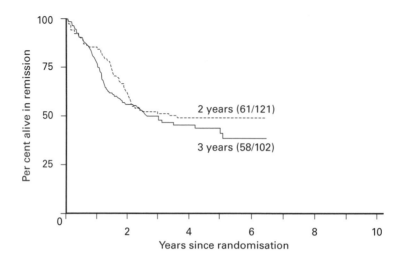

Figure 15.4 Disease free survival for males in UKALL-II and UKALL-III combined, ignoring testicular recurrence, according to allocation to stop or continue maintenance

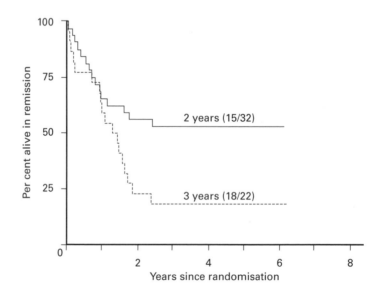

Figure 15.5 Disease free survival according to allocated treatment duration (including testicular relapse) among poor prognosis males, UK ALL-II and UK ALL-III intensive

Table 15.1 Site of first relapse following treatment allocation to stop at 1½ or 2 years (S) or continue to 3 years (C)[a]

Trial	Sex	S/C	Site of first relapse			Death in remission	No. of patients randomised to S/C
			Marrow	CNS not marrow	Isolated testicular		
No CNS prophylaxis (UKALL I only)	M	S	7	4 (4)	0	0	13
	M	C	3	4 (0)	0	0	12
	F	S	2	0 (0)	–	0	8
	F	C	1	6 (1)	–	0	14
CNS prophylaxis (UKALL I, II, and III)	M	S	46	4 (2)	31 (18)	0	141
	M	C	35	7 (4)	22 (11)	2	113
	F	S	17	1 (0)	– –	0	97
	F	C	19	1 (1)	– –	3	95

[a] First relapses in bone marrow are listed as such, irrespective of involvement of other sites, and coincident CNS and testicular relapses are listed as CNS. The numbers of patients who suffered CNS or testicular relapse without marrow involvement but suffered a later marrow relapse are shown in parentheses.

recurrences in relation to duration of treatment were observed in either the UKALL-II or III trial (Figure 15.4).

The relapse rate for boys in UKALL-II and UKALL-III intensive was lower in those randomised to the shorter maintenance arm (Figure 15.5; $p = 0.02$) and additionally relapse rate beyond 2 years after diagnosis was unrelated to the prognostic category in both sexes (O/E, standard risk; high risk was 120/125·9: 40/34·1 for boys and 43/43·7: 9/8·3 for girls; combined $p = 0.26$).

Relapses and deaths that occurred after randomisation to stop or continue treatment are shown in Table 15.1.

Among girls, there was no significant difference in relation to duration of treatment within any trial or in any comparison of overall results between trials.

Conclusion

It was concluded that 18 months or 2 years of maintenance treatment was as effective as 3 years of treatment for girls, but for boys 18 months was inferior to 3 years of treatment, although there was no significant difference between 2 or 3 years of treatment.

Comment

See also Chapter 16, Study 2 (Henze *et al*) which demonstrates the equivalence of 2 years versus 2·5 years of therapy.

Study 2

Nesbitt ME, Jr, Sather HN, Robison LL, Ortega JA, Denman Hammond G and the Children's Cancer Study Group.
Randomised study of 3 years versus 5 years of chemotherapy in childhood acute lymphoblastic leukaemia.
J Clin Oncol 1983;**1**:308–16.

CCG-101 and CCG-143 were prospective randomised multicentre trials that were conducted between June 1972 and February 1975.

Objectives

The objectives of the trial were to determine the optimum duration of maintenance chemotherapy in children with acute lymphoblastic leukaemia (3 *v* 5 years of therapy).

Details of the study

Previously untreated patients with ALL < 18 years who were in continuous complete remission (CCR) for 3 years after start of maintenance therapy were eligible for randomisation to stop or continue treatment.

Induction chemotherapy consisted of vincristine (VCR), prednisone (PDN) and L-asparaginase (ASP). All who achieved remission were randomised to one of six CNS prophylaxis regimens and were maintained on 6-mercaptopurine (6-MP), methotrexate (MTX), VCR and PDN. Those remaining in CCR for 3 years were eligible for randomisation either to stop or continue treatment for a further 2 years. Examination of bone marrow and CSF were mandatory prior to randomisation. Testicular biopsies were not required prior to randomisation.

Outcome measures were bone marrow relapse rate, testicular relapse rate, overall survival and relapse free survival (RFS).

Outcome

Analysis was on intention to treat (except in the 7 non-compliant patients). A total of 486 were eligible for randomisation (after 3 years of CCR), of whom 170 were excluded (non-randomly continued or stopped), 316 (65%) were randomised with the result that 156 continued treatment (5 years) and 160 stopped treatment (3 years).

Seven randomised patients were non-compliant: 5 who were randomised to continue treatment stopped, and 2 who were to stop continued treatment.

There were 22 bone marrow relapses in patients who had 3 years of treatment (n = 160) versus 12 bone marrow relapses in the 5 year group (*n* = 156) (p = 0·09). Median time to relapse was 323 days in the 3 year group, with only one patient relapsing after stopping treatment in the 5 year group. Probability of bone marrow remission at 60 months after randomisation was 86% in the 3 year group versus 91% in the 5 year group (Figure 15.6).

Eleven isolated testicular relapses occurred in the group that discontinued therapy at 3 years and 5 testicular relapses (2 relapsed after therapy had been discontinued) in the group randomised to 5 years of therapy (p = 0·13). Of the 13 who relapsed after discontinuing treatment (3 year group, 11; 5 year group 2), only 8 remained free of disease at a median follow-up of 31 months, while the other 5 died of leukaemia.

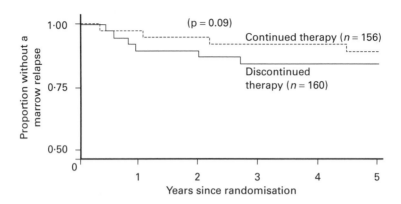

Figure 15.6 Time to bone marrow relapse from randomisation

Results for isolated CNS relapse were that 4 of 6 patients who relapsed on treatment (5 year group) later relapsed in the marrow and died, while one of the 2 patients who relapsed off treatment (3 year group) died after a subsequent marrow relapse.

At 5 years after randomisation no significant difference was seen in survival between patients who received 3 years of therapy and those treated for 5 years (93% v 89% respectively, $p = 0.27$).

No statistically significant differences in RFS were observed between patients treated for 3 years and those treated for 5 years ($p = 0.24$), neither were any differences seen in RFS according to sex in patients treated for 3 years

compared to those treated for 5 years respectively (males: 81% v 75%, $p = 0.14$; females: 89% v 89%, $p = 0.95$).

Both sexes in the 3 year group had a risk of marrow relapse 1·7 times that of patients who discontinued therapy at 5 years but this was not statistically significant. The survival of females in the 5 year group was poorer but not statistically significant (relative risk of death 3·6; $p = 0.08$).

Conclusion

It was concluded that no demonstrable difference was evident in survival or relapse free survival between 3 years or 5 years of total ALL treatment.

Study 3

Chessells JM, Durrant J, Hardy RM and Richards S.
Report to the Council by the Working Party on Leukaemia in Childhood. Medical Research Council Leukaemia Trial UKALL-V: an attempt to reduce the immunosuppressive effects of therapy in childhood acute lymphoblastic leukaemia.
J Clin Oncol 1986;**4**:1758–64.

UKALL-V was a prospective randomised multi-centre trial with three built in randomisations. It ran from January 1976 to March 1979.

Objectives

The objective of the study was to compare and evaluate 2 years versus 3 years of maintenance chemotherapy in children with acute lymphoblastic leukaemia.

Details of the study

All children with previously untreated ALL between the ages of 1 and 14 and with a diagnostic WBC count $< 20 \times 10^9/\ell$ were enrolled in the trial. Patients with CNS involvement or mediastinal enlargement at diagnosis were excluded from the trial.

Remission induction consisted of vincristine (VCR) 1·5 mg/m^2/week $\times 4$, prednisolone (PDN) 40 mg/m^2/d $\times 4$ weeks and L-asparaginase (ASP) 10 000 U/m^2/dose $\times 4$ doses in 1 week. 6-Mercaptopurine (6MP) was administered through-out the phase of cranial irradiation and this was followed by a 2 week course of VCR and PDN.

Randomisation for CNS irradiation (CRT) was between 24 Gy in 12 fractions and 21 Gy in seven fractions. Five intrathecal (IT) doses of methotrexate (MTX) were given during CRT.

Patients were randomised to one of three maintenance regimens given below:

Regimen I: 210 mg/m^2/d $\times 5$days of 6-MP and MTX 10 mg alternating with 12·5 mg over 3 days every 3 weeks. The doses were increased over the next two cycles to a maxi-mum dose of 300 mg/day of 6-MP and to 5 days of MTX as permitted by blood counts or presence of oral ulceration.

Regimen C: 6-MP 50 mg/day and MTX 20 mg/week. 6-MP was increased as tolerated to 70 mg/day.

Regimen G: MTX similar to regimen C, but 6-MP started at a higher dose of 70 mg/day and increased to 100 mg/day if tolerated.

All three regimens delivered the same total dose of 6-MP and MTX per metre body surface area over a 12 week cycle.

At the end of 96 weeks of treatment, patients were randomised either to stop treatment or continue till week 144, if bone marrow and CSF were normal and in boys if testicular biopsy was normal. The schema of treatment shown in Figure 15.7.

Analysis were done by log-rank method and only first relapses were counted. All analysis was based on intention to treat.

Outcome measures were disease free survival (DFS), bone marrow relapse rate and CNS relapse rate.

Outcome

A total of 550 patients were registered on the trial, of whom 22 were excluded (previous chemotherapy, diagnostic error). Of the 528 who were evaluable, 496 were in remission after

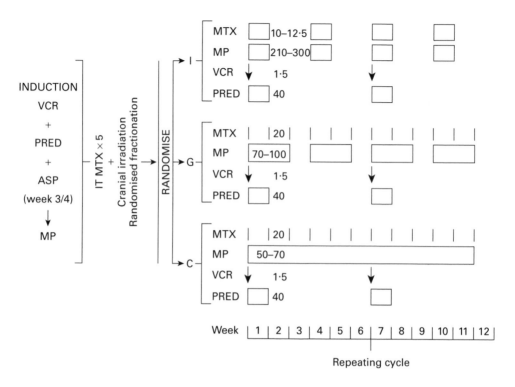

Figure 15.7 Design of the UKALL-V trial. The drug doses are in mg/m^2 surface area. Details of the maintenance schedules are described in the text

induction chemotherapy and 348 were in remission at 2 years. Two hundred and ninety-two patients were randomised to stop or continue treatment for a further four cycles (144 weeks).

There was a statistically significant higher haematological relapse rate in girls who received only 2 years of treatment (28 v 17; p = 0·01).

There was a slightly increased rate of testicular and bone marrow relapse in boys who received only 2 years of maintenance treatment but this did not reach statistical significance. Though bone marrow relapses were higher in patients receiving 2 years of therapy in groups C and G,

there was no significant difference in disease free survival between patients receiving 2 or 3 years of maintenance treatment in either groups C and G. This was due to three remission deaths in group C during the third year of treatment.

Overall, there was an apparent benefit for patients who received 3 years of maintenance treatment (Table 15.2).

Conclusion

It was concluded that 3 years of maintenance chemotherapy was superior to 2 years.

Table 15.2 Two years v 3 years of chemotherapy

Event	Relapse and/or death in remission[a]			Marrow relapse as first event[b]			CNS relapse as first event[c]			Testicular relapse as first event		
	Obs.	Exp.	P	Obs.	Exp.	P	Obs.	Exp.	P	Obs.	Exp.	P
Duration of therapy												
2 yr	62	48·6	0·005	47	35·4	0·005	7	5·5	0·2	10	8·1	0·2
3 yr	47	60·4		33	44·6		5	6·5		9	10·9	
Sex												
M (2 yr)	28	22·8	0·08	19	15·0	0·09	2	1·8	0·4	10	8·1	0·2
M (3 yr)	25	30·2		16	20·0		2	2·2		9	10·9	
F (2 yr)	34	25·6	0·01	28	20·4	0·01	5	3·8	0·2			
F (3 yr)	22	30·4		17	24·6		3	4·2				
Chemotherapy												
C (2 yr)	14	10·6	0·1	11	6·7	0·02	2	1·4	0·2	2	1·8	0·4
C (3 yr)	11	14·4		5	9·3		1	1·6		2	2·2	
G (2 yr)	23	18·5	0·07	18	13·7	0·05	0	0·5	0·5	4	3·7	0·4
G (3 yr)	15	19·5		10	14·3		1	0·5		6	6·3	
I (2 yr)	25	19·4	0·05	18	15·1	0·2	5	3·5	0·1	4	2·4	0·1
I (3 yr)	21	26·6		18	20·9		3	4·5		1	2·6	
C and G (2 yr)	37	28·8	0·02	29	20·1	0·003	2	1·9	0·5	6	5·6	0·4
C and G (3 yr)	26	34·2		15	23·9		2	2·1		8	8·4	
Total no. of events	107			80			12			19		

Abbreviations: Obs. observed event; Exp. expected event.

[a] Four deaths in remission.

[b] One combined bone marrow and CNS relapse, five bone marrow and testis.

[c] Two combined CNS and testis relapses.

Study 4

Bleyer WA.
Remaining problems in the staging and treatment of childhood lymphoblastic leukaemia.
Am J Pediatr Hematol/Oncol 1989;**11**:371–9.

CCG-161, 162 and 163 were prospective multicentre randomised trials of the Children's Cancer Study Group. No details regarding the period of the study are given in the report.

Objectives

The objectives of the study were to ascertain the optimal duration of treatment in children with ALL: 2 years versus 3 years of therapy.

Details of the study

According to risk status, children with low risk ALL were assigned to CCG study 161, those with intermediate risk to CCG study 162, and high risk children to CCG study 163.

Treatment details are not available in the report. Children, who were in continuous clinical remission 2 years after diagnosis, were randomised either to stop treatment or to continue maintenance therapy for an additional year. Boys underwent bilateral testicular biopsies prior to randomisation and were randomised only if they had no evidence of occult disease.

Outcome measures were relapse free survival (RFS) and overall survival (OS).

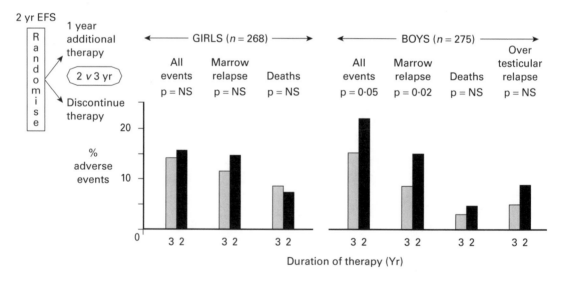

Figure 15.8 Comparison of adverse events after randomisation to 2 years versus 3 years of maintenance chemotherapy of ALL

No details of randomisation methodology are given in the report.

Outcome

The 2 versus. 3 year randomisation was conducted in 1082 children, of whom 539 were randomised to stop treatment (2 years) and 545 to 3 years of treatment.

Figure 15.8 shows the outcome of only 543 of the 1082 randomised children.

Girls had no benefit in extending treatment beyond 2 years. There were decreased bone marrow and testicular relapses in boys who had 3 years of therapy.

Toxicity

There were no increased deaths in remission in either sex in the 3 year treatment arm.

Conclusion

It was concluded that, in boys, the disease free survival was superior in the group given 3 years of treatment. This benefit was not evident in girls.

Study 5

Miller DR, Leikin SL, Albo VC, Sather H and Denman Hammond G.

Three versus five years of maintenance therapy are equivalent in childhood acute lymphoblastic leukaemia: a report from the Children's Cancer Study Group.

J Clin Oncol 1989;**7**:316–25.

The Children's Cancer Study Group conducted the CCG-141 trial from February 1975 to February 1977. It was a prospective multicentre randomised trial.

Objectives

The aim of the study was to determine whether 3 years and 5 years of maintenance therapy in childhood ALL were equivalent.

Details of the study

All children and adolescents with ALL less than 18 years of age, who were in 3 years of continuous complete remission (CCR) from initial CNS prophylaxis therapy ("primary maintenance") or in CCR 3 years after having had an isolated extramedullary relapse with negative testicular biopsy ("secondary maintenance") were eligible for randomisation.

Boys with occult testicular leukaemia after 3 years of CCR were ineligible for randomisation.

In those with a WBC count $< 20 \times 10^9/\ell$ with no mediastinal mass the induction treatment consisted of vincristine (VCR), prednisone (PDN) and asparaginase (standard regimen). CNS prophylaxis consisted of 24 Gy cranial irradiation plus 6-weekly intrathecal injections of methotrexate

(MTX). Maintenance treatment during the first year consisted of 6-mercaptopurine (6-MP), oral MTX and monthly pulses of PDN and VCR. During the second and third years of maintenance, the pulses of VCR and PDN were omitted.

Children with a WBC count $> 20 \times 10^9/\ell$ and or mediastinal mass were randomised to either the standard induction regimen or to an intensive regimen in which oral cyclophosphamide was also added to the standard regimen. During CNS prophylaxis, the dose of 6-MP was increased while during the first year of maintenance treatment; alternating cycles of VCR, PDN, 6-MP and MTX or PDN, VCR, cytosine arabinoside and doxorubicin were administered. The second and third year of maintenance were identical to the standard treatment patients.

After 3 years of CCR patients were randomised:

Regimen A: stop treatment.
Regimen B: 4 weeks of re-induction with VCR, PDN and asparaginase and stop.
Regimen C: continue maintenance for 2 more years and stop.

No details of the randomisation methodology are given in the report. Analysis was on the basis of intention to treat.

Outcome

CCG-141 registered 880 children, of whom 827 (94%) achieved CR. Five hundred and seven patients completed 3 years of primary or secondary maintenance. Twenty-six boys had occult testicular disease on biopsy at the end of 3 years of CCR and were excluded. A total of 481 patients were eligible for randomisation (boys 229; girls 252). Three hundred and ten

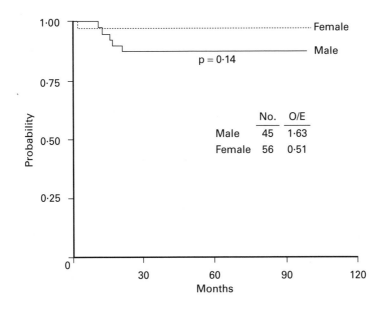

Figure 15.9 DFS in males and females randomly assigned to regimen A (discontinue therapy after 3 years continuous clinical remission)

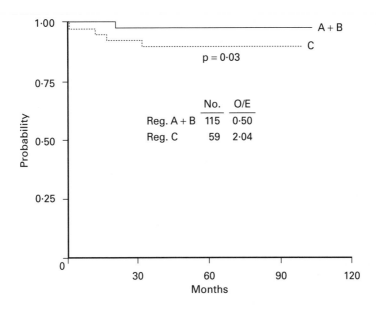

Figure 15.10 Survival in females randomly assigned to discontinue (regimens A and B) or continue chemotherapy (regimen C)

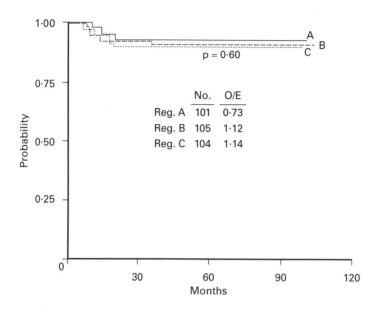

Figure 15.11 DFS of patients randomly assigned to regimens A, B and C

patients were randomised while 171 non-randomly continued or stopped treatment. Details of the randomisation methodology are not given in the report, neither are reasons for non-randomisation specified.

Randomisation distribution was as follows: regimen A 101; regimen B 105; regimen C 104.

Patient characteristics in the three regimens were similar with respect to age, sex, WBC count, day 14 bone marrow status and maintenance treatment as well as prior extramedullary relapses. Seventy per cent had WBC count $< 20 \times 10^9/\ell$ (low count group). Of the high WBC count group (30%), 54% had standard treatment while 46% had intensive treatment. The median follow up was 72 months from randomisation.

Outcome measures were disease free survival (DFS) and non-leukaemia related deaths.

No significant differences were seen in either the duration of haematological remission, recurrent disease, overall survival (OS), CNS relapse or isolated testicular relapse. There were five isolated CNS relapses with an overall incidence of 3·1% and there were two isolated testicular relapses among the 137 boys (1·5%).

DFS (p = 0·10) and OS (p = 0·83) were not significantly different in boys and girls. Though the relative event rate in boys randomised to regimen A was 3·2 times that in girls, this was not statistically different (p = 0·14) (Figure 15.9). Girls randomised to regimen C had a significantly worse survival than those randomised to the combined regimens A and B (p = 0·03); their relative death rate was 3·9 times higher (Figure 15.10).

Disease free survival (DFS) at 6 years from randomisation was as follows:

Regimen A 93%; regimen B 89·2%; regimen C 89·1% (p = 0·60) (Figure 15.11).

Of the 10 deaths in CCR, 5 occurred off therapy (regimen A 2; regimen B 1; regimen C 2) and 5 occurred on therapy: 3 children in regimen C died while on maintenance treatment due to disseminated varicella pneumonia while 2 children on regimen B died due to pneumonia and second malignant tumour respectively.

Conclusion

It was concluded that prolongation of maintenance therapy beyond 3 years does not improve survival or decrease risk of relapse.

Study 6

ALL steering committee of the Associazone Italiana Ematologia Oncologica Paediatrica (AIEOP): Paolucci G, Massera G, Vecchi V, Marsoni S, Pession A, Zurlo MG.
Treating childhood acute lymphoblastic leukaemia (ALL): summary of 10 years' experience in Italy.
Med Paediatr Oncol 1989;**17**:83–91.

This report summarises the results of three AIEOP multicentre trials that were conducted between 1976 and 1986. Trial 79–01/02 had two randomised components; low and average risk patients were randomised to a total length of 2 versus 3 years of treatment while high risk patients were randomly assigned two different chemotherapy regimens.

Objectives

The objective was to determine whether 2 years versus 3 years of maintenance therapy in low risk/average ALL patients was equivalent.

Details of the study

All children with previously untreated ALL aged between 1 and 14 years (inclusive), were included in the three studies. Though children with CNS disease at diagnosis or B-ALL were eligible for enrolment in the early trials, they were excluded from analysis. Patients were categorised into three prognostic groups; low (LR), average (AR) and high (HR) and treatment was stratified according to risk groups:

LR: Non-T, Non-L3 ALL, WBC $< 10 \times 10^9/\ell$, age 3–6 years, FAB $\leq$ 25% L2 blasts.
AR: Non-T, Non-L3 ALL, WBC $< 10 \times 10^9/\ell$, age 3–6 years, FAB $>$ 25% L2 blasts.
or WBC $10–50 \times 10^9/\ell$, age 3–6 years or WBC $< 50 \times 10^9/\ell$, age $<$ 3 or $\geq$ 7, years.
HR: T-ALL and or FAB L3 and or WBC $> 50 \times 10^9/\ell$.

The AIEOP treatment protocols are outlined in Table 15.3. To summarise briefly, all studies consisted of an induction, intensification and maintenance phase. A second re-intensification was

Table 15.3 AIEOP ALL protocol

Protocol	Induction	Intensification	CNS prophylaxis	Maintenance	Duration
1979 LR	V, P, MTX IT	L-ASP	18 Gy	6-MP, MTX + V/P pulses	2 years
1979 SR	V, P, MTX IT	L-ASP, 6-TG, AC, A	18 Gy	6-MP, MTX + V/P pulses	3 years

V, vincristine; P, prednisolone; MTX, methotrexate; L-ASP, L-asparaginase; 6-TG, 6-thioguanine; AC, cytosine arabinoside; A, doxorubicin; R, randomise.

introduced in the 82 Trial. CNS prophylaxis was mainly with cranial irradiation and intrathecal methotrexate. In the 79 Trial, LR and AR patients were randomised to a total duration either 2 or 3 years of treatment.

The log-rank test was used to compare disease free survival (DFS) rates. Significance level of 5% was adopted in all the two-tailed tests. The median follow up was 61 months at the time of the analysis.

Details of randomisation methodology are not specified in the report.

Outcome measure was disease free survival.

Outcome

Of the 815 patients who were enrolled on the AIEOP 79 trial, 545 patients were categorised as either low or average risk. Only 540 were eligible for analysis. Of the 540 eligible patients, 464 were assigned to correct risk groups and analyses refer to this latter group. A total of 177 patients were randomised to either 2 or 3 years of total treatment.

Five year DFS for patients randomised to 3 years of treatment was 70% versus. 68·3% for the 2 year group, $\chi^2_1 = 0·55$. The duration of total treatment (2 or 3 years) did not affect final outcome.

Conclusion

Two years of total treatment was concluded to be adequate in children with low or average risk ALL.

Study 7

Eden OB, Lilleyman JS, Richards S, Shaw MP, Peto J.

Results of Medical Research Council Childhood Leukaemia Trial UKALL-VIII (Report to the Medical Research Council on behalf of the Working Party on Leukaemia in Childhood).
Br J Haematol 1991;**78**:187–96.

UKALL-VIII was a prospective multicentre randomised trial and ran from September 1980 to December 1984.

Objectives

The study addressed the question of whether an additional year (third year) of maintenance treatment improves survival outcome in children with acute lymphoblastic leukaemia.

Details of the study

All children aged 0–14 years inclusive, irrespective of initial presenting features, were eligible for enrolment on the study.

All patients received a three drug induction regimen of weekly vincristine (1·5 mg/m²/dose) × 5, 28 days of oral prednisone (40 mg/m²/d) and nine intramuscular injections of L-asparaginase (6000 U/m²/dose). From September 1981, all children were randomised to receive two doses of daunorubicin (45 mg/m²/dose) during induction or not. Cranial prophylaxis consisted of intrathecal methotrexate (*n* = 4) and cranial irradiation (18 Gy) given immediately after achieving remission. Those not in remission by 4 weeks were given a further 2 weeks of vincristine and

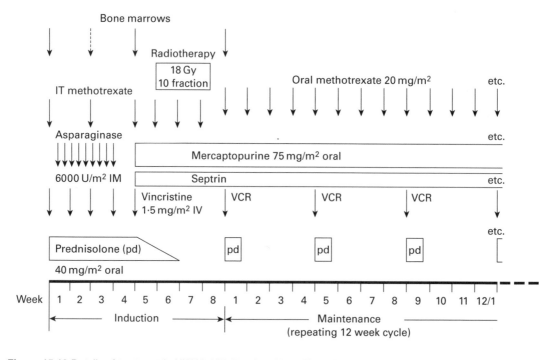

Figure 15.12 Details of treatment in UKALL-VIII. Reprinted from Eden OB *et al*, *Br J Haematol* (full reference above) with permission from Blackwell Science Ltd.

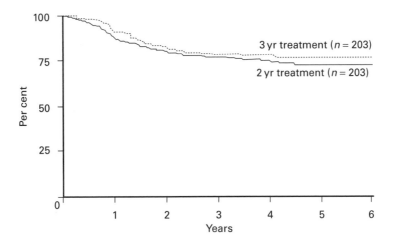

Figure 15.13 Disease free survival from the time of second randomisation: 3 years, DFS = 77%; 2 years, DFS = 73%. Reprinted from Eden OB *et al*, *Br J Haematol* (full reference p 386) with permission from Blackwell Science Ltd.

oral prednisone, but were taken off protocol if they failed to achieve remission. Maintenance therapy consisted of oral methotrexate (20 mg/m² weekly) and 6-mercaptopurine (75 mg/m²/d) with monthly pulses of vincristine (1·5 mg/m²/dose) and 5 days of oral prednisone (40 mg/m²/d). From January 1983 to the close of the trial in December 1984, there was a further randomisation for those still in remission at 2 years, between 2 or 3 years of maintenance therapy (Figure 15.12).

Outcome measures were disease free survival (DFS) and overall survival (OS) in the two groups of randomised patients according to duration of maintenance therapy.

Details of the randomisation method were not specified in the report.

Outcome

Of the 829 patients registered in the trial, only 826 were available for analysis (3 did not have ALL).

Four hundred and six patients were randomised with regard to the duration of maintenance treatment (2 years *n* = 203 *v* 3 years. *n* = 203).

Five year DFS for the entire cohort was 55%. There was no difference between 2 years and 3 years of maintenance therapy for the whole group and also irrespective of sex. Five year DFS for 3 years of treatment was 77% versus 73% for 2 years treatment (Figure 15.13).

More relapses were seen after stopping treatment at 2 than 3 years (17% versus 25%; p for RFS = 0·04), however, there was 4% increased remission deaths in the 3 year arm.

Conclusion

It was concluded that there was no significant survival benefit for those receiving 3 years of maintenance therapy.

Study 8

Childhood ALL Collaborative Group.
Duration and intensity of maintenance chemotherapy in acute lymphoblastic leukaemia: overview
of 42 trials involving 12,000 randomised children.
Lancet 1996;**347**:1783–8.

This report is a meta-analysis of 42 randomised
trials in childhood ALL that were performed
worldwide before 1987.

Objectives/methodology

Individual patient data of approximately 3900,
3700, 1300 and 3150 patients were retrieved
and analysed with regard to the duration of
maintenance therapy, the efficacy of re-
induction therapy during maintenance, effectiveness of regular pulses of vincristine and
predni-sone during maintenance and various
other questions.

Table 15.4 Randomised comparisons with outcome data available that began before 1987 of
the duration or intensity of maintenance chemotherapy in childhood ALL

Treatment comparison	Trials	Patients	Relapse or death
Longer v shorter maintenance	16	3861	984
Addition of pulses of vincristine and prednisolone during maintenance	5	1251	447
Addition of intensive re-induction treatment during maintenance	6	3696	1246
Other drug additions during maintenance			
Higher v lower dose	2	476	276
Cytosine arabinoside + cyclophosphamide + doxorubicin	1	711	263
Cytosine arabinoside + cyclophosphamide	2	365	284
Cyclophosphamide	4	990	446
L-asparaginase + cytosine arabinoside	1	191	131
Cytosine arabinoside	2	296	182
Prednisolone	1	33	29
Vincristine	1	31	26
6-Mercaptopurine	1	40	22
All studies with data available	42	11941	4336

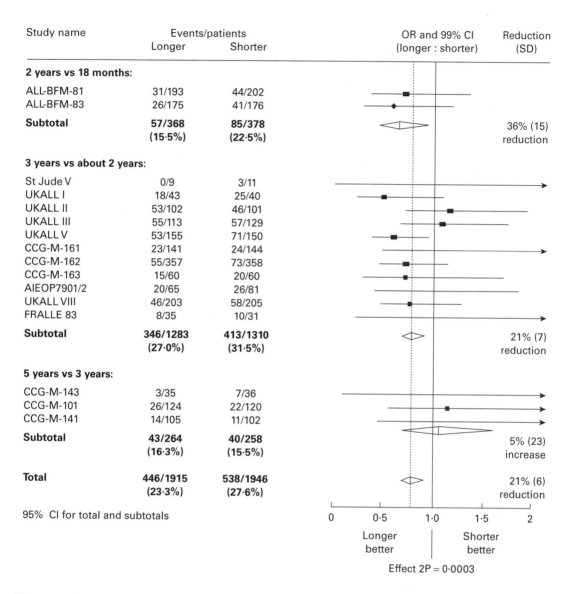

Study name	Events/patients		OR and 99% CI (longer : shorter)	Reduction (SD)
	Longer	Shorter		
2 years vs 18 months:				
ALL-BFM-81	31/193	44/202		
ALL-BFM-83	26/175	41/176		
Subtotal	**57/368**	**85/378**		36% (15)
	(15·5%)	**(22·5%)**		reduction
3 years vs about 2 years:				
St Jude V	0/9	3/11		
UKALL I	18/43	25/40		
UKALL II	53/102	46/101		
UKALL III	55/113	57/129		
UKALL V	53/155	71/150		
CCG-M-161	23/141	24/144		
CCG-M-162	55/357	73/358		
CCG-M-163	15/60	20/60		
AIEOP7901/2	20/65	26/81		
UKALL VIII	46/203	58/205		
FRALLE 83	8/35	10/31		
Subtotal	**346/1283**	**413/1310**		21% (7)
	(27·0%)	**(31·5%)**		reduction
5 years vs 3 years:				
CCG-M-143	3/35	7/36		
CCG-M-101	26/124	22/120		
CCG-M-141	14/105	11/102		
Subtotal	**43/264**	**40/258**		5% (23)
	(16·3%)	**(15·5%)**		increase
Total	**446/1915**	**538/1946**		21% (6)
	(23·3%)	**(27·6%)**		reduction

95% CI for total and subtotals

0   0·5   1·0   1·5   2

Longer better   Shorter better

Effect 2P = 0·0003

Figure 15.14 Duration of maintenance chemotherapy in childhood ALL; effects on survival in first remission. Larger squares indicate more informative trials and hence shorter CIs. If square is to the left of solid line, survival in first remission is better in group allocated longer maintenance treatment, but if CI crosses this line, this result is not of extreme statistical significance (2p > 0·01). Subtotals and overall total are represented as diamonds centred on OR estimate, with 95% CI shown by width of diamond and with odds reduction also given as percentage along with its SD

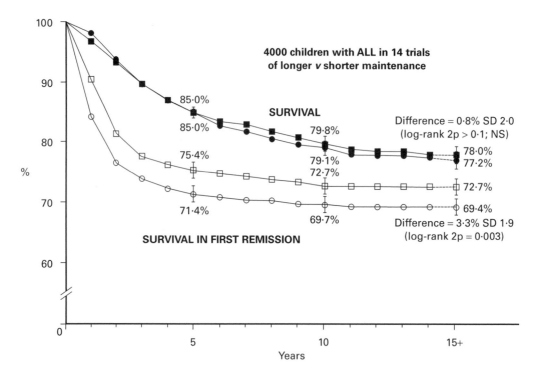

Figure 15.15 Duration of maintenance chemotherapy in childhood ALL: effects on survival and on survival in first remission. Upper pair of lines describe survival, and lower pair (open symbols) survival in first remission from time of randomisation: both pairs derive from stratified analyses. Squares and circles denote active and control, respectively

Analyses were of survival in first remission, overall survival and cause specific mortality.

Only randomised trials (prior to 1987 only) were evaluated. All the trials were identified by Medline and clinical trials database search, hand searching of meeting abstracts, reference lists of trials, review articles or by personal communication. Analysis was on an intention to treat basis. Trials were excluded only if randomisation was deemed unsatisfactory.

The main analysis was survival and survival in first remission from date of randomisation. An event was defined as relapse death in remission or death without remission. In some analyses, mortality was subdivided into death in first remission and death after relapse.

Statistics

The statistical methods involved comparison of the observed number of patients in one treatment group (O) who suffered a particular event with the log-rank expected number (E), which was based on the average experience of both treatment groups. From the log-rank (O–E), its variance was calculated (odds ratio), including 99% confidence interval. Information from different trials is then combined by summing the separate O-E values, one per trial.

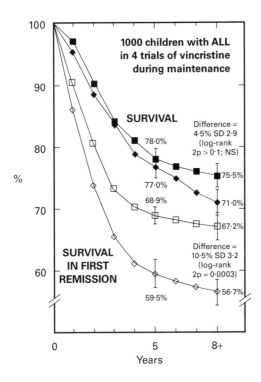

Figure 15.16 Addition of pulses of vincristine plus prednisolone during maintenance chemotherapy in childhood ALL: effects on survival, and on survival in first remission

The risk of relapse or death was 27·6% (n = 538/1946) for patients who had a shorter duration of maintenance (usually 2 years) compared to 23·3% (n = 446/1915) with longer maintenance. The overall odds reduction was 21% with standard deviation (SD 6) (2p = 0·0003) (Figure 15.14). Longer maintenance halved the relapse rate but did not translate into improved long term survival (Figure 15.15). Deaths during first remission were increased by longer maintenance (2·7% v 1·2%).

Reinforcement with vincristine and prednisone (VP) during seven maintenance trials compared maintenance therapy with and without pulses of VP. A total of 1251 patients were randomised to receive or not VP pulse (patient data available from five trials). Overall, VP pulses during maintenance reduced the absolute risk of relapse or death by 9·2%. Deaths in remission were slightly higher (4·0% v 3·2%) while deaths after relapse were lower (both non-significant) among patients allocated reinforcement VP pulses. Overall survival was better in patients who were randomised to receive VP pulse therapy but this was not statistically significant (Figure 15.16).

Additional re-induction therapy during maintenance therapy

Of the seven trials that addressed this issue, data were available from only six. Of the 3696 patients randomised, individual patient data was available from all except 254 patients. The median follow up (where patient data were available) was at least 5 years.

Patients who were randomised to receive the additional intensification block had highly significant difference in relapse rate that resulted in improved survival in first remission – absolute

Outcome

Table 15.4 shows the 42 trials of maintenance therapy. Information from seven trials was not available.

Duration of maintenance therapy

Of the 17 trials that compared the duration of maintenance therapy (commonest being 2 v 3 years), data was not available in one trial (BFM). All trials were between 1970 and 1983, with the last patients randomised in 1990. In the 16 trials together, 3861 patients were randomised either to the shorter or longer maintenance arm. The median follow-up was > 5 years for all but one trial.

difference in survival in first remission by the fifth year was 7·6% (71·1% *v* 63·5%). There was a significant reduction of relapses at all sites and a non-significant increase in deaths in remission (4·8% *v* 3·3%) in this group of patients.

Conclusion

- Longer maintenance reduced the risk of haematological and testicular relapse during the third year, however, this did not translate into improved overall survival due to a slight increase in deaths during first remission.
- Intensive re-induction therapy improved overall survival as well as survival in first remission due to reduction in leukaemia relapses and leukaemia related deaths.
- Reinforcement VP pulse therapy reduced relapses but did not result in any significant improvement in overall survival.

Study 9

Schrappe M, Reiter A, Zimmermann M, Harbott J, Ludwig WD, Henze G, Gadner H, Odenwald E, Riehm H.
Long-term results of four consecutive trials in childhood ALL performed by the ALL–BFM study group from 1981 to 1985.
Leukaemia 2000;**14**:2205–22.

ALL-BFM 81 and ALL BFM 83 were multicentre prospective randomised studies with treatment stratified according to the BFM risk criteria. ALL BFM 81 began in April 1981 and was closed in September 1983 and ALL BFM 83, which commenced in October 1983 and closed in September 1986, followed this.

Objectives

The study objectives were to determine whether the total duration of ALL treatment could be shortened from 24 months to 18 months in all risk groups of patients.

Details of the study

The study was open to all patients below 18 years of age with previously untreated leukaemia. Children with Down's syndrome who had severe cardiac defects were excluded, as were children who developed ALL as a second malignancy.

Patients were categorised as standard risk (SR: RF < 1·2), medium risk (MR: RF 1·2–1·7) or high risk (HR: RF ≥ 1·7) according to the leukaemic cell mass (BFM risk factor: RF) at diagnosis. SR patients were further subdivided in ALL BFM 83 into low SR (RF < 0·8 and no CNS disease or mediastinal mass) and high SR (RF 0·8 – < 1·2) groups.

The duration of induction therapy ranged from 8 (BFM 81) to 11 (BFM 83) weeks. ALL BFM 83 induction therapy commenced with a 1 week prednisone window with a stepwise increase to full dose of 60 mg/m²/d. The other drugs used during induction therapy consisted of vincristine (VCR), prednisone (PDN), daunorubicin (DNR) and L-asparaginase (ASP): phase A and phase B included cyclophosphamide (CPM), cytosine arabinoside (ARA-C), 6-mercaptopurine (6-MP) and intrathecal methotrexate (IT MTX). For BFM 83 HR patients, two blocks of dexamethasone (DEX), IV MTX, tenoposide (VM-26), ARA-C and CPM – 'Element B', followed the PDN prophase. All patients (except SR patients not randomised to cranial RT) in BFM 81 had cranial irradiation after induction therapy – 18 or 24 Gy.

Consolidation therapy in BFM 81 consisted of 6-MP and oral MTX alone except in SR patients who did not receive cranial irradiation (SR-B). SR-B of BFM 81 and all patients of BFM 83 received 6-MP and IV MTX during the consolidation phase.

Re-intensification consisted of two phases: phase A – DEX/VCR/doxorubicin (DOX)/ASP – and phase B – ARA-C/6-thioguanine (6-TG)/IT MTX (Protocol III, 4 weeks) with CPM for the MR group (Protocol II, 6 weeks) only and was similar in both the trials. Low SR patients in BFM 83 were either to receive protocol III or not. HR patients in BFM 81 received the same drugs as in Protocol II plus VM-26 and additional ARA-C (Protocol IV, 8 weeks) (BFM 83) while HR patients in BFM 83 received Protocol II chemotherapy. High SR patients were randomised to either 18 Gy or 12 Gy cranial irradiation while MR (18 Gy) and HR (24 Gy) patients in BFM 83 had cranial irradiation during this phase.

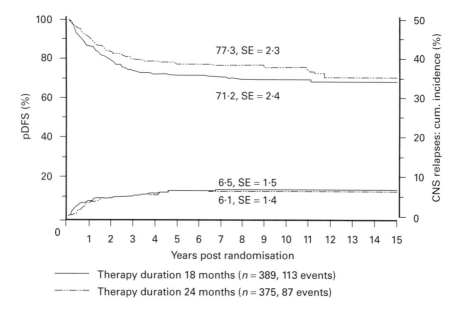

Figure 15.17 Evaluation of treatment duration in studies ALL-BFM 81 and 83. Adapted and reprinted from Schrappe M *et al, Leukaemia* with permission from Nature Publishing Group (full reference p 393).

Maintenance phase consisted of daily oral 6-MP and weekly oral MTX in both trials for 18 months.

Intrathecal chemotherapy comprised seven courses in BFM 81 and eight courses in BFM 83.

Patients in continuous clinical remission were randomised either to stop therapy (18 months) or to continue maintenance treatment for a further 6 months and stop (24 months).

Outcome measures were CNS relapse rate, disease free survival (DFS) and overall survival.

Randomisation details are not specified in the report. Comparisons between the treatment groups were made using the log-rank test.

All analyses were performed on the basis on intention to treat.

Outcome

Of the 1264 patients enrolled on both studies together, 764 patients were randomised to evaluate the impact of duration of treatment (18 months *v* 24 months) on DFS. The report does not give the exact numbers of registered patients who were excluded from analysis, remission deaths, toxic deaths, non-compliant patients, numbers of patients who relapsed prior to randomisation etc.

The 8 year DFS for patients randomised (*n* = 375) for 24 months and 18 months (*n* = 389) of therapy were 77·3% ± 2·3% and 71·2% ± 2·4% respectively. Log-rank test (p = 0·11) did not show any significant difference because of late events occurring 10 years from diagnosis (Figure 15.17).

The cumulative incidence of CNS relapses at 10 years from randomisation was similar, however, there was a trend for lesser relapses at other sites in the group that received 24 months of therapy (p = 0·07).

There was also a significant difference in overall survival at 10 years for patients who had 24 months of treatment (p = 0·025).

No details of toxicity have been specified.

Conclusion

It was concluded that 2 years of treatment was superior to 18 months of therapy.

16

Modification of continuing chemotherapy in acute lymphoblastic leukaemia

Studies

Pulsed vincristine and prednisolone

Study 1

Bleyer WA, Sather HN, Nickerson HJ, Coccia PF, Finklestein JZ, Miller DR, Littman PS, Lukens JN, Siegel SE, Denman Hammond G.
Monthly pulses of vincristine and prednisone prevent bone marrow and testicular relapse in low-risk childhood acute lymphoblastic leukaemia: a report of the CCG-161 study by the Children's Cancer Study Group.
J Clin Oncol 1991;**9**:1012–21.

Trial CCG-161 by the Children's Cancer Study Group extended from April 1978 till May 1983. It was a prospective randomised multicentre study. In October 1982, regimens containing CRT were closed to patient accrual.

A single randomisation was performed with a two by two multifactorial design (four treatment arms). One factor was the use of cranial radiotherapy (CRT) or intrathecal methotrexate (IT MTX) and the second factor was the use of monthly vincristine and prednisone pulses or not during maintenance treatment.

Objectives

The objectives of the study were to determine whether the addition of monthly pulses of vincristine and prednisone to methotrexate (MTX) and 6-mercaptopurine (6-MP) during the maintenance phase of treatment, improves overall and disease free survival.

Details of the study

Children between 3 and 6 years of age and WBC count at diagnosis of $< 10 \times 10^9/\ell$ with $< 25\%$ L2 morphology cells in bone marrow were enrolled on the study.

All patients received vincristine (VCR) 1·5 mg/m^2/week IV $\times$ 5, prednisone 40 (PDN) mg/m^2/d orally $\times$ 28 days and tapered thereafter, L-asparaginase 6000 U/m^2/dose IM 3 times per week $\times$ 9 doses, and IT MTX on days 0, 14, 28, 35 42, 49. Intrathecal methotrexate doses were

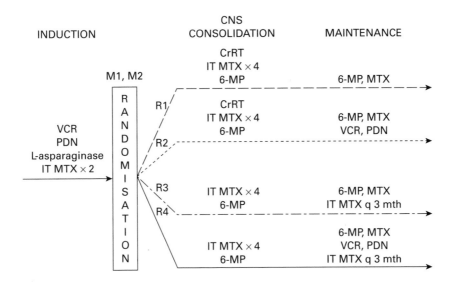

Figure 16.1 Study design of CCG-161

age adjusted – 6 mg, 8 mg, 10 mg and 12 mg for ages < 1, 1, 2 and 3 years or greater respectively (Figure 16.1). At the end of induction, patients were randomised to either cranial irradiation 18 Gy given over 10 fractions or intrathecal Methotrexate (IT MTX) and maintenance IT MTX.

Maintenance treatment was MTX 20 mg/m^2/week and 6-MP 75 mg/m^2/d, given to all patients and modified according to absolute neutrophil and platelet counts. In addition, one half also received monthly pulses of VCR 1·5 mg/m^2 and PDN 40 mg/m^2 × 5 days. Children randomised to IT MTX also received additional IT treatment during the maintenance phase.

No details are given in the report of the randomisation method used.

Outcome measures for analysis were disease free survival (DFS), overall survival, haematological remission, CNS remission and testicular remission. Analysis was based on actual treatment received.

Outcome

The number of patients registered on the trial was 698, of whom 679 reached consolidation. Forty-eight refused randomisation and the number randomised to maintenance was 631. There were 26 protocol violations, leaving 605 correctly randomised. The number receiving 6-MP/MTX plus VCR and PDN was 302; 303 received 6-MP/MTX alone. There were 163 boys randomised to VCR/PDN/6-MP/MTX and 166 to 6-MP/MTX alone.

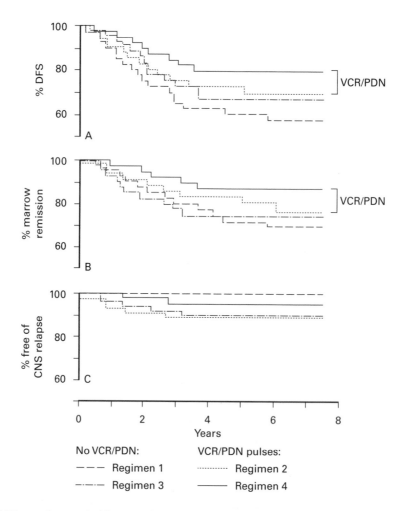

Figure 16.2 (A) Disease free survival (p = 0·032); (B) haematologic remission (p = 0·034) and (C) CNS remission (p = 0·035) from randomisation in patients on CCG-161 who were randomised to receive or not to receive VCR-PDN pulses during maintenance therapy. For details of regimens, see Figure 16.1

Five year DFS in the 6-MP/MTX/VCR/PDN arm was 76·7% versus 63·9% (p = 0·003) in the 6-MP/MTX alone arm, regardless of CNS therapy.

This difference was due to increased bone marrow – 38 (12·6%) v 69 (22·7%) – and testicular relapses (in boys).

The difference between VCR/PDN pulses and no pulses was most pronounced in the group who received IT MTX rather than CRT.

Five year continuous haematological remission in the VCR/PDN arm was 86·3% versus 74·5% in the 6-MP/MTX alone arm (p = 0·0008). (Figure 16.2)

Both irradiated boys and girls had a higher CNS relapse rate with VCR/PDN pulses than without them (10·2% v 0% in girls; 5·6% v 0% in boys). However, in both sexes who received IT MTX there were lower CNS relapses in those treated with VCR/PDN pulses than in those who were not (2·5% v 9·2% in girls; 5·6% v 6·3% in boys, p = 0·11)

Five year DFS for boys randomised to VCR/PDN was 74·7% versus 55·1% for those who were not (p = 0·001). Bone marrow (BM) and testicular relapses were significantly lower in boys randomised to VCR/PDN: BM 23/163, testicular 10/163 compared to 44/166 and 30/166 respectively, in the boys who did not receive it (p = 0·0006 and p = 0·003 respectively). The effect of VCR/PDN was stronger in the non-irradiated boys: 2·59 times higher risk of bone marrow relapse in the 6-MP/MTX alone group as compared to 1·59 times higher in the irradiated boys.

Five year DFS for girls randomised to VCR/PDN was 78·9% compared to 74·9% for the girls who did not receive VCR/PDN pulses.

The effect of VCR/PDN pulses was more evident in the non-irradiated group.

Survival was not significantly different for VCR/PDN or CNS therapy at the time of analysis.

Toxicity

There were 10 excess deaths in remission in the VCR/PDN arm, which were equally distributed between the cranial irradiation and IT MTX regimens. These were mostly due to viral or *Pneumocystis Carinii* infections.

Conclusion
Monthly pulses of vincristine and prednisone decreased the incidence of testicular and bone marrow relapses and improved DFS. This was most evident in the non-irradiated group of patients.

Study 2

Henze G, Langermann HJ, Fengler R, Brandeis M, Evers KG, Gadner H, Hinderfeld L, Jobke J, Kornhuber B, Lampert F, Lasson U, Ludwig R, Müller-Weihrich S, Neidhardt M, Nessler G, Niethammer D, Rister M, Ritter J, Schaaff A, Schellong G, Stollmann B, Treuner J, Wahlen M, Weinel P, Wehinger H, Riehm H.

Therapiestudie BFM 79/81 zur Behandlung der akuten lymphoblastischen Leukämie bei Kindern und Jugendlichen: intensivierte Reinduktionstherapie für Patientengruppen mit unterschiedlichem Rezidivrisiko.

Klin Pädiat 1982;**194**:195–203.

The BFM 79/81 study ran from April 1979 to March 1981. It was a multicentre prospective randomised study.

Objectives
The aims of this trial were to:

- Determine whether treatment outcome for non-high risk ALL patients could be improved by the introduction of an intensive re-induction block early in remission.
- To evaluate the efficacy of regular pulses of vincristine and prednisone during

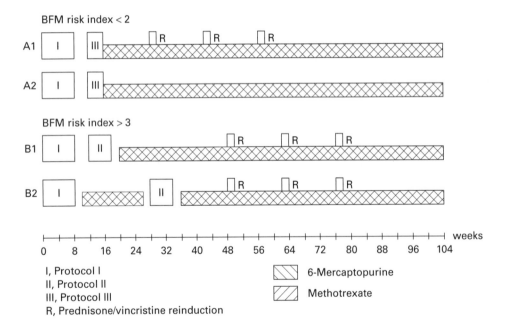

Figure 16.3 Treatment plan of study BFM 79/81

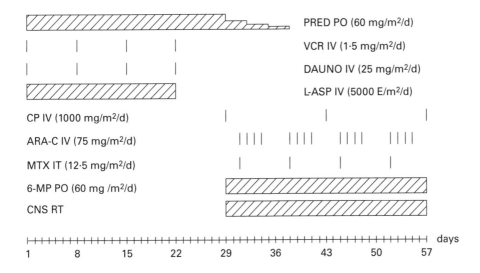

Figure 16.4 Protocol I for study BFM 79/81. PRED, prednisone; VCR, vincristine; DAUNO, daunorubicin; L-ASP, asparaginase; CP, cyclophosphamide; ARA-C, cytosine arabinoside; MTX, methotrexate; 67-MP, 6-mercaptopurine; PO, orally; IV, intravenous; IT, intrathecal; RT, radiotherapy

maintenance therapy in improving disease free survival in standard risk ALL patients.

- To compare and evaluate 2·5 years with 2 years of treatment in children with high risk ALL.

Here we focus primarily on the duration of treatment for high risk ALL and efficacy of regular pulses of vincristine and prednisone in improving DFS in standard risk patients.

Details of the study

Patients were categorised into standard and high risk groups as per the BFM (Berlin–Frankfurt–Murster) risk index and treatment was stratified according to risk status as shown in Figure 16.3 and 16.4.

Details regarding randomisation are not reported.

Outcome measures were relapse free survival (RFS).

Outcome

There were no differences in the outcome in children treated with regular pulses of vincristine and prednisone compared to those who were not: RFS 0·83 (SD = 0·06) v 0·83 (SD = 0·05) respectively.

Reducing the duration of treatment from 2·5 years to 2 years in children with high risk ALL did not adversely affect outcome.

Conclusions

- Regular pulses of vincristine and prednisone during maintenance therapy were
  unnecessary in patients with standard
  risk ALL.
- In children with high risk ALL, a total of
  2 years' treatment was satisfactory.

See also Study 8, Chapter 15: meta-
analysis by Richards *et al.*

Dose and route of methotrexate

Study 3

Lange BJ, Blatt J, Sather HN, Meadows AT. Randomised comparison of moderate dose methotrexate infusions to oral methotrexate in children with intermediate risk acute lymphoblastic leukaemia: a Children's Group study. *Med Paediat Oncol* 1996;**27**:15–20.

CCG-139, which ran from November 1984 till January 1989, was a prospective randomised limited institution study.

Objectives

The aim of the study was to compare the efficacy of moderate dose intravenous methotrexate against oral methotrexate in improving overall and disease free survival in children with intermediate risk acute lymphoblastic leukaemia.

Details of the study

Children and adolescents between 1 and 19 years of age who had no bulky lymphomatous disease and with a WBC count $10 < 50 \times 10^9/\ell$ or WBC $<10 - \times 10^9/\ell$ but with > 10% blasts with L2 morphology were categorised as intermediate risk and were enrolled on the study.

All patients were randomised prior to commencement of induction therapy. Details of the randomisation method are not specified.

Induction and CNS prophylaxis were identical for both the randomised regimens and comprised vincristine (VCR) 1·5 mg/m^2/week × 5, prednisone (PDN) 40 mg/m^2/day × 28 days and tapered to stop over a week, L-asparaginase 6000 U/m^2 × 9 doses and intrathecal methotrexate (IT MTX) on days 1, 15 and 28. IT MTX doses were age adjusted – 8 mg, 10 mg and 12 mg for ages 1, 2 and 3 years or greater respectively.

Consolidation and maintenance for regimen 1 included infusions of methotrexate at 500 mg/m^2. A third of the total dose was given as a bolus and the remainder as a 24 hour infusion. This was given three times during consolidation and 6-weekly during maintenance. Folinic acid rescue was at 48 and 72 hours. Maintenance therapy consisted of oral 6-mercaptopurine (6-MP) 75 mg/m^2/day and oral MTX 20 mg/m^2/week (during the 5 weeks when there was no IV MTX). VCR and PDN pulses were given 6-weekly during maintenance therapy.

Patients on regimen 2 received standard oral MTX 20 mg/m^2/week, oral 6-MP 75 mg/m^2/d with pulses of VCR and PDN given every 4 weeks during maintenance.

Duration of maintenance therapy lasted for 2 years (114 weeks) for girls and 3 years (166 weeks) for boys. The total cumulative dose of methotrexate in regimen 1 was 16 240 mg/m^2 and 11 749 mg/m^2 while in regimen 2 it was 3120 mg/m^2 and 2080 mg/m^2 in regimen 2 for boys and girls respectively.

Median follow-up was 75 months.

Outcome measures were event free survival (EFS) and overall survival.

Outcome

Though analysis was on the basis of intention to treat, the first 16 patients were non-randomly

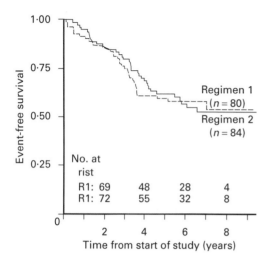

Figure 16.5 Event free survival in CCG-139

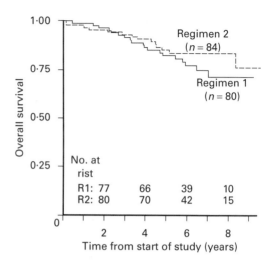

Figure 16.6 Overall survival in CCG-139

assigned to either regimen 1 ($n = 10$) or 2 ($n = 6$). The number of patients registered on the study was 168. Three patients in regimen 1 were removed from the study because of parent or physician preference and 1 because of CNS toxicity.

Of the 164 eligible patients, 80 were randomised to regimen 1 and 84 to regimen 2. A higher proportion of patients in regimen 1 were above 10 years of age.

There were 34 events among 80 regimen 1 patients (IV MTX arm): 33 relapses and 1 early death. Relapse sites were: 12 bone marrow 14 CNS, 2 testicular, 4 combined bone marrow and CNS and 1 CNS and testis.

Thirty-six events occurred in regimen 2 (standard arm) patients: 33 relapses, 1 induction failure and 2 early deaths. Sites of relapses were similar, with 14 bone marrow, 10 CNS relapses and 5 combined bone marrow and CNS relapse, 2 testicular, 1 combined bone marrow and testis and in one

patient site of relapse was not specified.

Six year event free survival for regimen 1 was 58·4% (± 5·6); regimen 2, 57·4% (± 5·6) (p = 0·92) (Figure 16.5).

Relative event rate is 1·02 for regimen 1 compared to Regimen 2. The frequency and distribution of relapses did not differ between the two regimens.

Six year overall survival for regimen 1 was 76·9% (± 5·0); regimen 2, 83·1% (± 4·3) (p = 0·31) (Figure 16.6). Relative death rate was 1·43 for regimen 1 compared to regimen 2.

There were no significant differences in toxicity in the two arms.

Conclusion

It was concluded that use of IV methotrexate in this dose and schedule did not confer any advantage over standard therapy.

Study 4

Lilleyman JS, Richards S, Rankin A on behalf of the Medical Research Council's Working Party on Childhood Leukaemia.
Medical Research Council leukaemia trial, UKALL VII: a report to the Council by the Working Party on Leukaemia in Childhood.
Arch Dis Childh 1985;**60**:1050–54.

UKALL-VII was a prospective randomised multi-centre trial with enrolment open from April 1979 to March 1980.

Objectives

The aim of the study was to evaluate the efficacy of a reduction in the dose of cranial irradiation and its impact on the treatment outcome in children with acute lymphoblastic leukaemia. The study also had other objectives, which included the need for prophylactic testicular irradiation, the number of doses asparginase during induction, need for extra intrathecal methotrexate (IT MTX) during maintenance and the use of oral versus intramuscular methotrexate during maintenance.

This review focuses on the comparative efficacy of oral (OP MTX) versus intramuscular methotrexate (IM MTX) during maintenance therapy.

Details of the study

Eligibility criteria are detailed in Chapter 13 Study 2.

There were two randomisations during maintenance therapy and both were independent of each other. Specifically, these were:

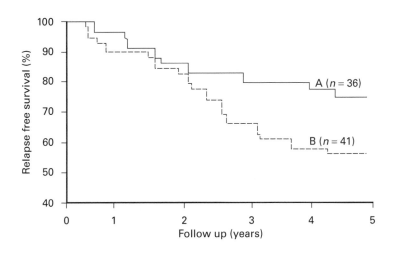

Figure 16.7 Relapse free survival for UKALL-VII. A, intramuscular maintenance methotrexate: relapses = 5; deaths in remission = 4. B, oral maintenance methotrexate: relapses = 17, deaths in remission = 1. Difference: p < 0·05 (log-rank)

1   The giving of extra doses of intrathecal methotrexate (IT MTX) at 6 weekly intervals during maintenance treatment or not.

2   Maintenance systemic methotrexate given intramuscularly or orally.

The treatment schema is shown in Chapter 13, Figure 13.4.

The method of randomisation is not specified in the report.

The outcome measure was relapse free survival (RFS).

Results

Of the 87 patients enrolled on the study, 8 were excluded due either to ineligibility ($n = 5$) or failure to remit ($n = 3$). Analysis was performed on the basis of intention to treat as well on the basis of treatment actually received (see Table 13.1).

Forty children were randomised to IM MTX and 39 to PO MTX. As shown in Table 13.1, only 36 patients received IM MTX while 41 received PO MTX.

When the analysis was performed by the actual treatment received by the patient groups, then patients in the IM MTX group ($n = 36$) had fewer relapses ($n = 5$) compared to 17 in the PO MTX ($n = 41$) group. In contrast, deaths in remission were lower in the PO MTX group ($n = 1$) compared to 4 in the IM MTX group (Figure 16.7). This difference was statistically significant (log-rank $p < 0.05$). This difference was lost when the analysis was based on the allocated treatment ($p = 0.11$) as 3 of the 4 patients who should have received IM MTX subsequently relapsed.

Of 36 patients given IM MTX, 27 (75%) were alive compared with 23 of 41 (56%) given PO MTX.

Conclusion

It was concluded (analysed according to actual treatment received) that IM MTX was more effective than PO MTX during maintenance treatment.

Schedule of therapy

Study 5

Koizumi S, Fujimoto T, Takeda T, Yatabe M, Utsumi J, Mimaya J, Ninomiya T, Yanai M, and the Japanese Children's Cancer and Leukaemia Study Group.
Comparison of intermittent or continuous methotrexate plus 6-mercaptopurine in regimens for standard risk acute lymphoblastic leukaemia in childhood (JCCLSG-S811).
Cancer 1988;**61**:1292–1300.

Study JCCSLG-S811 ran between (January 1981 and December 1983). It was a prospective randomised study conducted by the Japanese Children's Cancer and Leukaemia Study Group for children with standard risk acute lymphoblastic leukaemia.

Objectives

The aim of the study was to compare and evaluate the efficacy of intermittent cycles of 6-mercaptopurine (6-MP) and methotrexate (MTX) combined with pulses of vincristine (VCR) and prednisone (PDN) against the continuous administration of 6-MP and MTX during the maintenance phase of ALL treatment in children.

Details of the study

Previously untreated children with standard risk ALL were enrolled on the study. Patients were stratified into prognostic risk groups according to the initial WBC count and age at diagnosis (Table 16.1).

Remission induction therapy consisted of either (VCR) 2 mg/m^2/week (max. 2 mg) ×4, or vindesine (VDS) 3 mg/m^2/week (max. 3 mg) × 4 plus (PDN) 60 mg/m^2/d (max. 60 mg) × 4 weeks. Patients not in remission at 4 weeks were given an additional 2 weeks of treatment and were withdrawn from the study if remission was not achieved at 6 weeks.

CNS prophylaxis consisted of 18 Gy cranial irradiation (15 Gy for children aged <1 year) plus three doses of intrathecal MTX 12 mg/m^2 (max. 15 mg) and hydrocortisone 50 mg/m^2 during cranial irradiation.

On completion of CNS prophylaxis, all patients in remission were randomised to maintenance therapy of either oral 6-MP 175 mg/m^2/d × 5 days alternating with MTX 225 mg/m^2 IV at 2-weekly intervals and combined with pulses of VCR 2 mg/m^2 and PDN 120 mg/m^2/day × 5 days (intermittent cycle: regimen A) or oral 6-MP 50 mg/m^2/d plus oral MTX 20 mg/m^2/week combined with VCR and PDN every 4 weeks at the same dosage as regimen A. (continuous cycle: regimen B).

Details of the method of randomisation are not given in the report.

Patients who remained in clinical remission for 2 years were given five courses of high dose MTX with folinic acid rescue (late intensification therapy).

Treatment was complete after 3 years of maintenance therapy. Boys also had testicular biopsies prior to discontinuation of treatment.

Table 16.1 Stage of acute lymphoblastic leukaemia according to age and WBC count at diagnosis

WBC count (×10⁹/ℓ)	Age (Yr)				
	<1	1–<4	4–<6	6–<10	≥10
≤ 5000	II	I	I	II	III
5– ≤10	II	I	II	III	III
10– ≤ 50	III	II	II	III	III
50+	III	III	III	III	III

I plus II: standard risk group; I: low risk group; II: intermediate risk group; III: high risk group.

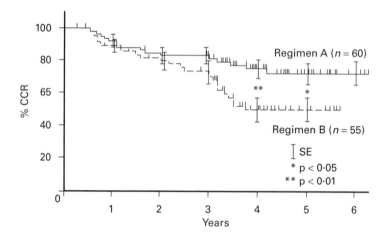

Figure 16.8 Kaplan–Meier analysis of duration of initial continuous complete remission (CCR). The CCR was significantly longer among patients on regimen A (Z = 2·0983; p < 0·05 by the generalised Wilcoxon test)

The outcome measure was continuous clinical remission (CCR).

Outcome

Of the 131 patients enrolled on the study, 119 patients were considered eligible for analysis (12 were excluded due to incorrect diagnosis, wrong treatment stratification, major protocol violations, early death or due to refusal of treatment). A total of 115 patients achieved clinical remission and completed CNS prophylaxis treatment. Sixty patients were randomised to regimen A maintenance therapy and 55 patients to regimen B.

The median duration of initial CCR for patients in regimens A and B was 46 (5–75) and 39 (2–68) months respectively.

The CCR rate for patients in regimens A and B was 75·1% ± 5·8% (mean ± 1 SE) and 49·7% ± 7·3% at 4 years (p = 0·001) and 72·1% ± 6·3% and 49·7% ± 7·3% at 5 years (p<0·05) respectively (Figure 16.8).

There was an increased incidence of bone marrow, CNS and testicular relapses in regimen B patients especially, after 3 years of CCR.

Toxicity

Patients treated on regimen B had a higher incidence of infective episodes compared to regimen A patients. Two regimen B patients died of viral encephalitis during CR and 17 patients developed varicella zoster infections compared to none in regimen A.

Conclusion

It is concluded that intermittent administration of 6-MP and MTX was superior to the continuous administration of both drugs during maintenance therapy in children with standard risk ALL.

Study 6

Chessells JM, Durrant J, Hardy RM, Richards S. Report to the Council by the Working Party on Leukaemia in Childhood. Medical Research Council Leukaemia Trial UKALL-V: an attempt to reduce the immunosuppressive effects of therapy in childhood acute lymphoblastic leukaemia. *J Clin Oncol* 1986;**4**:1758–64.

UKALL-V ran from January 1976 to March 1979 and was a prospective randomised multicentre trial with three built-in randomisations (see study 3 in Chapter 15).

Objectives/Details of the study

The study aimed to compare the relative efficacy of maintenance treatment with oral 6-mercaptopurine and methotrexate given as:

- A continuous regimen.
- A semi-continuous regimen.
- A 5 day pulse every 3 weeks.

For details of patient eligibility criteria, treatment and statistical analysis, refer to Study 3 in Chapter 15.

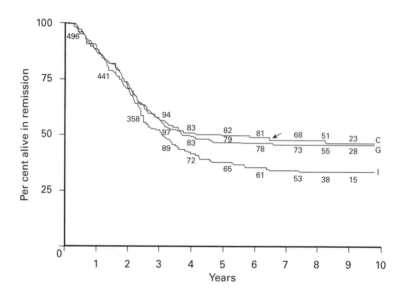

Figure 16.9 Disease free survival in patients receiving continuous (C), intermediate (G) or intermittent (I) chemotherapy. The arrow represents the child with a brain tumour. The numbers refer to patients at risk at the start of each year. Up to 2 years, the numbers represent all patients; thereafter, those in the individual groups. Standard error at 7 and 8 years: ± 3·9, groups C and G; ± 3·7, group I. At 9 years, SE ± 4·0 for group C, ± 3·9 for group G and ± 3·7 for group I

Table 16.2 Prognostic variables and maintenance chemotherapy

Event	Relapse and/or death in remission[a]			Marrow relapse as first event[b]			CNS relapse as first event[c]			Testicular relapse as first event		
	Obs.	Exp.	p	Obs.	Exp.	p	Obs.	Exp.	p	Obs.	Exp.	p
Sex												
M	165	140·1	0·001	107	98·9	0·1	16	16·0	0·5	7	8·6	0·3
F	118	142·9		93	101·1		16	16·0		30	28·4	
Age												
< 3	57	57·2	0·5	42	40·4	0·4	6	6·4	0·4	7	8·6	0·3
≥ 3	226	225·8		158	159·6		26	25·6		30	28·4	
WBC($10^9/\ell$)												
< 10	196	217·6	0·002	137	153·8	0·003	22	24·5	0·2	27	28·2	0·3
≥ 10	87	65·4		63	46·2		10	7·5		10	8·8	
Chemotherapy												
C	84	93·5	0·02	53	66·2	0·002	10	10·5	0·3	11	11·4	0·5
G	89	96·8		61	68·5		9	10·9		14	13·3	
I	110	92·7		86	65·3		13	10·6		12	12·3	
Chemotherapy												
C and G	173	190·3	00·2	114	134·7	0·001	19	21·4	0·2	25	24·7	0·5
I	110	92·7		86	65·3		13	10·6		12	12·3	
Total no. of events	283			200			32			37		

Abbreviations: Obs. observed event; Exp., expected event.

[a] Twenty-three deaths in remission, 3 relapses of other type.

[b] Four combined bone marrow and CNS relapses, 5 bone marrow and testicular relapses.

[c] Three combined CNS and testicular relapses.

The outcome measure was disease free survival (DFS). All analysis was based on intention to treat.

Outcome

Of the 550 patients rigistered on the trial, 22 were excluded (previous chemotherapy, diagnostic error). All 496 patients who achieved remission after induction chemotherapy were randomised to one of three maintenance regimens: regimen C (continuous) $n = 161$, regimen G (semi-continuous) $n = 166$ and regimen I (intermittent) $n = 169$.

Patients randomised to either to regimen C or G had significantly lower bone relapses and superior DFS compared to the patients randomised to regimen I (Table 16.2). The 7 year DFS was (95% CI) 48·4% ± 7·64% in group C 46·4% ± 7.64% in group G and 35·1% ± 7·25% in group I (Figure 16.9).

Remission deaths were more common in regimen C and G patients compared to regimen I patients (p = < 0·025).

Conclusion

It was concluded that intermittent continuing (maintenance) therapy was less effective than conventional continuing therapy in the treatment of childhood ALL.

Study 7

Vilmer E, Suciu S, Ferster A, Bertrand Y, Cave H, Thyss A, Benoit Y, Dastugue N, Fournier M, Souiller G, Manel A-M, Robert A, Nelken B, Millot F, Lutz P, Rialland X, Mechinaud F, Boutard P, Behar C, Chantraine J-M, Plouvier E, Laureys G, Brock P, Uyttebroeck A, Margueritte G, Plantaz D, Norton L, Francotte N, Gyselinck JL, Waterkeyn C, Solbu G, Philippe N, Otten J.

Long term results of three randomised trials (58831, 58832, 58881) in childhood acute lymphoblastic leukaemia: a CLCG-EORTC report. *Leukaemia* 2000;**14**:2257–66.

Trial 58881 was a prospective randomised trial carried out from 1989 to 1998.

Objectives

The aim of the trial was to determine:

- The toxicity and efficacy of two types of L-asparaginase, *E.coli* (standard arm) and Erwinia (experimental arm) when administered at equal dosage.
- Whether high dose cytosine arobinoside (1 g/m^2 12 hourly × 2) combined with high dose methotrexate during interval therapy reduced the incidence of CNS relapse and improved outcome.
- Whether the addition of monthly intravenous (IV) 6-mercaptopurine (1 g/m^2) during maintenance therapy to conventional maintenance improved disease free survival.

Here we focus primarily on the use of intravenous 6-mercaptopurine during acute lymphoblastic leukaemia maintenance therapy and its effect in improving DFS.

Details of the study

All patients below 18 years of age were eligible to be registered on this study. Patients were categorised into two risk groups: standard risk (SR) and very high risk (VHR). VHR patients were those who had >1000 blasts/mm^3 in the peripheral blood at the end of 7 days of prednisone monotherapy and one intrathecal dose of methotrexate, those who die not achieve complete remission or those with a t(4; 11) or t(9; 22) translocation present in the leukaemic clone. All others were considered standard risk.

All patients received the same induction regimen. Tables 16.3 and 16.4 show the treatment schema for SR and VHR patients respectively. For SR patients a total of 10 intrathecal methotrexate (IT MTX) injections were scheduled during the intensive phases of treatment but none planned during maintenance.

VHR patients received an intensified treatment for 1 year followed by two series of three BFM type chemotherapy regimens (R1, R2 and R3). CNS prophylaxis consisted of ten injections of IT MTX and six injections of triple IT chemotherapy (methotrexate, cytosine arabinoside and steroids), including ten courses of high dose MTX during the first year of treatment.

Maintenance therapy commenced 2 weeks after protocol II or after the last R3 block and consisted of daily oral mercaptopurine (initial dose 50 mg/m^2) and methotrexate (20 mg/m^2 weekly). For all patients the total duration of treatment was 2 years.

The outcome measure was disease free survival (DFS).

Table 16.3 EORTC-CLCG 58881: treatment protocols for standard risk patients

Treatment phase/drug	Dose	Days given
Induction – consolidation		
Protocol IA		
Prednisolone	60 mg/m²	1–28
Vincristine	1·5 mg/m²	8, 15, 22, 29
Daunorubicin	30 mg/m²	8, 15, 22, 29
Methotrexate (IT)	12 mg (age dependent)	1, 8, 22, 38, 52
L-Asparaginase[a]	10 000 IU/m²	12, 15, 18, 22, 25 29, 35, 38
Protocol IB		
Cyclophosphamide	1 mg/m²	36, 63
Cytosine arabinoside	75 mg/m²	38–41, 45–48, 52–55, 59–62
6-Mercaptopurine	60 mg/m²	36–63
Interval therapy		
6-Mercaptopurine	25 mg/m²	1–56
Methotrexate (24 h infusion)	5 g/m²	8, 22, 36, 50
Methotrexate (IT)	12 mg (age dependent)	9, 23, 37, 51
according to randomisation[b]		
Cytosine arabinoside	1 g/m² (twice 12 h interval)	9, 23, 37, 51
Reinduction: protocol II		
Dexamethasone	10 mg/m²	1–21
Vincristine	1·5 mg/m²	8, 15, 22, 29
Doxorubicin	30 mg/m²	8, 15, 22, 29
L-Asparaginase[a]	10 000 IU/m²	8, 11, 15, 18
Methotrexate (IT)	12 mg (age dependent)	38
Cyclophosphamide (IV)	1 mg/m²	36
Cytosine arabinoside	75 mg/m²	36–41, 45–48
6-Thioguanine	60 mg/m²	36–49

[a] Patients, regardless of their risk group, were randomly assigned to receive *E. coli* asparaginase or Erwinia asparaginase at equal dosages.

[b] Patients in CR, with an initial RF > 0·8 or with a T-lineage ALL and without VHR features, were eligibile for this randomisation.

Table 16.4 EORTC-CLCG 58881: treatment protocol for VHR patients

Treatment element/drug	Dose	Days given
Protocol IB		
Cyclophosphamide	1 g/m^2	43 and 85
Methotrexate (24 h infusion)	5 g/m^2	43, 57, 71
Cytosine arabinoside	1 g/m^2	50, 51, 64, 65, 78, 79
L-Asparaginase	25 000 IU/m^2	44, 51, 58, 65, 72, 79
6-Mercaptopurine (PO)	25 mg/m^2	43–84
Methotrexate (IT)	12 mg (age dependent)	44, 58, 72
VANDA		
Dexamethasone	20 mg/m^2	1–5
Cytosine arobinoside	2 g/m^2 (twice, 12 h interval)	1, 2
Mitoxantrone	8 mg/m^2	3, 4
Etoposide	150 mg/m^2	3, 4, 5
L-Asparaginase	10 000 IU/m^2	7, 9, 11, 13
Methotrexate (IT)	12 mg (age dependent)	5
Interval therapy		
6-Mercaptopurine (PO)	25 mg/m^2	1–42
Methotrexate (24 h infusion)	5 g/m^2	8, 22, 36
Cytarabine (10 min infusion)	1 g/m^2 (twice, 12 h interval)	9, 23, 37
Methotrexate (IT)	12 mg (age dependent)	9, 23, 37
Bloc R1		
Dexamethasone	20 mg/m^2	1–5
6-Mercaptopurine	100 mg/m^2	1–5
Vincristine	1·5 mg/m^2	1,6

Continued

Table 16.4 Continued

Treatment element/drug	Dose	Days given
Methotrexate (24 h infusion)	5 g/m^2	1
Cytosine arabinoside	2 g/m^2 (twice 12 h interval)	5
L-Asparaginase	25 000 IU/m^2	6
Methotrexate/cytosine arabinoside/prednisone (IT)	12 mg/30 mg/10 mg	1
Bloc R2		
Dexamethasone	20 mg/m^2	1–5
6-Thioguanine	100 mg/m^2	1–5
Vincristine	3 mg/m^2	1
Methotrexate (24 h infusion)	5 g/m^2	1
Ifosfamide	400 mg/m^2	1–5
Daunorubicin	50 mg/m^2	5
L-Asparaginase	25 000 IU/m^2	6
Methotrexate/cytosine arabinoside/prednisone (IT)	12 mg/30 mg/10 mg	1
Bloc R3		
Dexamethasone	20 mg/m^2	1–5
Cytosine arabinoside	2 g/m^2 (twice, 12 h interval)	1, 2
Etoposide	150 mg/m^2	3, 4, 5
L-Asparaginase	25 000 IU/m^2	6
Methotrexate/cytosine arabinoside/prednisone (IT)	12 mg/30 mg/10 mg	5

No details of the randomisation method are given in the report.

Outcome

Of the 2078 patients registered on the trial, only 2065 were evaluable, of whom 2019 patients (97·8%) achieved complete remission. Eight hundred and twenty patients were randomised to either to the conventional maintenance therapy (without IV mercaptopurine) or to the experimental arm with monthly IV mercaptopurine added to conventional maintenance treatment. There were no differences on either the prognostic factors or the in type of asparaginase received by both groups of patients.

The 5 year DFS in the group that received IV mercaptopurine was 71·2% ± 2·3% compared to 78·6% ± 2·1% of the conventional maintenance group (lon-rank p < 0·027). The difference was more marked in those who were also randomised to the less potent Erwinia asparaginase (59·2% ± 4·8% v 74·5% ± 4·3%; Hazard Ratio (HR) 1·71) compared to the group randomised to *E. coli* asparaginase (78·2% ± 3·9% v 78·4% ± 3·9%; HR 1·08).

Conclusion

The addition of IV 6-mercaptopurine to conventional maintenance during maintenance therapy was deleterious and increased the risk of late relapse.

417

Type of thiopurine

Study 8

Harms DO, Janka-Schaub GE on behalf of the COALL Study Group.
Co-operative Study Group for childhood acute lymphoblastic leukaemia (COALL): long-term follow up of trials of 82, 85, 89 and 92.
Leukaemia 2000;**14**:2234–8

COALL-92 trial was a prospective randomised multicentre study that ran from February 1992 to July 1997.

Objectives

The aim of the study was to determine whether the use 6-thioguanine (6-TG) during maintenance therapy offered a therapeutic advantage over 6-mercaptopurine (6-MP).

Details of the study

Children and adolescents between the ages of 1 and 18 with previously untreated ALL were enrolled on the study.

Table 16.5 summarises the COALL-92 treatment schedule. Detailed information of the chemotherapy schedule has been previously published[1-5]. Cranial irradiation was given to high risk patients only. Patients were randomised to either 6-MP or 6-TG during the maintenance phase of treatment.

Log-rank tests were used to evaluate the differences in the event free survival (EFS) between the patient groups.

Outcome measures were event free survival (EFS) and overall survival (OS).

All analyses were performed on an intention to treat basis.

Outcome

Randomisation details were not given in the report. A total of 578 patients were enrolled on the study. Forty were excluded because of previous treatment elsewhere. Of the 538 eligible patients, 474 (88%) were randomised between 6-TG ($n = 236$) and 6-MP ($n = 238$) during maintenance therapy.

Five year EFS for the entire cohort was 76·9% ± 1·9%. The 5 year EFS for patients on 6-TG was 80·1% ± 2·9% versus 82·8% ± 2·6% for patients on 6MP. Analysis according to risk status (LR and HR) showed no significant differences. The use of 6-TG during maintenance was not significantly superior to 6-MP.

Toxicity

Haematological toxicity, especially thrombocytopenia, was greater with 6-TG. Non-haematological toxicity was similar for both drugs.

Conclusion

It was concluded that maintenance treatment with 6-TG had no impact on outcome, whether stratified for risk status or lineage.

Table 16.5 Protocols COALL-92

	High risk	Low risk
Prephase induction	VD ×4 + P PO ×28	VD ×4 + P PO ×28
Intensification	CYC ×2 + ID MTX ×2 + ASP ×4 + MP PO	IDMTX + ASP ×2 + MP PO
	IDMTX ×2 + VM-26 ×2 + AC ×2 + TG PO	IDMTX + VM-26 + AC + TG PO
	HDAC 2×4 + ASP ×4	HDAC ×4 + ASP ×2
		IDMTX + ASP ×2 + MP PO
CNS prophylaxis	C-/Pre-B-ALL+ WBC <25/50 ×10^9/l MIT + MP PO all others + CRT 12–18 Gy	MIT + MP PO
Reinduction	VA ×4 + ASP ×4 + DEX PO ×28	VA ×2 + ASP ×2 + DEX PO ×14
	CYC ×2 + AC 4×4 + TG PO	CYC + AC ×4 + TG PO
Maintenance	MP or TG + MTX	MP or TG + MTX PO

V, vincristine; D, daunorubicin; P, prednisone; ASP, L-asparaginase; CYC, cyclophosphamide; HDMTX, high dose methotrexate; AC, cytosine arabinoside; MP, mercaptopurine; ITMX, intrathecal methotrexate; CR, cranial irradiation; VA, doxorubicin; VM-26, teniposide; TG, thioguanine; IDMTX, intermediate dose methotrexate; HDAC, high dose cytosine arabinoside; DEX, dexamethasone; PO, orally

References

1   Janka GE, Winkler K, Juergens H *et al.* Acute lympho-blastic leukaemia in childhood: the COALL therapy studies. *Klin Pädiatr* 1986;**198**:177–7.

2   Janka GE, Winkler K, Juergens H *et al.* Early intensifica-tion therapy in high risk childhood lymphoblastic leukaemia: lack of benefit from high dose methotrexate. *Haematol Blood Transfus* 1987;**30**:456–60.

3   Janka GE, Harms D, Goebel U *et al.* Randomised comparisons of rotational chemotherapy in high risk acute lymphoblastic leukaemia of childhood: follow up after 9 years. *Eur J Pediatr* 1996;**155**:640–8.

4   Janka GE, Winkler K, Goebel U *et al.* The COALL-85 co-operative study for high risk patients with acute lymphatic leukaemia: initial results. *Klin Pädiatr* 1988;**200**:17–16.

5   Janka GE, Harms D, den Boer ML *et al.* In vitro drug resistance as independent prognostic factor in the study COALL-05-92. Treatment of childhood acute lym-phoblastic leukaemia; two-tiered classification of treat-ments based on accepted risk criteria and drug sensi-tivity profiles in study COALL-06-97. *Klin Pädiatr* 1999;**211**:233–8.

Index